Drug Delivery and Targeting
for Pharmacists and Pharmaceutical Scientists

Drug Delivery and Targeting
for Pharmacists and Pharmaceutical Scientists

Edited by

Anya M. Hillery
Department of Health Sciences
Saint Louis University
Madrid Campus, Spain

Andrew W. Lloyd
School of Pharmacy and Biomolecular Sciences
University of Brighton
UK

and

James Swarbrick
President, PharmaceuTech Inc
Pinehurst, NC
USA

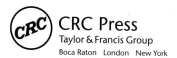

CRC Press
Taylor & Francis Group
Boca Raton London New York

CRC Press is an imprint of the
Taylor & Francis Group, an **informa** business

Published in 2001by
CRC Press
Taylor & Francis Group
6000 Broken Sound Parkway NW, Suite 300
Boca Raton, FL 33487-2742

© 2001 by Taylor & Francis Group, LLC
CRC Press is an imprint of Taylor & Francis Group

No claim to original U.S. Government works
Printed in the United States of America on acid-free paper

International Standard Book Number-10: 0-415-27198-3 (Softcover)
International Standard Book Number-13: 978-0-415-27198-1 (Softcover)

Library of Congress Cataloging-in-Publication Data

Catalog record is available from the Library of Congress

Visit the Taylor & Francis Web site at
http://www.taylorandfrancis.com

and the CRC Press Web site at
http://www.crcpress.com

Contents

Section 2: Routes of Drug Delivery

Section 3: Future Directions of Drug Delivery and Targeting

Preface

The phenomenal advances in the fields of biotechnology and molecular biology over recent years have resulted in a large number of novel molecules with the potential to revolutionize the treatment or prevention of disease. The "new biotherapeutics" include such moieties as novel peptide and protein drugs and vaccines, genes and oligonucleotide therapies. However, their potential is severely compromised by the significant delivery and targeting obstacles which prevail *in vivo*. These obstacles are often so great that effective drug delivery and targeting is now recognized as the key to the effective development of many therapeutics.

In response, the field of advanced drug delivery and targeting has seen an explosion of activity, as researchers address these obstacles and try to facilitate or enhance the action of the new biotherapeutics, as well as conventional drugs.

Activity in the field includes the development of novel drug delivery systems to circumvent the various pharmacokinetic obstacles that can result in zero or minimal drug absorption, unwanted distribution, and premature inactivation and elimination. Technologies are also addressing ways to minimize drug toxicity or immunogenicity, or to enhance vaccine immunogenicity. The importance of drug targeting to the site of action is the subject of intense research interest, as are considerations of the importance of drug timing to optimize therapeutic regimens, with the ongoing development of controlled, pulsatile and bio-responsive release systems. Novel routes of drug delivery are also under investigation.

Although this is an expanding field of crucial importance to therapeutics, there is currently no single text that covers all aspects of advanced drug delivery and targeting, at an appropriate level for undergraduate and continuing education courses. General pharmacy textbooks, concerned with the rudimentaries, are of necessity limited to conventional pharmaceutical formulations such as tablets, capsules and topical creams. At the other extreme, existing texts relating to this field tend to focus on a single aspect of drug delivery and targeting, or constitute the proceedings of specialized conferences and are, as such, invariably complex and esoteric. This book aims to bridge this gap, by providing a single, comprehensive text which describes the fundamental technological and scientific principles of advanced drug delivery and targeting, their current applications and potential future developments.

This book is primarily intended for undergraduate and postgraduate students taking courses in relevant aspects of the biological sciences. In particular, it should prove useful to students undertaking programs in pharmacy, pharmaceutical science, medicine, dentistry, biochemistry, bioengineering, biotechnology, or other related biomedical subjects. It is hoped it will also serve as an introductory text and source of reference for those employed in the (bio)pharmaceutical sector, professions allied to medicine and pharmacists in practice.

Considerable attention has been paid to the overall layout and content of the text. Section 1 serves as an introduction to the field of advanced drug delivery and targeting. The opening chapter introduces such concepts as bioavailability, the pharmacokinetic processes, the importance of timing for optimal therapy and the special delivery considerations for the new biotherapeutics. In doing so this chapter also highlights the necessity for advanced drug delivery and targeting systems in order to optimize therapeutic efficacy. The therapeutic impetus for advanced delivery systems is further compounded by commercial interests, which are described in Chapter 2. A broad overview of advanced drug delivery and targeting is then provided (Chapter 3), which introduces the terminology and various key concepts pertinent to this subject.

Advanced drug delivery and targeting is particularly concerned with two key concepts: rate-controlled drug release and effective drug targeting. Parenteral drug delivery is the route in which the greatest progress has been made with respect to these concerns. The introductory section therefore continues with a chapter on implantable drug delivery systems (Chapter 4), which also serves as a general introduction to the different methods of controlled release achievable with drug delivery systems. Similarly, Chapter 5 specifically describes parenteral drug delivery and targeting systems but also provides a general description of the state-of-the-art methods currently available to achieve drug targeting to the site of action.

Section 2 of the book is concerned with the major individual routes of drug delivery currently under investigation. This section begins with a chapter on the oral route (Chapter 6) which is the most common and convenient of the existing administration methods for introducing drugs to the bloodstream. The limitations associated with oral drug delivery are also described, which paves the way for the subsequent chapters on other routes which are currently being explored as alternative portals of drug entry to the systemic circulation.

The chapters in Section 2 concerning the various routes of drug delivery have been edited with particular care to ensure that the treatment of each particular route follows a common format. This has been undertaken not only to ease understanding and facilitate learning but also to highlight the many similarities that exist between the various routes, as well as the unique attributes associated with each specific route.

Section 3 deals with the future directions of drug delivery and targeting in the new millennium. The new and exciting possibilities of plasmid-based gene therapy are described in Chapter 14. The importance of rationally integrating the drug discovery process with that of drug delivery is discussed in Chapter 15 and emphasizes that in the future this alliance offers the best, and indeed the only, way forward for effective therapeutics. Finally Chapter 16 describes the new generation technologies, which include such advances as the use of biosensors, microchips and stimuli-sensitive hydrogels in drug delivery and targeting.

In keeping with our aim to produce an accessible, easy-to-read book we have endeavored to ensure that the text is clear, concise and easily comprehensible. Each individual chapter is written by one or more distinguished authors from the relevant field and careful editing has ensured an overall style and continuity throughout the text. European and American trade names are given where appropriate to avoid any possible conflicts of terminology and phraseology which may arise from multinational readership and authorship.

A series of *Objectives* is included at the beginning of each chapter, which serve as an introductory outline. A list of titles is provided as *Further Reading* at the end of each chapter. These titles are predominantly review articles serving as a useful starting point for further study. A series of *Self-Assessment Questions* are also provided, allowing students to test their knowledge of the content of each chapter. Ample usage of figures and tables has been included to facilitate the pedagogic approach.

The successful completion of this text has been made possible by the assistance of a large number of people to whom we are most grateful. The individual chapter contributors are acknowledged overleaf, as are the chapter and book reviewers. We would also like to acknowledge the support of the Publishers and thank Helen Courtney for illustrative support. We are grateful for the generous educational grant provided by 3M Pharmaceuticals.

Finally, AMH would also like to thank Mike Pinkney, for his steadfast support during the preparation of this text.

We welcome readers' suggestions, comments and corrections on the text, which should be sent to us c/o Taylor and Francis (Life Sciences Division), 11 New Fetter Lane, London EC4P 4EE, UK.

Anya M. Hillery
Andrew W. Lloyd
James Swarbrick

Acknowledgements

The editors gratefully acknowledge the individual chapter contributors and also the advice and assistance of the following colleagues who served on chapter/book reviews:

Professor A. Florence, London School of Pharmacy
Professor J. Robinson, University of Wisconsin Madison
Dr G. Martin, Kings College London
Professor Y. Barenholz, The Hebrew University-Hadassah-Medical School
Dr F. Martin, Alza Corporation
Dr P. Gard, University of Brighton

Corresponding Authors

David Bailey
De Novo Pharmaceuticals Ltd
Cambridge
UK

Yie W. Chien
Controlled Drug-Delivery Research Center
Rutgers University College of Pharmacy
Piscataway, NJ
USA

Daan Crommelin
Department of Pharmaceutics
Utrecht Institute for Pharmaceutical Sciences
Utrecht University
Utrecht
The Netherlands

Paul Evers
Weaver Shipyard
Northwich
UK

Richard H. Guy
Centre Interuniversitaire de Recherche et d'Ensegnement
"Pharmapeptides"
Archamps
France

Anya M. Hillery
Department of Health Sciences
Saint Louis University
Madrid
Spain

Janet Hoogstraate
Biopharmaceutics Concept Division
Astra Pain Control AB
Sodertalje
Sweden

Alison B. Lansley
Cellective Ltd
Lewes
UK

Vincent H.L. Lee
Department of Pharmaceutical Sciences
School of Southern California
Los Angeles CA
USA

Andrew W. Lloyd
School of Pharmacy and Biomolecular Sciences
University of Brighton
Brighton
UK

Gary P. Martin
Department of Pharmacy
Kings College London
London
UK

Hiroaki Okada
Pharmaceutical Business Development Department
DDS Research Laboratories
Takeda Chemical Industries Ltd
Osaka
Japan

William M. Pardridge
Department of Medicine
UCLA School of Medicine
Los Angeles CA
USA

Kinam Park
School of Pharmacy
Purdue University
West Lafayette
Indianapolis, IN
USA

Hongkee Sah
Department of Pharmaceutical Sciences
The University of Tennessee College of Pharmacy
Memphis TN
USA

Isabelle Seyler
Research and Development
Laboratoires 3M Sante
Pithiviers Cedex
France

Glyn Taylor
The Welsh School of Pharmacy
Cardiff University
Cardiff
UK

Eric Tomlinson
35 Holymead
The Woodlands
Texas
USA

Clive G.L. Wilson
Department of Pharmaceutical Sciences
University of Strathclyde
Glasgow
UK

I Drug Delivery: The Basic Concepts

Anya M. Hillery

OBJECTIVES

On completion of this chapter the reader should be able to:

- Describe the limitations of conventional drug delivery
- Explain the concept of bioavailability
- Describe the various pharmacokinetic processes, with particular reference to drug absorption
- Explain the importance of timing for optimal drug therapy
- Describe the special delivery considerations for the "new biotherapeutics"

1.1 INTRODUCTION

When a drug is taken by a patient, the resulting biological effects, for example lowering of blood pressure, are determined by the pharmacological properties of the drug. These biological effects are usually produced by an interaction of the drug with specific receptors at the drug's site of action.

However, unless the drug can be delivered to its site of action at a rate and concentration that both minimize side-effects and maximize therapeutic effects, the efficiency of the therapy is compromised. In some cases, delivery and targeting barriers may be so great as to preclude the use of an otherwise effective drug candidate. The purpose of any delivery system is to enhance or facilitate the action of therapeutic compounds. Ideally, a drug delivery system could deliver the correct amount of drug to the site of action at the correct rate and timing, in order to maximize the desired therapeutic response.

Specialized drug delivery systems constitute a relatively recent addition to the field of pharmaceutical technology. Up until the 1940s conventional dosage forms essentially comprised:

- injections;
- oral formulations (solutions, suspensions, tablets and capsules);
- topical creams and ointments.

Such simple dosage forms possess many inherent disadvantages for drug delivery. Parenteral delivery is highly invasive, generally requires intervention by clinicians and the effects are usually short-lived. Although oral administration is highly convenient, many drugs, such as insulin, cannot be given by this route due to poor absorption characteristics and/or propensity to degrade in the gastrointestinal tract. Topical creams and ointments were limited to *topical* rather than *systemic* effects.

Dosage forms became more advanced during the 1950s and 1960s; however, drug delivery technology was mainly limited to sustained-release delivery via the oral route. An example of an oral sustained-release formulation from this period is the Spansule capsule technology developed by Smith Kline and French Laboratories. The Spansule consists of hundreds of tiny coated pellets of drug substance. As the pellets travel down the gastrointestinal tract, the coating material dissolves to release the drug. By using a capsule containing pellets incorporating a spectrum of different thickness coatings (and thus dissolution rates), sustained drug release of a given pattern is possible.

It was not until the 1970s, with the advent of dedicated drug delivery research companies, that significant advances in drug delivery technology were made. The recognition that specific research had to be undertaken in order to overcome the problems of conventional drug delivery led to the evolution of modern-day pharmaceutical science and technology. The phenomenal advances in the fields of biotechnology and molecular biology gave an additional impetus to drug delivery research in the 1980s and early 1990s. These advances provided large quantities of new biopharmaceuticals, such as peptides, proteins and antisense oligonucleotides, which generally possess inherent disadvantages for drug delivery. Disadvantages include such properties as large molecular size, hydrophilicity and instability, making these "new biotherapeutics" unsuitable for oral delivery. Generally such drugs must be given by the parenteral route, which has many associated disadvantages, as mentioned above.

Recent research has been directed towards the use of alternatives to the parenteral route, for drugs (including the "new biotherapeutics") that cannot be delivered orally. Potential alternative portals of drug entry to the systemic circulation include the buccal, sublingual, nasal, pulmonary and vaginal routes. These routes are also being studied for the local delivery of drugs directly to the site of action, thereby reducing the dose needed to produce a pharmacological effect and also possibly minimizing systemic side-effects.

Drug delivery technology is becoming increasingly sophisticated and current approaches take into account such factors as the influence of pharmacokinetic processes on drug efficacy, as well as the importance of drug timing and of drug targeting to the site of action. Emerging technologies are addressing a variety of issues, including bio-responsive drug release and the delivery of nucleic acid therapeutic entities. This book is concerned with the various routes of delivery under investigation, and these new and emerging delivery technologies. However, a full appreciation of these concerns cannot be gained without first understanding:

- the concept of bioavailability;
- the process of drug absorption;
- the pharmacokinetic processes;
- the importance of timing for optimal drug therapy;
- delivery considerations for the "new biotherapeutics";
- the limitations of conventional therapy.

This chapter provides an overview of these considerations and highlights the necessity for advanced drug delivery systems, in order to optimize drug efficacy.

1.2   THE CONCEPT OF BIOAVAILABILITY

Bioavailability is defined as the *rate* and *extent* to which an active agent is absorbed and becomes available at the site of action and therefore gives a therapeutic response. In terms of drug efficacy, the bioavailability of a drug is almost as important as the potency of the active agent itself.

Measuring a drug's bioavailability thus involves measuring the rate and extent of drug absorption. This is ideally measured in terms of the clinical response of a patient; however, only a minority of clinical responses, such as blood pressure, can provide accurate quantitative data for analysis. A further method of assessment is the measurement of the drug concentration at the site of action; however, this cannot be achieved practically. For clinical purposes, it is generally accepted that a dynamic equilibrium exists between the concentration of drug at the site of action (C_s) and the concentration of drug in blood plasma (C_p). Thus C_p is generally used as an indirect indicator of the concentration of drug at its site of action[#] and the most commonly used method of assessing the bioavailability of a drug involves the construction of a Cp versus "Time" curve (Cp vs T curve).

A typical Cp vs T curve following the administration of an oral tablet is given in Figure 1.1(a). At zero time (when the drug is first administered), the concentration of drug in the plasma is zero. As time proceeds, more and more of the drug starts to appear in the plasma, as the drug is gradually absorbed from the gut. Following peak levels, the concentration of drug in the plasma starts to decline, as the processes of drug distribution and drug elimination predominate. Thus a profile of the rate and extent of drug absorption from the formulation over time is obtained. The area under the (Cp vs T) curve (Area Under the Curve: AUC) is related to the total amount of drug absorbed after a specific dose.

The utility of this approach is shown in Figure 1.1 (b), in which the oral bioavailability of a drug from three different formulations is assessed by comparing their respective Cp vs T curves. Formulations A and B have similar AUCs, indicating that the drug is absorbed to a similar *extent* from both formulations; however, formulation A has a faster *rate* of absorption, indicating that this formulation shows a rapid onset of therapeutic action. Formulation B has a slower onset of therapeutic action, but the therapeutic effect is sustained longer than that obtained with formulation A. Formulation C demonstrates both a slow rate and extent of absorption, in comparison to the other two formulations.

Figure 1.1 Typical plasma concentration-time curves obtained by administering various formulations of a drug by either the oral or intravenous route (see text for details)

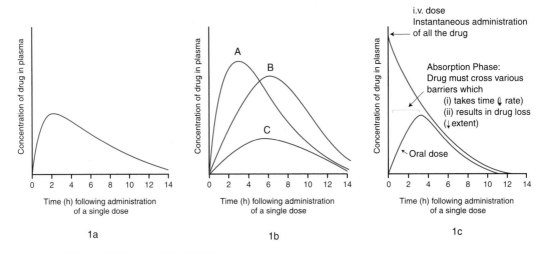

1a

1b

1c

[#] Using C_p as an indicator of C_s is obviously a simplification that is not always valid and the relationship cannot be used without first establishing that C_p and C_s are consistently related. As many drugs bind in a reversible manner to plasma proteins, a more accurate index of C_s is the concentration of the drug in protein-free plasma C_{pfp}. However, this measurement is more difficult to carry out practically than measuring the total concentration of both unbound and bound drug in total plasma, thus C_p is often used in preference to C_{pfp} as an index of C_s

Relative Bioavailability is the comparison of the rate and extent of absorption of two formulations given by the *same* route of administration. A study of relative bioavailability generally involves the comparison of a "test" product to a "standard" product, to determine if the test formulation has equivalent, lower, or higher bioavailability to the standard product. For example, the bioavailability of a new tablet formulation of a drug for oral administration can be compared with the oral bioavailability of the brand leader tablet formulation. The relative bioavailabilities may be calculated from the corresponding Cp vs T curves as follows:

$$\text{Relative Bioavailability} = (AUC)_{test} / (AUC)_{standard}$$

(Equation 1.1)

Formulations showing superimposable Cp vs T curves are said to be bioequivalent.

In contrast, Absolute Bioavailability involves comparison of the drug's bioavailability with respect to the corresponding bioavailability after iv administration. Absolute bioavailability may be calculated by comparing the total area under the Cp vs T curve obtained from the absorption route in question (often the oral route, although the approach can be used for other routes, such as the nasal, buccal, transdermal routes etc.), with that of the Cp vs T curve following iv administration:

$$\text{Absolute Bioavailability} = (AUC)_{absorption\ route} / (AUC)_{iv\ route}$$

(Equation 1.2)

After IV injection, the drug is delivered immediately and totally into the blood (100% bioavailability). In contrast, a drug administered via any other route (intramuscular, subcutaneous, intestinal, rectal, buccal, sublingual, nasal, pulmonary and vaginal) will have to circumvent various physical and chemical barriers (discussed below), so that the bioavailability will be lower in comparison to that obtained after iv administration. For example, to achieve 100% bioavailability via the oral route requires the drug to:

- be completely released from the dosage form into solution in the gastrointestinal fluids;
- be completely stable in solution in the gastrointestinal fluids;
- pass through the epithelium of the gastrointestinal tract;
- undergo no first-pass metabolism in the gut wall or liver, prior to reaching the systemic circulation.

The bioavailable dose (F) is the fraction of the administered dose that reaches the systemic circulation. For example, if a drug is given orally and 90% of the administered dose is present in the systemic circulation, F = 0.9. As can be seen from Figure 1.1 (c), the bioavailability of a drug may be substantially reduced because of the absorption process. This process is discussed in detail in the following section.

1.3   THE PROCESS OF DRUG ABSORPTION

Drugs administered orally must cross the GI tract epithelium to be absorbed and enter the systemic circulation. Similarly, drugs administered by alternative routes, such as the buccal, sublingual, nasal, pulmonary and vaginal routes, must all cross the appropriate epithelial interfaces to reach the general circulation. The types of epithelial interfaces, the barriers they pose to drug absorption, and the routes and mechanisms of drug absorption across these interfaces, are described below.

1.3.1   Epithelial interfaces

The epithelia are a diverse group of tissues, which, with rare exceptions, line all body surfaces, cavities and glands. They consist of one or more layers of cells, separated by a minute quantity of intercellular material. All epithelia are supported by a basement membrane of variable thickness, which separates the epithelium from underlying connective tissues.

Epithelial interfaces are involved in a wide range of activities such as absorption, secretion and protection; all these major functions may be exhibited at a single epithelial surface. For example, the epithelial lining of the small intestine is primarily involved in absorption of the products of digestion, but the epithelium also protects itself from potentially harmful substances by the secretion of a surface coating of mucus.

Epithelia are classified according to three morphological characteristics:

- the number of cell layers;
- the cell shape;
- the presence of surface specializations.

A single layer of epithelial cells is termed simple epithelium, whereas those composed of more than one layer are termed stratified epithelia. Stratified epithelia are found in areas which have to withstand large amounts of wear and tear, for example the inside of the mouth, or the skin. Epithelial cells may be, for example, squamous (flattened), columnar (tall), cuboidal (intermediate between squamous and columnar) and may contain surface specializations, such as cilia in the nasal epithelium and keratin in the skin.

Detailed descriptions of the epithelia present in the various routes of drug delivery are given in the relevant chapters; a generalized summary is given here in Table 1.1.

1.3.2   Epithelial barriers to drug absorption

The absorption of drugs, although dependent on the particular absorption site in question, is often controlled by the same set of epithelial barriers, which include:

Mucus

The majority of the epithelia discussed in this book are covered by a layer of mucus (Table 1.1). Mucus is synthesized and secreted by

Table 1.1 The nature of the epithelia associated with various sites of drug delivery

Absorption Route	Epithelial Type	Surface Specialization	Presence of Mucus	Primary Role
Oral (stomach and intestinal)	Simple columnar	Brush border (microvilli)	Yes	Absorption
Buccal and sub-lingual	Stratified squamous	May be keratinized	Yes	Protection
Vaginal	Stratified squamous	May be keratinized	"Vaginal fluids"	Protection
Transdermal	Stratified squamous	Keratinized	No	Protection
Nasal	Pseudostratified columnar	Cilia	Yes	Protection
Pulmonary	Simple cuboidal (in the bronchioles)	Cilia	Yes	Protection
	Simple squamous (in the alveolar region)	No	No	Gaseous exchange
Ocular (the cornea)	Stratified Squamous	Not normally keratinized	No	Protection

modified columnar epithelial cells known as goblet cells (so named because of their resemblance to drinking goblets). In man, goblet cells are scattered amongst cells of many simple epithelial linings, particularly of the respiratory and gastrointestinal tracts.

Mucus is mainly composed of long, entangled glycoprotein molecules known as mucins, which vary in length from 0.5 to 10 μm and are composed of sub-units (monomers) each about 500 nm in length. Each monomer consists of a protein backbone, approximately 800 amino acids long, rich in serine, proline and threonine. Oligosaccharide side chains, generally up to 18 residues in length, composed of N-acetyl-galactosamine, N-acetylglucosamine, galactose, fucose and N-acetyl-neuraminic acid are attached to the protein monomers.

Mucus serves as a lubricant and protective layer. Its most important property is its viscoelasticity, which enables it to act as a mechanical barrier, but also allows it to flow. The presence of a mucus layer has important implications for drug delivery. Mucus acts as a physical barrier through which drug molecules must diffuse, prior to reaching the absorbing surface. The rate of diffusion through the mucus will be dependent upon such factors as the thickness of the mucus layer, mucus viscosity and any interactions which may occur between the drug and mucus.

In the respiratory tract, mucus is also involved in the process of mucociliary clearance, which contributes to the epithelial barrier properties by entrapping potentially hazardous substances, such as dust and microorganisms, within a viscoelastic mucus blanket. The mucus is then propelled by the claw-like tips of "hair-like" cilia towards the throat (movement occurs in a downwards direction from the nasal epithelium, or in an upwards direction from the lungs), where the mucus and any entrapped particulates are either swallowed or expectorated. Although this process is beneficial if inhaled particles are hazardous, drug particles may also be cleared by this mechanism.

Hydrophobic membranes and cell junctions

Membranes surround all living cells and cell organelles. They are essential for maintaining and protecting the cell and its compartments. In the fluid mosaic model of the plasma membrane, the surfaces of the membrane are composed of tightly packed lipoidal molecules (including phospholipids, sphingolipids and sterols), interspersed with proteins. The proteins were originally thought to float in a sea of lipid, resulting in a rather ill-defined mixed membrane. However, it is now accepted that the membrane is a highly organized structure. Proteins in specific conformations act as structural elements, transporters of nutrients and environmental monitors.

The plasma membrane of epithelial cells, in common with other cell types, is *selectively permeable*, allowing the penetration of some substances but not others. The construction of the membrane from amphipathic lipid molecules forms a highly impermeable barrier to most polar and charged molecules, thereby preventing the loss of most water-soluble contents of the cell. This selective permeability presents a physical barrier to drug absorption, limiting absorption to specific routes and mechanisms, as described below (see Section 1.3.3).

A further important feature of epithelia for drug delivery is that the epithelial cells are bound together by several types of plasma membrane specializations, including desmosomes, gap junctions and junctional complexes (Figure 1.2). Desmosomes (macula adherens) are the commonest type of cell junction and are found at many intercellular sites, including cardiac muscle, skin epithelium and the neck of the uterus. They also occur as part of the junctional complexes (see below). At the desmosome, the opposing plasma membranes are separated by a gap in which many fine, transverse filaments are present. Desmosomes provide strong points of cohesion between cells and act as anchorage points for the cytoskeleton of each cell.

Gap junctions (nexus) are broad areas of closely opposed plasma membranes, but there is no fusion of the plasma membranes and a narrow gap, of about 2 to 3 nm wide, remains. The "gap" is crossed by cytoplasmic filaments, which allow intracellular cytoplasm to transfer between cells. This type of cell junction not only functions as an adherent zone, but also permits the passage of ions and other small molecules (sugars, amino acids, nucleotides and vitamins). Thus the gap junctions are sites of intercellular information exchange.

Junctional complexes comprise intercellular membrane specializations which encircle the cells, preventing access of luminal contents to the intercellular spaces. They are found between the cells of simple cuboidal (for example in the lungs) and simple columnar (for example in the gastrointestinal tract) epithelia, and lie immediately below the luminal surface. They are made up of three components:

Figure 1.2 Epithelial cell junctions and junctional complexes

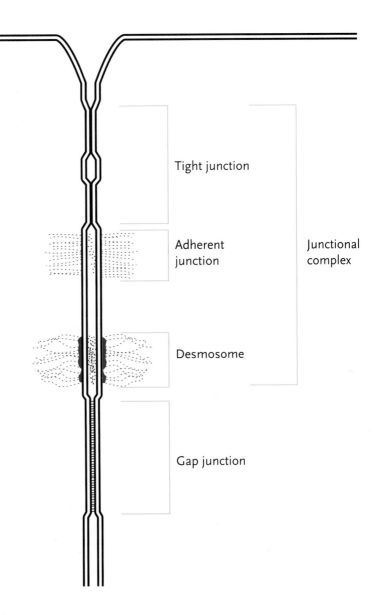

Tight junction

Adherent junction

Junctional complex

Desmosome

Gap junction

(i)   tight junctions (zonula occludentes), which consist of small areas where the outer lamina of opposing plasma membranes are *fused* with one another, via specific proteins which make direct contact across the intercellular space. The tight junction forms a complete circumferential band around each cell.

(ii) adherent junctions (zonula adherentes), which are located beneath the tight junctions, consist of areas where the opposing plasma membranes diverge. A fine mat of filamentous material is present on the cytoplasmic aspect of these junctions.

(iii) desmosomes, which form the third component of junctional complexes, have been described above.

The presence of the various types of cell junctions in epithelia means that neighboring cells are sealed together, to create a continuous sheet of cells, further compounding the physical barrier of the epithelium to drug absorption.

Biochemical barriers

In addition to a physical barrier, the epithelia also present a biochemical barrier to drug absorption, in the form of degradative enzymes. For example, the gastrointestinal tract contains a wide array of enzymes, which are present in a variety of locations:

- the lumen;
- adsorbed to the mucus layer;
- the brush-border (microvilli) of the enterocytes;
- intra-cellular (free within the cell cytoplasm and within cellular lysosomes);
- the colon (colonic microflora).

Enzymes in the gut lumen include proteases, glycosidases and lipases, which are highly efficient at breaking down proteins, carbohydrates and fats from foodstuffs, so that they can be absorbed to make energy available to the body. However, these enzymes (and the enzymes present in the other locations in the gastrointestinal tract) can also degrade drug molecules, deactivating them prior to absorption. For example, the metabolizing enzyme cytochrome P450 on the microvillus tip is associated with a significant loss of drugs. Drugs that are orally absorbed must also first pass through the liver, via the portal circulation, prior to reaching the systemic circulation. The loss of drug activity due to metabolism in the gut wall and liver prior to reaching systemic circulation is termed the "first-pass" effect. In some cases this pre-systemic metabolism accounts for a significant, or even total, loss of drug activity.

Thus the gastrointestinal tract poses a formidable challenge to the delivery of enzymatically labile drugs, such as therapeutic peptides and proteins. The extremely high metabolic activity of the gastrointestinal tract has been a major impetus in the exploration of alternative routes for systemic drug delivery. In comparison to the oral route, much less is known about the nature of the enzymatic barrier presented by the buccal, nasal, pulmonary, dermal and vaginal routes. However, it is generally accepted that such routes have a lower enzymatic activity, particularly towards drugs such as peptides and proteins. Furthermore, such routes also offer the advantage of avoiding first-pass metabolism by the liver.

Efflux systems

In recent years, it has been found that the barrier function of the intestinal epithelium cannot be adequately described by a combination of metabolic and physical barriers alone. Apically polarized efflux systems are known to be present in cancer cells and represent a major barrier to the uptake of a wide variety of chemotherapeutic agents (i.e. in multi-drug resistance). Efflux systems have also now been identified in normal intestinal and colonic cells, and also at other epithelial sites.

Some of these efflux systems seem to involve P-glycoprotein, the principal component of multidrug resistance in a variety of cell types. P-glycoprotein is a 170–180 kDa membrane glycoprotein acting as an ATP-dependent efflux pump that reduces the intracellular accumulation and/or the transcellular flux of a wide variety of drugs, including peptides such as gramicidin D, valinomycin and cyclosporin.

As these efflux systems are located on the apical surface of the plasma membrane, it can be assumed that their physiological role is to restrict transcellular flux of some molecules.

1.3.3 Routes and mechanisms of drug absorption

The organization and architecture of epithelial mucosa restrict drug permeation across the barrier to two main routes (Figure 1.3):

- paracellular: *between* adjacent epithelial cells;
- transcellular: *across* epithelial cells.

1.3.3.1 *Paracellular route*

The paracellular route is a passive, diffusional transport pathway, taken by small, hydrophilic molecules, for example mannitol, which can pass through the various types of junctions between adjacent epithelial cells. The rate of passive diffusion follows Fick's Law, which is described in detail below. Passive diffusion is driven by a concentration gradient and is inversely related to molecular weight. This route is therefore not suitable for large molecular weight drugs, which are too large to cross between cell junctions.

One approach to enhancing drug absorption via this route is to temporarily damage the integrity of the tight junctions using certain types of penetration enhancers. Obviously this approach has considerable toxicological implications, both directly, by damaging the epithelial interface and also indirectly, by increasing the permeability of the epithelium, thereby increasing the possibility of entry of potentially harmful substances.

1.3.3.2 *Transcellular route*

The transcellular pathway involves the movement of the drug across the epithelial cell, by active and/or passive processes (Figure 1.3), which are discussed in detail below.

Transcellular passive diffusion

Low molecular weight and lipophilic drug molecules are usually absorbed transcellularly, by passive diffusion across the epithelial cells. With respect to passive diffusion, the outer membrane of the epithelial cell may be regarded as a layer of lipid, surrounded on both sides by water (Figure 1.4). Thus for transport through the apical membrane, there are three barriers to be circumvented:

- the external water-lipid interface;
- the lipid membrane;
- the internal lipid-water interface.

Figure 1.3 Routes and mechanisms for drug transport across epithelia*

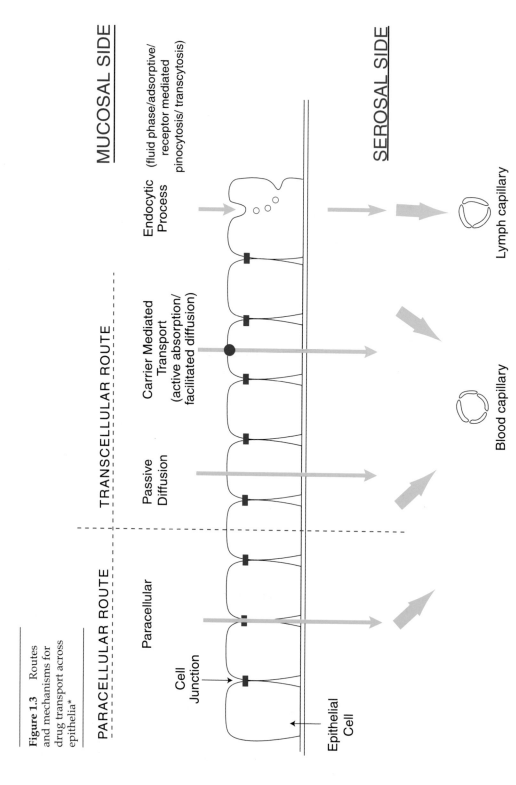

*As discussed in the text, various types of epithelia exist; however, the routes and mechanisms of absorption depicted here are generally applicable to all epithelial types.

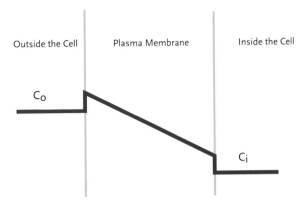

Outside the Cell   Plasma Membrane   Inside the Cell

C_o

C_i

Figure 1.4 The process of passive diffusion across membranes

C_o = concentration of drug on the outside of the membrane,
C_i = concentration of drug on the inside of the membrane.

In the process of passive diffusion:

- lipid-soluble substances move into the lipid membrane according to their lipid/water partition coefficient;
- molecules then diffuse across the lipid phase according to the concentration gradient established between the apical and basolateral sides of the membrane;
- the molecules distribute out at the other side of the membrane, according to their lipid/water partition coefficient.

The rate of diffusion through the membrane follows Fick's Law, which states that the rate of diffusion across a membrane is proportional to the difference in concentration on each side of the membrane:

$$dm/dt = (Dk/h) . A . \Delta C$$

(Equation 1.3)

where dm/dt = the rate of diffusion across the membrane

D = the diffusion coefficient of the drug in the membrane

k = the partition coefficient of the drug into the membrane

h = the membrane thickness

A = the available surface area

ΔC = the concentration gradient, i.e. $C_o - C_i$ where C_o and C_i denote the drug concentrations on the outside and the inside of themembrane, respectively.

Thus a drug molecule, driven by the concentration gradient, diffuses through the apical cell membrane and gains access to the inside of the cell. The molecule then diffuses through the epithelial cell and subsequently diffuses out through the basolateral membrane, to be absorbed by the underlying blood capillaries (Figure 1.3).

Another possibility is that certain drugs, of appropriate partition coefficients, would preferentially remain within the lipid bilayer of the plasma membrane, rather than partitioning out into the cell cytoplasm. Such moieties could thus diffuse along the lipid bilayer of the membrane, down the *side* of the cell (rather than *through* it), emerging finally at the basolateral surface of the cell. However this scenario is limited by the fact that the lipid membrane constitutes a minute proportion of the available surface area of the cell; also cell junctions can act as diffusion barriers within the lipid bilayer of the plasma membrane.

From Figure 1.3 it can be seen that in order to reach the underlying blood capillaries to be absorbed, the drug must pass through at least two epithelial membrane barriers (the apical and basolateral epithelial cell membranes) and also the endothelial membrane of the capillaries. In some cases, for example in stratified epithelia such as that found in the skin and buccal mucosa, the epithelial barrier comprises a number of cell layers rather than a single epithelial cell. Thus the *effective* barrier to drug absorption is not diffusion across a single membrane as described above, but diffusion across the entire epithelial and endothelial barrier, which may comprise several membranes and cells in series.

The driving force for absorption is, again, the concentration gradient and the process is governed by Fick's Law. However, in this case, the concentration gradient driving absorption comprises the gradient established across the entire *effective* barrier, from the epithelial surface to the circulating blood. Similarly, the parameters D, K, h and A of Equation 1.3 refer to the entire "barrier" (i.e. the overall effective barrier to drug absorption, which may comprise several membranes and cells in series) rather than simply the apical plasma membrane.

It should be noted, however, that even though the barrier to drug absorption may actually comprise several membranes and cells in series, it would appear that, generally, it is ultimately the *apical plasma membrane* which is rate-limiting for drug absorption. Thus in transcellular passive diffusion, the epithelium is assumed to act as a simple lipophilic barrier through which drugs diffuse and the rate of diffusion correlates with the lipid solubility of the drug.

The circulating concentration of the drug is reduced by one or more of the following factors:

- distribution into body tissue and other fluids of distribution;
- binding to plasma proteins;
- metabolism and excretion.

As a consequence, the concentration of drug in systemic circulation is negligible in comparison to the drug concentration at the absorption surface. In this case, the blood is said to act as a "sink" for absorbed drug. When sink conditions occur, it ensures that a large concentration gradient is maintained throughout the absorption phase, thereby enhancing the driving-force for absorption. The maintenance of sink conditions means that:

$C_0 > C_i$, thus $\Delta C \approx C_0$.

and Equation 1.3 is reduced to:

$$dm/dt = (Dk/h) . A . C_0$$

(Equation 1.4)

Substituting further into Equation 1.4 gives:

$$dm/dt = P . A . C_0$$

where P, the permeability constant, is defined as Dk/h and has the units cm/s.

This can be simplified further to give:

$$dm/dt = K_1 C_0$$

(Equation 1.5)

Equation 1.5 is the familiar form of first-order rate equation and indicates that the rate of absorption is proportional to drug concentration. K_1 is a pseudo-rate constant and is dependent on the factors D, A, k and h.

Fick's Law is often described in any of the three different forms given above. Hence:

$$dm/dt = (Dk/h).A.C_0 = P.A.C_0 = K_1 C_0$$

(Equation 1.6)

Carrier-mediated transport

In this situation (Figure 1.3), specialized membrane protein molecules transport substrates across the cell membranes, either against the concentration gradient (active absorption), or with the concentration gradient (facilitated diffusion).

In active absorption, carriers may transport substrates *against* a concentration gradient, in an energy-consuming process. This form of transport may occur through "dynamic pores", consisting of proteins or protein systems which span the plasma membrane. Alternatively, the proteins may be located on the apical surface of the membrane and active absorption is associated with a series of steps:

1 The substrate forms a complex with the carrier in the membrane surface.
2 The substrate-carrier complex moves through the membrane.
3 The substrate is released from the complex at the other side of the membrane.
4 The carrier molecule (now free) then returns to the apical surface of the membrane, and is ready to bind with further substrates.

Substrates may include drugs, small ions, and other endogenous substances. The best-studied systems of this type are the ATPase transport proteins which are particularly important in maintaining concentration gradients of small ions in cells, such as nerve cells. The major substances that are believed to be actively transported across membranes are sodium and calcium ions. Absorption of many molecules occurs by co-transport, a variation of active transport in which absorption into the cell against the concentration gradient is linked to the secretion of a cellular ion such as sodium down its concentration gradient. This process is important for the absorption of glucose and amino acids in the small intestine.

The small intestine contains a wide variety of transporters (amino acid transporters, oligopeptide transporters, glucose transporters, lactic acid transporters etc.) on the apical membrane of the epithelial cells, which serve as carriers to facilitate nutrient absorption by the intestine. On the basolateral membrane, the presence of amino acid and oligopeptide transporters has been demonstrated. Active transport mechanisms for di- and tri-peptides have also been demonstrated in the nasal and buccal epithelia.

Facilitated diffusion involves carrier-mediated transport *down* a concentration gradient. The existence of the carrier molecules means that diffusion down the concentration gradient is much greater than would be expected on the basis of the physicochemical properties of the drug. A much larger number of substances are believed to be transported by facilitated diffusion than active transport, including vitamins such as thiamine, nicotinic acid, riboflavin and vitamin B6, various sugars and amino acids.

Both processes exhibit classical saturation kinetics, since there are only a finite number of carrier molecules. Thus unlike passive absorption (paracellular or transcellular), where the rate of transport is directly proportional to the drug concentration (Figure 1.5, A), carrier-

Figure 1.5 Kinetics of (A) passive diffusion and (B) active transport

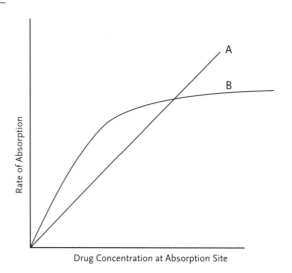

Chapter One

mediated transport is only proportional to the drug concentration at low concentrations of drug. At higher concentrations, the carrier mechanism becomes saturated and the rate of absorption remains constant (Figure 1.5, B).

If a drug is sufficiently similar to a substance naturally transported by a carrier-mediated system, the drug may also be transported by the same system. For example, the drugs levodopa, methyldopa and penicillamine are all absorbed via various amino acid transporters. Serine and threonine derivatives of nitrogen mustard, which have been investigated for antitumor activity, are also absorbed by a carrier-mediated process. Digitalis and other cardioselective glycosides also demonstrate behavior not compatible with simple partition theory, which suggests the involvement of carrier-mediated transport.

Considerable attention is being focused on the identification of the structural requirements necessary for the binding and transport via the di- and tri-peptide transporters present in the gastrointestinal tract, in order to exploit this route for the oral delivery of peptides. Critical structural features that have been found to influence transport include stereoisomerism, side-chain length and net charge. Several drugs including a pGlu-L-dopa prodrug, as well as angiotensin-converting enzyme inhibitors and various thrombin inhibitors, have all demonstrated success in targeting endogenous transporters and enhancing transport across the intestinal mucosa.

Endocytic processes

All the above transport mechanisms are only applicable to the absorption of small molecules, less than approximately 500 Da. There is evidence that larger molecules can be absorbed with low efficiency due to endocytosis. Endocytosis is defined as the internalization of plasma membrane with concomitant engulfment of extracellular material and extracellular fluid. The process can be divided into two types, pinocytosis and phagocytosis.

Pinocytosis is a non-specific process that goes on continually in all cell types, in which the plasma membrane invaginates and forms an inward channel, into which extracellular fluid flows (Figure 1.6).

Solutes dissolved in the extracellular fluid, including large (soluble) macromolecules, may flow with the extracellular fluid into the invaginations and become internalized. This process, i.e. the uptake of macromolecules in solution, is known as fluid-phase pinocytosis. Alternatively, uptake may involve:

- adsorptive pinocytosis, in which macromolecules bind to non-specific membrane receptors, prior to pinocytosis;
- receptor-mediated pinocytosis, in which macromolecules bind to specific membrane receptors, prior to pinocytosis.

The invaginated membrane then "pinches off" to form detached vesicles. The pinocytic vesicles (endosomes) migrate inwardly and fuse with lysosomes, which contain many lysosomal enzymes, to form secondary lysosomes. The ligand is degraded by the lysosomal enzymes, the degraded products are released and the membrane is recycled

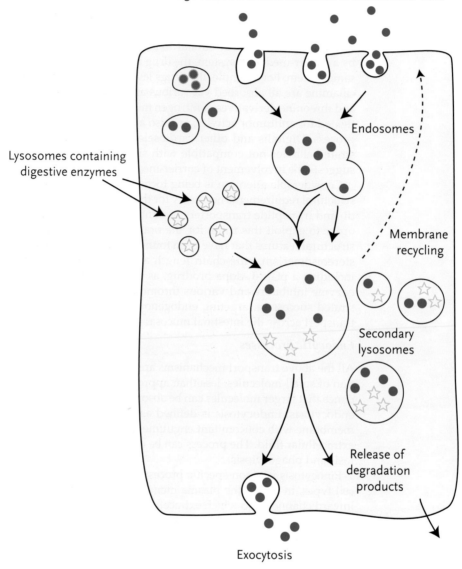

Drug macromolecules dissolved in extracellular fluid

Endosomes

Lysosomes containing
digestive enzymes

Membrane
recycling

Secondary
lysosomes

Release of
degradation
products

Exocytosis

● Drug molecule dissolved in the extracellular fluid
☆ Lysosomal digestive enzymes

Figure 1.6 Schematic representation of fluid-phase pinocytosis and exocytosis

back to the plasma membrane. Alternatively, the secondary lysosomes can fuse with the cell membrane, leading to exocytosis of their contents, and the membranes are recycled back to the plasma membrane.

Thus pinocytosis offers a pathway through which large macromolecules, which are otherwise incapable of passing through the membrane, may be taken up by cells. In some cases, following uptake of a

Chapter One

drug via receptor-mediated pinocytosis, the endosomes carrying the drug actually bypass the lysosomes and migrate toward the basolateral membrane, resulting in the release of the undegraded drug into the extracellular space bounded by the basolateral membrane. This process, known as *transcytosis*, represents a potentially useful and important pathway for the absorption of high molecular weight drugs such as peptides and proteins. Indeed, some peptides and proteins are known to enter intestinal mucosal cells through pinocytosis; furthermore, a few peptides and proteins (including immunoglobulin G, nerve growth factor and epidermal growth factor) have been reported to reach blood vessels in the lamina propria and the portal venous circulation.

The process of phagocytosis involves the internalization of particulate matter. The phagocytic process occurs in a number of stages (See Chapter 5, Figure 5.2):

- *Adsorption*: the drug/particulate adsorbs to the phagocytic cell surface. This process may be facilitated by serum proteins knows as opsonins, which cover the particulate and promote adsorption and ingestion. The extent and pattern of opsonization depends highly on antigen surface characteristics such as charge and hydrophilicity.
- *Ingestion*: the cell membrane moves outwards, surrounding the particle surface, and forms a vesicle, known as a phagosome, which detaches from the plasma membrane to float freely within the cytoplasm.
- *Digestion*: the internalized phagosome eventually fuses with intracellular lysosomes and degradation by lysosomal enzymes again takes place. When digestion is complete, the lysosomal membrane may rupture, discharging its contents into the cytoplasm.

Phagocytosis is only carried out by the specialized cells ("professional phagocytes") of the mononuclear phagocyte systems (MPS; also known as the reticuloendothelial system, RES), which include the circulating blood monocytes and both fixed and free macrophages. Fixed macrophages are found lining certain blood and lymph-filled spaces, such as the sinusoids of the liver (these cells are commonly referred to as Kupffer cells), bone marrow and spleen. The MPS constitutes an important part of the body's immune system, being responsible for the removal of particulate antigens such as damaged blood cells, microbes, denatured proteins and other foreign particulates.

For the purpose of completeness, the process of phagocytosis has been described briefly here. However, it should be remembered that phagocytosis is not generally relevant to the transport of drugs across epithelial interfaces, as it is only carried out by the professional phagocytes of the MPS.

The process of phagocytosis is of particular relevance when particulate delivery systems, such as microspheres, liposomes and other advanced delivery systems (described in Chapter 5), are used. Such particulate carriers are susceptible to MPS clearance. Sequestration by the MPS is useful in some cases, for example in the treatment of certain microbial diseases. However, if the drug is to be delivered to sites other than the MPS, it is highly undesirable. Therefore considerable research effort is being directed towards methods of avoiding MPS uptake of drug delivery systems. Strategies to both exploit and avoid MPS uptake are described in detail in Chapter 5 (see Section 5.1.4).

Phagocytic processes are also finding applications in oral drug delivery and targeting. Specialized epithelial cells known as M cells, which overly lymphoid sections of the gastrointestinal tract, may be involved in the phagocytic uptake of macromolecules and microparticles from the gut (see Section 6.2.2).

Pore transport

A further mechanism of transcellular transport is via the aqueous pores which exist in many lipid membranes. The pores are of the order of 0.4 nm in diameter, thus very small hydrophilic molecules such as water, urea and low molecular weight sugars can diffuse through these channels and thus be absorbed by epithelial cells. However, most drugs are generally much larger (≥ 1 nm in diameter) than the pore size, and this route is therefore of minor importance for drug delivery.

1.3.4 Physicochemical properties of the drug influencing drug absorption

Physicochemical properties of a drug which influence drug absorption include such properties as:

- lipid solubility and partition coefficient;
- pKa;
- molecular weight and volume;
- aqueous solubility;
- chemical stability.

These properties will influence the route and mechanism of drug absorption through the mucosa. For example, it is not unreasonable to assume that:

- low molecular weight hydrophilic compounds would tend to be absorbed via the paracellular route, moving between the epithelial cells;
- lipid-soluble drugs would usually absorbed via transcellular passive diffusion, diffusing through the lipidic membrane barrier;
- macromolecules may be absorbed via endocytic processes;
- drugs bearing structural similarities to endogenous nutrients may be absorbed via carrier-mediated mechanisms.

However, this is a rather simplistic view and it is important to realize that these considerations are only broad generalizations. Thus although a drug molecule may be *predominantly* absorbed via one particular route/mechanism, it is also likely that *suboptimal* transport will occur via other routes and mechanisms. In particular, drugs that are absorbed via active mechanisms are often also absorbed, to a (much) lesser extent, via passive diffusion mechanisms.

A brief description of the effect of the physicochemical properties of the drug on the absorption process is given below and is discussed in more detail in the relevant chapters.

1.3.4.1 *Lipid Solubility and Partition Coefficient*

For most conventional drug molecules, which tend to be small and lipophilic, absorption occurs transcellularly, via passive diffusion across the epithelial cells. In this case, where the GI tract (or other epithelial interface) is assumed to act as a simple lipophilic barrier, absorption occurs down a concentration gradient according to Fick's Law, and the rate of absorption correlates with the lipid solubility of the drug (see Section 1.3.3.2).

A measure of the lipid solubility of a drug is given by its oil/water equilibrium partition coefficient. This is determined by adding the drug to a mixture of equal volumes of a lipophilic liquid (often octanol, but other solvents also used) and water and shaking the mixture vigorously to promote partitioning of the drug into each phase. When equilibrium is attained, the phases are separated and assayed for drug. The partition coefficient (P) is given by:

$$P = C_{oil}/C_{water}$$

(Equation 1.7)

where C_{oil} = concentration of drug in the oil phase
and
C_{water} = concentration of drug in the water phase

Often, the logarithm of the partition coefficient, (log P), of a compound is quoted.
For a given drug:

if log P = 0 , there is equal distribution of the drug in both phases
if log P > 0, the drug is lipid soluble
if log P < 0, the drug is water soluble

Thus in general, the higher the log P, the higher is the affinity for lipid membranes and thus the more rapidly the drug passes through the membrane via passive diffusion. This is exemplified in Table 1.2 for five different barbiturate compounds, in which an almost perfect rank correlation exists between the partition coefficient and the extent of absorption.

Values of log P that are too high (> 6) or too low (< 3) may be associated with poor transport characteristics. Drugs with very high log P values have poor aqueous solubility, which is partly the reason for their poor absorption properties, as some degree of aqueous solubility is required for drug absorption (see Section 1.3.4.4). Furthermore, if a drug is too lipophilic, it will remain in the lipidic membrane and never partition out again into the underlying aqueous environment.

Very polar compounds (with very low log P values) are not sufficiently lipophilic to be able to pass through lipid membrane barri-

Barbiturate	Structure	Partition Coeff.	% Absorbed
Barbital		0.7	12
Phenobarbital		4.8	20
Cyclobarbital		13.9	24
Pentobarbital		28	30
Secobarbital		50.7	40

Table 1.2   Comparison of barbiturate absorption in rat colon and partition coefficient (chloroform/water) of undissociated drug.

Data from Schanker, L. S. (1959) Absorption of drugs from the rat colon. *J. Pharmacol. Exp. Ther.*, 126:283–290.

ers. If a drug molecule forms hydrogen bonds with water, desolvation and breaking of the hydrogen bonds is required, prior to partitioning into the apical membrane of the epithelial cell. If the number of hydrogen bonds between the drug and water is > 10, too much energy is required and there will be minimal drug transport across the membrane. The number of hydrogen bonds a drug forms with water can be estimated by inspection of the drug structure (Table 1.3).

The lipid solubility of a drug molecule can be increased by blocking the hydrogen bonding capacity of the drug. This may be achieved by, for example, substitution, esterification or alkylation of existing groups on the molecules and will decrease the drug's aqueous solubility, favoring partitioning of the drug into the lipid membrane. The development of clindamycin, which differs from lincomycin by the single substitution of a chloride for a hydroxyl group, is such an example. Alternatively, the drug may be covalently bound to a lipid carrier, such as long-chain fatty acids.

Table 1.3   Number of hydrogen bonds formed per type of functional group on a molecule

Functional Group	Number of Hydrogen Bonds
Ester group	1/2
Carbonyl group	1
Hydroxyl group	2
Primary amino or amide group	3
Terminal amide group	4

However, these approaches involve modifying the existing structure of the drug, forming a new chemical entity. Altering the structure of the drug carries the concomitant risks of:

- compromising the activity of the drug;
- increasing the toxicity of the drug;
- increasing the molecular weight to such an extent that the molecule will be too large to cross the membrane barrier (see Section 1.3.4.3).

An alternative strategy, which overcomes these limitations, is to use the prodrug approach (Figure 1.7). This involves the chemical transformation of the active drug substance to an inactive derivative (prodrug), which is subsequently converted to the parent compound *in vivo* by an enzymatic or non-enzymatic process. Thus a prodrug of a drug, because of its increased lipid solubility, may demonstrate enhanced membrane permeability in comparison to the parent drug. Enzymatic or chemical transformation converts the inactive prodrug to the pharmacologically active drug, after absorption has taken place.

A further important point, discussed in detail in the next section, is that lipid solubility must be considered in the context of the degree of ionization of the drug.

1.3.4.2 Degree of ionization

Many drugs are weak electrolytes and their degree of ionization depends on both their pKa and the pH of the solution. Assuming, for transcellular passive diffusion, that the GI tract is acting as a simple lipophilic barrier, the ionized form of a molecule will be more water-

Figure 1.7 The prodrug approach to drug delivery

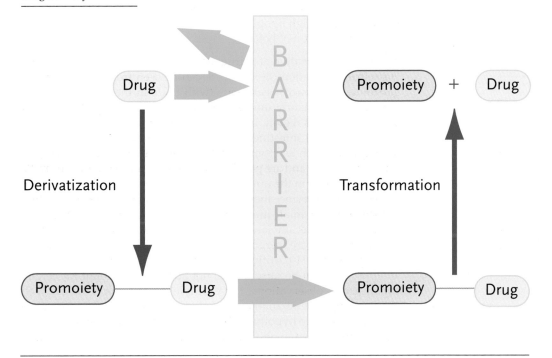

soluble and will have negligible lipid solubility in comparison with the unionized, lipid-soluble form, i.e.:

- Unionized form of the drug = lipophilic $\Rightarrow$ membrane transport;
- Ionized form of the drug = hydrophilic $\Rightarrow$ minimal membrane transport.

Therefore the pH of the solution will affect the overall partition coefficient of an ionizable substance. The barbiturate example given above (Table 1.2) is a simplified case, in which all three compounds have approximately equivalent pKa values, so that the degree of ionization is similar for all the drugs, allowing a direct correlation of lipophilicity with absorption. For ionizable drugs log P is pH dependent and hence log D, the log distribution coefficient of the drug at different pHs, is usually employed instead of log P, as an estimation and/or prediction of absorptive potential. The pH at which the log D is measured should be reported but values normally correspond to determinations carried out at a physiological pH of 7.4. Log D is effectively the log partition coefficient of the unionized form of the drug at a given pH. The relationship between the observed overall partition coefficient and the distribution coefficient is given by the equation:

$$D = P(1-\alpha)$$

where α is the degree of ionization of drug.

The interrelationship between the dissociation constant and lipid solubility of a drug, as well as the pH at the absorption site, is known as the pH-partition theory of drug absorption. Accordingly, rapid transcellular passive diffusion of a drug molecule may be due to:

- a high proportion of unionized molecules;
- a high log P (high lipophilicity);
- or a combination of both.

The extent of ionization of a drug molecule is given by the Henderson-Hasselbalch Equation (Box 1.1). As can be seen from Box 1.1, in the gastrointestinal tract, weak acids (with pK_a's in the range 2.5 to 7.5) will be predominantly unionized in the stomach, which favors their absorption in this region. In contrast, a very low percentage is unionized in the small intestine, which suggests unfavorable absorption. Strong acids, such as cromoglycate, are ionized throughout the gastrointestinal tract and are poorly absorbed. The reverse is true for weak bases (with pK_a's in the range 5 to 11), which are poorly absorbed, if at all, in the stomach since they are largely ionized at low pH, but are well absorbed in the small intestine, where they are unionized. Strong bases, such as mecamylamine, are ionized throughout the gastrointestinal tract and are therefore poorly absorbed.

Although the pH-partition hypothesis is useful, it must be viewed as an approximation because it does not adequately account for certain experimental observations. For example, most weak acids are well absorbed from the small intestine, which is contrary to the predictions of the pH-partition hypothesis. Similarly, quaternary ammonium compounds are ionized at all pHs but are readily absorbed from the gas-

The Henderson-Hasselbalch Equation:

Acid

$$pH = pKa + \log \frac{[A-]}{[HA]}$$

Base

$$pH = pKa + \log \frac{[B]}{[BH+]}$$

To illustrate the concept of the pH-partition hypothesis, consider the absorption of the weak electrolytes, aspirin and codeine, from the gastrointestinal tract.

Weakly Acidic Drug: Aspirin (pKa = 3.5)

Unionized [HA]   Ionized [A⁻]

In the stomach, assume the pH of the gastric fluid = 1. The Henderson-Hasselbalch equation gives:

$$1 = 3.5 + \log \frac{[A^-]}{[HA]}$$

$$\log \frac{[A-]}{[HA]} = -2.5$$

$$\text{Therefore } \frac{[A^-]}{[HA]} = 10^{-2.5} = 0.003$$

Thus at the low pH in the stomach, [HA] is far greater than [A⁻], i.e. the drug is predominantly unionized = absorbable form.

In the intestine, assume the pH of the intestinal fluid = 6.5. The Henderson-Hasselbalch equation gives:

$$6.5 = 3.5 + \log \frac{[A^-]}{[HA]}$$

$$\log \frac{[A-]}{[HA]} = 3$$

$$\text{Therefore } \frac{[A^-]}{[HA]} = 10^3 = 1000$$

Thus at the high pH in the small intestine, [A⁻] is 1000 times greater than [HA], i.e. the drug is predominantly ionized = unabsorbable form

Weakly Basic Drug: Codeine (pKa = 8)

Unionized [B]   Ionized [BH⁺]

In the stomach, assume the pH of the gastric fluid = 1. The Henderson-Hasselbalch equation gives:

$$1 = 8 + \log \frac{[B]}{[BH^+]}$$

$$\log \frac{[B]}{[BH^+]} = -7$$

$$\text{Therefore } \frac{[B]}{[BH^+]} = 10^{-7} = 0.0000001$$

Thus at the low pH in the stomach, [BH⁺] is 10^7 greater than [B], i.e. the drug is predominantly ionized = unabsorbable form

In the intestine, assume the pH of the intestinal fluid = 6.5. The Henderson-Hasselbalch equation gives:

$$6.5 = 8 + \log \frac{[B]}{[BH^+]}$$

$$\log \frac{[B]}{[BH^+]} = -1.5$$

$$\text{Therefore } \frac{[B]}{[BH^+]} = 10^{-1.5} = 0.03$$

Thus at the high pH in the small intestine, the drug is much less ionized than in the stomach and is therefore more readily adsorbed.

trointestinal tract. These discrepancies arise because the pH-partition hypothesis does not take into account the following:

- the large mucosal surface area of the small intestine, which compensates for ionization effects;
- the relatively long residence time in the small intestine, which also compensates for ionization effects;
- even the ionized form of a drug displays limited absorption;
- charged drugs, such as quaternary ammonium compounds, may interact with organic ions of opposite charge, resulting in a neutral species, which is absorbable;
- bulk transport of water from the gut lumen to the blood, or *vice* versa, can drag water-soluble molecules with it, resulting in an increase or decrease in the absorption of water-soluble drugs respectively. Solvent drag can arise due to differences in osmotic pressure (e.g. due to the presence of salts) between the lumen and the blood;
- the presence of unstirred water layer and the binding of some drugs to mucins in the mucus layer overlaying the epithelium affects the overall transport properties;
- some drugs are absorbed via active pathways.

1.3.4.3 *Molecular weight and molecular volume*

Drug diffusion in simple liquids is expressed by Stokes-Einstein equation:

$$D = R\,T/6\pi\eta r$$

where D = the diffusion of the drug
         R = gas constant = 8.314 J K^{-1} mol^{-1}
         T = temperature (kelvin)
         η = the viscosity of the solvent
         r = solvated radius of the diffusing solute

As: V = $(4/3)\pi r^3$
where V = volume
         r = radius,

drug diffusivity is inversely proportional to the cube-root of the molecular volume. A more complex relationship pertains for more complex and organized structures such as lipid bilayers, but again, drug diffusivity is inversely proportional (probably by an exponential relationship) to the molecular volume.

This means that drug diffusivity across membranes is sensitive to molecular weight, since molecular volume is determined by a number of factors, including the molecular weight of the molecule. Therefore, in general, large molecules will diffuse at a slower rate than small molecules.

However, molecular volume is also determined by:

- the overall conformation of the molecule;
- the heteroatom content that may be involved in inter- and intra-molecular hydrogen bonding.

Thus molecules which assume a compact conformation will have a lower molecular volume and thus a higher diffusivity. An important consequence of this property is that even if such molecules have a high molecular weight (i.e. above the molecular weight threshold of 500 Da normally the cut-off limit for transmembrane transport), their high diffusivity may nevertheless be able to facilitate absorption.

Molecular size and volume also have important implications for the paracellular route of drug absorption. It would appear that tight junctions bind cells together very efficiently and can block the passage of even relatively small molecules. Gap junctions are looser and molecules up to 1,200 Da can pass freely between cells. Larger molecules cannot pass through gap junctions, suggesting a functioning pore size for the connecting channels of about 1.5 nm.

1.3.4.4   Solubility

As described in detail in subsequent chapters, drugs can be administered via a variety of absorption routes, using a variety of dosage forms. For example, an orally administered drug can be given as a tablet, capsule or suspension; drugs for parenteral administration can be given as suspensions, emulsions and microparticulate systems; delivery systems for drugs administered via routes such as the transdermal, buccal, nasal and vaginal routes include suspensions, creams, gels and patches.

As described above, the epithelia present a significant physical and biochemical barrier to drug absorption. However, since drugs must generally be in solution before they can cross epithelia, in many cases the rate of absorption of the drug from the particular dosage form is controlled by how fast the drug dissolves in the fluids at the absorption site. When dissolution is the controlling step in the overall process, absorption is described as *dissolution rate limited*. Therefore the solubility of the drug constitutes an important physicochemical property affecting drug absorption. It has been estimated that 43% of new chemical entities are sparingly soluble in water, thus it is not surprising that methods to increase the solubility of poorly soluble drugs constitutes an important area of research.

Chapter 6 (Section 6.4) describes in detail the effect of drug solubility and dissolution rate on oral bioavailability. Further information is also given in the relevant chapters describing the various routes of drug delivery. To briefly summarize here, the general relationship describing the dissolution process is given by the Noyes-Whitney equation (Equation 6.1). One of the most important implications of this equation is that a drug dissolves more rapidly when its surface area is increased, which is usually accomplished by reducing the particle size of the drug. Many poorly soluble, slowly dissolving drugs for oral drug delivery are therefore marketed in micronized or microcrystalline form, as reducing the particle size of the drug increases the available surface area.

Drug solubility is also critically dependent on the pKa of the drug and the prevailing pH of the GI tract. The ionized form of a drug molecule is the more water-soluble form, therefore the dissolution rate of weak acids increases with increasing pH, whereas the dissolution rate of weak bases decreases with increasing pH.

Although it is the ionized form of a drug that is required for aqueous solubility, the *un*ionized form is required for lipid solubility and transcellular passive diffusion. However, the unionized form has poor aqueous solubility, which mitigates *against* membrane penetration. In practice, a balance between the lipid and aqueous solubility of a drug is required for successful absorption.

Various strategies to increase the solubility of a drug are given below; this subject is also discussed in detail in Chapter 6 (see Section 6.4) and in the further reading detailed at the end of this chapter.

Salt formation

Formation of a corresponding water-soluble salt increases the dissolution rate in the gastrointestinal tract. For weakly acidic drugs, increased dissolution is achieved by forming the corresponding sodium or potassium salt, whereas for weakly basic drugs increased dissolution is achieved by forming the corresponding HCl or other strong acid salt.

This phenomenon can be explained by considering that a weakly acidic drug is unionized in the stomach and therefore has a low dissolution rate. If the free acid is converted to the corresponding sodium or potassium salt, the strongly alkali sodium or potassium cations exert a neutralizing effect. Thus in the immediate vicinity of the drug the pH is raised to, for example, pH 5–6, instead of pH of 1–2 in the bulk medium of the stomach, resulting in an alkaline microenvironment around the drug particle. This causes dissolution of the acidic drug in this localized region of higher pH, which gives rise to overall faster dissolution rates. When dissolved drug diffuses away from the drug surface into the bulk of the gastric fluid where the pH is again lower, the free acid form may precipitate out. However, the precipitated free acid will be in the form of very fine wetted drug particles. These drug particles exhibit a very large total effective surface area in contact with the gastric fluids, much larger than would have been obtained if the free acid form of the drug had been administered. This increase in surface area results in an increased dissolution rate. Similarly, the HCl or other strong acid salts of weak bases cause a localized *drop* in pH around the drug, which enhances the dissolution of weak bases.

Examples of the use of soluble salts to increase drug absorption include novobiocin, in which the bioavailability of the sodium salt of the drug is twice that of the calcium salt and 50 times that of the free acid.

Soluble prodrugs

Although, as described above (see Section 1.3.4.1), most research efforts using prodrugs have been directed towards increasing the lipid solubility of the parent moiety, soluble prodrugs have also been developed for those drugs which are dissolution rate limited. For example, the minor tranquilizer clorazepate is a prodrug of nordiazepam and is marketed as a dipotassium salt that is freely soluble in water, in contrast to the poorly soluble parent, norazepam.

Polymorphic forms

Many drugs can exist in more than one crystalline form, for example chloramphenicol palmitate, cortisone acetate, tetracyclines and sulphathiazole, depending on the conditions (temperature, solvent, time) under which crystallization occurs. This property is referred to as polymorphism and each crystalline form is known as a polymorph. At a given temperature and pressure only one of the crystalline forms is stable and the others are known as metastable forms. A metastable polymorph usually exhibits a greater aqueous solubility and dissolution rate, and thus greater absorption, than the stable polymorph.

Amorphous forms

The amorphous form of a drug has no crystalline lattice and therefore less energy is required for dissolution, so that the bioavailability of the amorphous form is generally greater than that of the crystalline form. For example, the amorphous form of novobiocin is at least 10 times more soluble than the crystalline form.

Solvates

Many drugs can associate with solvents to produce crystalline forms called solvates. When the solvent is water, the crystal is termed a hydrate. Thus more rapid dissolution rates are often achieved with the anhydrous form of a drug. For example, the anhydrous forms of caffeine, theophylline and glutethimide dissolve more rapidly in water than do the hydrous forms of these drugs and the anhydrous form of ampicillin is about 25% more soluble in water at 37 °C than the trihydrate.

Formulation factors

The type of dosage form and its method of preparation or manufacture can influence drug dissolution and thus bioavailability. For example, there is no dissolution step necessary for a drug administered as a solution, while drugs in suspension are relatively rapidly absorbed because of the large available surface area of the dispersed solid. In solid dosage forms such as hard gelatin capsules or tablets, the processes of disintegration and deaggregation must occur before drug dissolution can proceed at any appreciable rate. Hence, the dissolution and thus bioavailability of a given drug generally tends to decrease in the following order of type of oral dosage form:

aqueous solutions > aqueous suspensions > hard gelatin capsules > tablets.

The effect of particle size on dissolution rate and bioavailability has been alluded to above and is discussed in detail in Section 6.4.2, as is the influence of formulation additives such as wetting agents, diluents, binders, surfactants, buffers etc. on the drug dissolution rate. These formulation additives may alter drug dissolution rates by such mechanisms as increasing the wetting of the dosage form, aiding rapid disintegration of the dosage form, forming poorly absorbable drug-excipient complexes and altering the pH. The effect of formulation factors on the dissolution rate for absorption routes other than the oral route is discussed in the relevant chapters.

1.3.4.5   *Stability*

The stability of a drug *in vitro* may be adversely affected by various environmental factors including temperature, pressure, light, moisture and pH.

Drug degradation is generally a first order process and can be described by the following equation:

$$Ln(C/C_0) = -kt$$
$$t_{1/2} = -0.693/k$$
$$t_{0.9} = -0.105/k$$

(Equation 1.8)

where C is the concentration at time t
C_0 is the initial concentration,
K is the rate constant
$t_{1/2}$ is the half-life
$t_{0.9}$ is the shelf life (i.e. the point where 90% of the original concentration is present, which is widely used as an indicator for the expiration date of the drug)

The most common degradation reactions are solvolysis and oxidation. Solvolysis involves drug decomposition through a reaction with the solvent present, for example water, ethyl alcohol or polyethylene glycol. These solvents act as nucleophilic agents and attack electropositive centers of the drug molecule. Drugs containing esters (e.g. aspirin, alkaloids, dexamethasone, estrone, nitroglycerin), lactones (e.g. pilocarpine, spironolactone), lactams (e.g. penicillins, cephalosporins) and amides (e.g. therapeutic peptides and proteins) are all prone to hydrolysis. Oxidation is another common degradation reaction. Functional groups that are subject to oxidation include phenols (e.g. phenols in steroids), catechols (e.g. dopamine, isoproterenol) and thioethers (e.g. phenothiazines such as chlorpromazine). Other degradation reactions include photolysis, racemization, and decarboxylation.

The stability of the drug to degradative enzymes is of particular importance *in vivo*, as discussed above.

1.4   PHARMACOKINETIC PROCESSES

Drugs differ in their intrinsic ability to produce an effect, in their ability to reach the site of action and in their rate of removal from that site. Pharmacodynamics is the study of the action of the drug on the body. Pharmacokinetics is the study of how drugs enter the body, reach the site of action and are removed from the body, i.e. the study of:

- drug absorption;
- drug distribution;
- drug metabolism;
- drug excretion.

Elimination is defined as the process of removal of the drug from the body, which may involve metabolism and/or excretion. These processes of absorption, distribution, metabolism and excretion (ADME) are called the pharmacokinetic processes (Figure 1.8). The pharmacokinetic aspects of a drug are obviously just as important as its pharmacodynamics, when considering therapeutic efficacy.

The process of drug absorption has been described above and a brief description of the processes of distribution, metabolism and excretion are given below, with particular reference to their influence on drug delivery.

1.4.1 Distribution

Figure 1.8 Schematic representation of the pharmacokinetic processes, absorption, distribution, metabolism and excretion (ADME)

Distribution is the process by which the drug is transferred from the general circulation into the tissues (including blood cells) and other fluids of distribution (for example, lymph and interstitial fluids). For many drugs this occurs by simple diffusion of the unionized form across cell membranes (see Section 1.3.3). When drugs are given by iv administration, there is an extremely high initial plasma concentration and the drug may rapidly enter and equilibrate with well-perfused tissues such as the lung, adrenals, kidneys, liver and heart. Subsequently, the drug enters poorly perfused tissues such as skeletal muscle, connective tissue and adipose tissue. As the concentration of

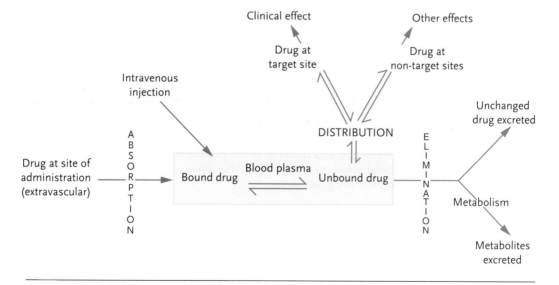

drug in the poorly perfused tissues increases, there is a corresponding decrease in the concentration in the plasma and well-perfused tissues.

Many drugs show an affinity for specific binding sites on plasma proteins such as albumin and α_1-acid glycoprotein, which results in a reversible association, with some important consequences in therapeutics:

- Drug binding lowers the concentration of free drug in solution, and thus the concentration of drug available to act at the receptor.
- Because of the reversible nature of protein binding, protein-bound drug can act as a drug depot *in vivo*.
- The competitive nature of protein binding means that other drug and endogenous ligands can compete for binding sites, in some cases displacing the drug and thereby increasing its concentration at the receptor.

A particular repercussion of the process of drug distribution is that after administration of a drug, *unwanted* drug disposition may occur, either:

- intra-vascular, by protein binding, or
- extra-vascular, at sites other than the target site.

This can result in the need to use high doses to compensate for drug wasteage, which is expensive. Unwanted deposition may also result in toxicity problems, arising from drug action at non-target sites.

Classic examples of toxic side-effects resulting from unwanted drug distribution are found in cancer chemotherapy. The chemotherapeutic agent, a cytotoxic poison, lacks specificity and has the potential to kill all cells, both normal and malignant. The drug exploits the difference in the turnover of cancer cells, which is very much greater than normal cells. However, rapidly dividing normal cells, for example the hair follicles, and the cells of the gastrointestinal tract, are also susceptible to attack. This gives rise to typical side-effects associated with cancer chemotherapy such as hair loss and acute gastrointestinal disturbances.

In the early 1900s Paul Ehrlich (who has been described as the father of drug delivery and therapeutics) pioneered the idea of the "magic bullet" approach, whereby therapy "could learn to aim". The inherent premise of this concept is to try to improve therapy by targeting the drug to the site of action, thereby removing unwanted toxic side-effects and minimizing drug wastage.

Methods to achieve drug targeting are introduced in Chapter 3 (Section 3.3), discussed in detail in Chapter 5 with respect to the parenteral route and also in further chapters concerning the various routes of drug delivery.

1.4.2 Metabolism

Drug metabolism involves the alteration of the chemical structure of the drug by an enzyme. It generally involves the transformation of a lipid-soluble drug (which can cross membranes and thus reach its site of action) into a more polar, water-soluble compound which can be rapidly eliminated in the urine.

Metabolic processes have considerable implications for successful drug delivery:

- Metabolic activity may result in premature degradation of the active moiety, prior to its arrival at the active site.
- Metabolites may be more active and have longer half-lives.
- Toxic metabolites of the active may be formed.
- In the case of prodrugs, enzymatic activity may be required to liberate the active species.

Metabolic activity may also constitute a considerable biochemical barrier to drug absorption. As described above, extensive enzymatic degradation of labile drugs in the gastrointestinal tract can severely limit their oral bioavailability. Other routes (nasal, buccal, transdermal etc.) are currently undergoing intensive investigations as possible sites of drug entry, partly, indeed often primarily, because these routes have lower enzymatic activity than the oral route and can avoid first-pass effects.

1.4.3 Excretion

Drugs are excreted via the urine either by:

- glomerular filtration: molecules less than 20 kDa are filtered out through pores in the glomerular membrane of the kidney, due to the positive hydrostatic pressure, or
- tubular secretion: the renal tubule has secretory mechanisms for both acidic and basic compounds; drugs and their metabolites may undergo an active carrier-mediated secretion mechanism.

Another process, tubular reabsorption, also takes place in the kidneys. Specific tubular uptake processes exist for carbohydrates, amino acids, vitamins etc. Drugs may pass from the tubule into the plasma if they are substrates for the uptake processes, or if they are lipid soluble (this process is highly dependent on the prevailing pH, see Section 1.3.4.2).

1.5   TIMING FOR OPTIMAL THERAPY

In addition to the ADME processes, another very important consideration for drug efficacy is the *timing* of drug therapy. Depending on the drug and the disease state, the timing of therapy may be optimal as either zero-order controlled release, or variable release. Considerable advances in controlling drug release from delivery systems have been made; such systems are described in detail in Chapters 3, 4 and 16.

1.5.1 Zero-order controlled release

For many disease states, an ideal dosage regimen is one in which:

- a therapeutic concentration of drug at the site of action is attained immediately;
- the therapeutic concentration remains constant for the desired duration of treatment.

By effective management of the dose size and the dose frequency, it is possible to achieve therapeutic steady-state levels of a drug by giving repeated doses. An example of the type of plasma profile obtained after repeated oral dosing of a drug is shown in Figure 1.9.

However, multiple oral dosing is associated with disadvantages:

- The drug concentration does not actually remain constant in the plasma, but fluctuates between maximum (peak) and minimum (trough) values (Figure 1.9). These fluctuations in plasma concentration may mean that drug levels may swing too high, leading to toxic side-effects; alternatively drug levels may fall too low, leading to a lack of efficacy.
- Drugs with short biological half-lives require frequent doses to maintain therapeutically effective plasma levels. Frequent dosing is likely to lead to poor patient compliance.

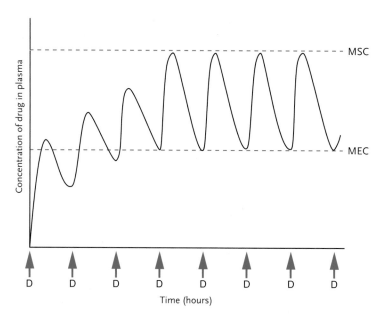

Figure 1.9 Plasma concentration-time(C_p vs T) curve following oral administration of equal doses, D, of a drug every 4 hours

MSC is the maximum safe plasma concentration of the drug.
MEC is the minimum effective plasma concentration of the drug.

An alternative approach to overcome these limitations is to use a delivery system which provides zero-order controlled release of the drug (Figure 1.10). A controlled release oral dosage form consists of two portions:

- a priming/loading dose: to attain therapeutic levels promptly;
- a maintenance/sustained dose to maintain therapeutic levels for a given period of time.

Zero-order controlled release offers the advantage of improved control over drug plasma levels: the peaks and troughs of conventional therapy are avoided and constant plasma levels are attained. The risk of side-effects is minimized since possible toxic peak drug plasma levels are never obtained and the total amount of drug administered is lower than with frequent repeated dosing. There is also a reduction in symptom breakthrough which can occur if plasma concentrations drop too low. Furthermore, patient compliance is also improved as a result of the reduction in the number and frequency of doses required to maintain therapeutic efficacy. For example, the problem of dosing through the night is eliminated since the drug is slowly released *in vivo*.

A wide variety of drug delivery systems have been developed to achieve zero-order controlled release and are discussed further in the relevant chapters.

1.5.2 Variable release

Although zero-order drug delivery may be very suitable for some drugs and specific clinical situations, in other cases a timed intermittent delivery system may be more appropriate. Situations in which changing levels of response may be required include:

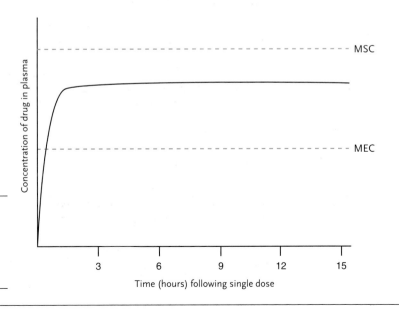

Figure 1.10 Plasma concentration-time curve following oral administration of a zero-order controlled release dosage form

Circadian rhythms

Biological processes are frequently associated with rhythms of a predictable period. Some of these rhythms have periods of less than a second, others are ultradian (a period ranging from a few minutes to a few hours), monthly, or seasonal. Most prominent are circadian rhythms, with periods approximating to 24 hours.

The intensity of the disease state and associated symptomatology may vary over a 24 h period. For example, in hypertension, blood pressure is lower during the night and increases early in the morning, therefore optimal therapy should facilitate maximum drug levels in the morning. Approximately 80% of insulin-dependent diabetics experience the dawn phenomenon, a rapid rise in serum glucose levels in the dawn hours. At this time interval, the insulin dose should be increased to meet the biological need. In nocturnal asthma, bronchoconstriction is worse at night.

Variation in the pharmacokinetics of a drug may also occur (chronopharmacokinetics) which is directly related to the time of day that the drug is administered. The responsiveness of the biological systems (chronopharmacodynamics) may also vary depending on the time of day that the drug is administered, thereby possibly resulting in altered efficacy and/or altered intensity of side-effects.

This in turn has created huge challenges, but also exciting opportunities for drug delivery. The goal is to tailor drug input to match these complex, newly defined time courses. There are already some examples of chronotherapeutics in the literature, including the timed administration of theophylline and corticosteroids to asthmatics, treatment of hypertension and, increasingly, the administration of cytotoxic drugs. However, this is still a new, and as yet, poorly understood area of study with much progress to be made. Further details of advances in this area are given in Chapter 16.

Fluctuating metabolic needs

Insulin causes a decrease in blood glucose concentrations. Physiologically, insulin delivery is modulated on a minute-to-minute basis as the hormone is secreted into the portal circulation and requirements vary widely and critically with nutrient delivery, physical activity and metabolic stress. Ideally, an insulin delivery system should be instantaneously responsive to these fluctuating metabolic needs. A variety of other drugs such as calcitonin and growth hormone also demand complex release requirements.

Pulsatile release

Many endogenous peptides and proteins are released in a pulsatile fashion and subject to complex feedback control mechanisms, consequentially, drug timing plays a crucial role in determining the observed effect.

For example, completely *opposite* effects can be obtained for gonadotrophin releasing hormone (GnRH) (also known as

Luteinizing hormone releasing hormone, LHRH) depending on the timing of the administration (Box 1.2). GnRH is responsible for the release of luteinizing hormone (LH) and follicle-stimulating hormone (FSH) from the anterior pituitary gland. In turn, LH and FSH stimulate the gonadal production of sex steroids and gametogenesis, respectively. If GnRH is given in a pulsatile manner, this mimics the endogenous hypothalmic secretion of GnRH and can be used to restore fertility in women with hypothalmic amenorrhea.

However, *chronic* administration (e.g. as a depot injection) evokes an initial agonist phase of several days to weeks, followed by a suppression of gonadotrophin secretion. The precise molecular site of action of this process is unclear, but it is thought to involve an initial loss of receptors, followed by an uncoupling of receptors from their effector systems. Chronic administration is used clinically in the treatment of sex-hormone responsive tumors such as prostate and breast cancer.

Again, the challenge for drug delivery is to match drug input with the desired therapeutic outcome.

1.6 DRUG DELIVERY CONSIDERATIONS FOR THE "NEW BIOTHERAPEUTICS"

The "new biotherapeutics" may be defined as the molecules being discovered and studied through the disciplines of biotechnology and molecular biology. Research is currently concentrated in two main areas:

- peptides and proteins;
- nucleic acid therapies.

Box 1.2   The effect of timing of the administration of GnRH on the subsequent pharmacological response and therapeutic indications.

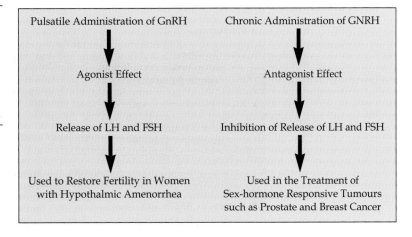

These new biotherapeutics are discussed briefly below, with particular reference to the problems associated with their successful drug delivery and targeting.

1.6.1 Peptides and proteins

Peptides and proteins are not strictly "new" therapeutic agents, indeed hormones, serum proteins and enzymes have been used as drugs ever since the commercial introduction of insulin in 1923. However, significant advances in recent years in the fields of biotechnology and molecular biology have led to the availability of large quantities of pure, potent and highly specific peptide and protein drugs, often with modified or "super-agonist" properties, for a wide variety of therapeutic and diagnostic indications (Box 1.3).

However, there exists a large number of barriers to their successful delivery:

In vitro *stability barriers*

Peptides and proteins possess an inherent instability due to the chemical reactivity of certain amino acids. This results in degradation reactions such as transpeptidation, side-chain hydrolysis, diketopiperazine formation, disulphide exchange, oxidation and racemization. Stability is affected by environmental factors, including pH, organic acids, ionic strength, metal ions, detergents, temperature, pressure, interfaces and agitation. Stability is also affected by manufacturing processes, for

Box 1.3 Peptide and protein biotechnology pharmaceuticals	• Colony stimulating factors
	
	• Biological response modifiers and other cytokines
	    – interferons
	    – interleukins
	
	• Enzymes
	    – clotting factors
	    – dismutases
	    – tissue plasminogen activators
	
	• Hormones
	
	• Growth factors
	    – tissue/bone growth factors
	    – neurotropic factors
	
	• Recombinant protein vaccines
	
	• Monoclonal antibodies
	    – diagnostic antibodies
	    – therapeutic antibodies
	
	• Recombinant soluble receptors
	
	• Fusion molecules
	
	• Peptides and peptidomimetics

example, susceptibility of proteins to thermal inactivation can seriously limit the range of methods that can be used in their sterilization, as well as in the fabrication of their delivery systems. Peptide and protein formulations are also highly susceptible to lyophilization. Freezing concentrates the protein, buffer salts, other electrolytes and may dramatically shift pH.

Peptide and protein instability *in vitro* is manifested by the tendency of such molecules to undergo self-association in solution, resulting in the formation of multimers and, in the extreme, aggregation and precipitation. For example, insulin at pH 7 exists predominantly as hexameric aggregates, which are too large to be absorbed.

Proteins tend to undergo denaturation *in vitro*, the rates of interfacial denaturation are strongly dependent on the specific protein and on such solution properties as temperature, pH and salt concentration. For example, human growth hormone undergoes only limited, and fully reversible, denaturation between pH 1.3 and pH 13, whereas human choriomammotropin undergoes substantial and irreversible interfacial denaturation above pH 11. Proteins also tend to adsorb at interfaces. Various approaches have been attempted to prevent loss of protein by adsorption to glass and plastic, including treating surfaces with proteins such as bovine serum albumin, fibrinogen and ovalbumin, or modifying the solvent by adding surfactants or glycerol.

Metabolic barriers

Stability problems also manifest *in vivo*. Potential peptide and protein drugs are subject to degradation by numerous enzymes or enzyme systems throughout the body. Degradation involves hydrolytic cleavage of peptide bonds by proteases (Figure 1.11):

- Endopeptidases cleave internal peptide bonds and include enkephalinase and cathepsin B. Small peptides are relatively resistant to the action of endopeptidases but their activity is significant for large peptides.

Figure 1.11 Generic peptide showing points of cleavage by exopeptidases and endopeptidases. Exopeptidases cleave at N- and C- termini and endopeptidases cleave at an internal peptide bond

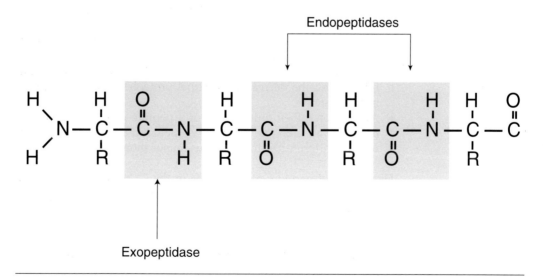

- Exopeptidases cleave peptides and proteins at their N and C termini and include aminopeptidases, carboxypeptidases and dipeptidyl peptidase.

Important features of peptide and protein enzymatic degradation include:

- Proteases and other proteolytic enzymes are ubiquitous;
- Biological degradation of even a single bond in a peptide or protein drug can destroy its biological activity;
- Several bonds are usually susceptible to enzyme attack;
- Each peptide bond may be degraded by a range of enzymes.

By considering these features, the enormous difficulties associated with overcoming the enzymatic barrier to peptide and protein delivery should be apparent. Degradation usually occurs at the site of administration and is possible in every anatomical site *en route* to the target receptor. Furthermore, protecting a single bond on a peptide or protein drug from a particular type of enzyme is insufficient to confer protection on the entire drug from enzymatic hydrolysis – other enzymes may attack the protected bond and the other unprotected bonds on the drug are still vulnerable.

Several methods of modifying peptide structure to improve metabolic stability have been investigated, including:

- substitution of an unnatural amino acid in the primary structure;
- introduction of conformational constraints;
- reversal of the direction of the peptide backbone;
- acylation or alkylation of the N-terminus;
- reduction of the carboxy-terminus; formation of an amide.

However, even extensive modifications of peptide structure can only afford relative, rather than absolute, protection from enzyme attack.

In the gastrointestinal tract, the enzymatic barrier is probably the most significant obstacle to the successful oral delivery of peptides and proteins, as demonstrated by the following observations:

- The rate of hydrolysis of peptides is inversely related to the amount transported across the intestine.
- The increased GI absorption of peptides observed in neonates correlates with the decreased intestinal proteolysis that exists in the neonatal state.
- Absorption (albeit quite small) of a peptide or protein generally occurs if an enzyme inhibitor is included in the formulation, whereas unprotected formulations do not show any absorption.

Hydrolysis of peptides and proteins in the GI tract can occur luminally, at the brush border and intracellularly. Luminal activity from the pancreatic proteases trypsin, chymotrypsin, elastase and carboxypeptidase A is mainly directed against large dietary proteins. The main enzymatic activity against small bioactive peptides is derived from the brush border of the enterocyte. Brush border proteases, such as aminopeptidase A and N, diaminopeptidease IV and Zn-stable Asp-Lys peptidase, preferentially cleave oligopeptides of up to 10 amino acid residues and are particularly effective in the cleavage of tri- and tetra-peptides.

Intracellular degradation is most specific against di-peptides and occurs mainly in lysosomes, but also in other intracellular organelles.

In comparison to the oral route, much less is known about the nature of the enzymatic barrier to therapeutic peptides and proteins in alternative routes such as the buccal, nasal, pulmonary, dermal and vaginal routes. As a first step in characterizing the proteolytic barrier, the proteolytic activity in various mucosal tissues can be determined by incubating a peptide or protein in epithelial tissue homogenates. However, care should be exercised in interpreting studies of this kind as peptides are often exposed to a wide range enzymes, including both extra- and intracellular enzymes, present in a homogenate of epithelial tissue. The actions of intracellular enzymes will not be significant if the peptide is absorbed by the paracellular route, never coming into contact with the inside of the cell.

Studies on characterizing the enzymatic barrier at each delivery site have investigated the pattern of cleavage of enkephalins, substance P, insulin and proinsulin, and have demonstrated the presence of both exo- and endo-peptidases in the various epithelial tissues. What distinguishes one route from another is probably the relative proportion of these proteases, as well as their subcellular distribution.

Absorption barriers

Absorption barriers to peptides and proteins arise from the enzymatic barrier described above and also from the physical barrier properties of the epithelium, arising from the hydrophobic membranes and tight intercellular junctions. The physicochemical properties of peptide and protein drugs generally make them unsuitable for absorption by any of the possible routes and mechanisms described above.

For example, these molecules are generally too large for transport via the paracellular route, unless the integrity of the tight junctions is disturbed by the use of penetration enhancers. Similarly, passive diffusion across lipidic membranes, the major route of absorption for conventional drug molecules, is also generally not possible, as the molecules tend to be too large and too hydrophilic to penetrate the lipidic membrane barrier. Again, the use of appropriate penetration enhancers can potentiate absorption via this route. Research is also being directed towards increasing the lipophilicity of these moieties, to enhance transport via this route.

Active transport mechanisms exist in the gastrointestinal tract and other epithelial sites, for the absorption of di- and tri-peptides. As described above, a greater understanding of the molecular specificity of this carrier could provide important leads for the delivery of peptides. Proteins and large peptides may be transported across cells via endocytic processes. Transcytosis is achieved if the endocytic vesicles can reach the basal membrane without fusion with lysosomes. However, various studies have shown that in the majority of cases the internalized protein is degraded, indicating that the transcytotic pathway is a minor one and most of the endocytosed protein is subject to lysosomal degradation.

Distribution and excretion barriers

As discussed above (see Section 1.4.1), a particular repercussion of drug distribution is that after administration of a therapeutic peptide or protein, *unwanted* drug disposition may occur, which can result in the need to use high doses to compensate for drug wastage, which can be costly given the expense involved in producing new biotherapeutics. Unwanted distribution may also cause toxic side-effects resulting from drug action at non-target sites.

Premature excretion may arise if small, highly potent, therapeutic peptides are cleared rapidly through the kidneys, before reaching the target site.

Chronopharmacological barriers

As discussed in Section 1.5, the timing of drug therapy is crucially important for the successful delivery of therapeutic peptides and proteins. For optimal drug therapy, drug delivery systems must tailor drug input in response to such factors as:

- circadian and other rhythms of predictable period;
- modulations on a minute-to-minute basis, in response to such factors as nutrient delivery, physical activity and metabolic stress;
- the pulsatile release patterns of many endogenous peptides and proteins;
- the complex feedback control mechanisms which affect the release and biological effects of many endogenous peptides and proteins

1.6.2 Nucleic acid therapies

Until recently, the term "biopharmaceutical" was virtually synonymous with therapeutic peptides and proteins. However, nucleic acid-based biopharmaceuticals are now becoming increasingly important therapeutic entities. Research into nucleic acid-based therapeutics is currently focused in two main areas:

- gene therapy;
- oligonucleotide therapy.

This whole field is still at a largely experimental stage, but holds great potential to revolutionize the treatment and prevention of disease if safe and effective delivery vectors can be found. The delivery of nucleic acid based-therapeutics is the subject of Chapter 14; the following discussion comprises a brief introduction to gene therapy.

1.6.2.1 *Gene therapy*

As described in detail in Chapter 14, gene therapy should prove useful in the treatment of a broad range of medical conditions, including:

Inherited diseases

Well over 4,000 genetic diseases have been characterized to date. Many of these are caused by the lack of production of a single gene product, or are due to the production of a mutated gene product incapable of carrying out its natural function. Some of the genetic conditions for which the defective gene has been pinpointed are summarized in Table 1.4. Gene therapy represents a seemingly straightforward therapeutic strategy to correct such diseases, which would be achieved by simply inserting a "healthy" copy of the gene in question into appropriate cells of the patient.

Cancer

To date, the majority of gene therapy trials have been directed towards cancer therapy rather than correcting inherited genetic defects. Various strategies have been investigated in an attempt to treat cancer using a gene therapy approach, including:

- modifying lymphocytes in order to enhance their antitumor activity;
- modifying tumor cells to enhance their immunogenicity;
- inserting tumor suppressor genes into tumor cells;
- inserting toxin genes into tumor cells in order to promote tumor cell destruction;
- inserting suicide genes into tumor cells.

Infectious diseases

A further disease target includes those caused by infectious agents, particularly intracellular pathogens such as HIV. The main strategy here is to introduce a gene into pathogen-susceptible cells. The gene product will subsequently interfere with pathogen survival/replication within those cells. For example, one anti-AIDS strategy currently being pursued is the introduction into viral-sensitive cells of a gene coding for an altered (dysfunctional) HIV protein, which is capable of inhibiting viral replication.

1.6.2.2 Basic approach to gene therapy

The basic approach to gene therapy involves (Figure 1.12):

- the genetic material to be transferred is usually packaged into some form of vector, which serves to deliver the nucleic acid to the target cell;

Table 1.4 Some examples of genetic diseases for which the defective gene responsible has been identified

Disease	Defective genes protein product
Haemophilia A	Factor VIII
Haemophilia B	Factor IX
Familial hypercholesterolaemia	Low-density protein receptor
Severe combined immunodeficiency	Adenosine deaminase
Cystic fibrosis	Cystic fibrosis transmembrane regulator

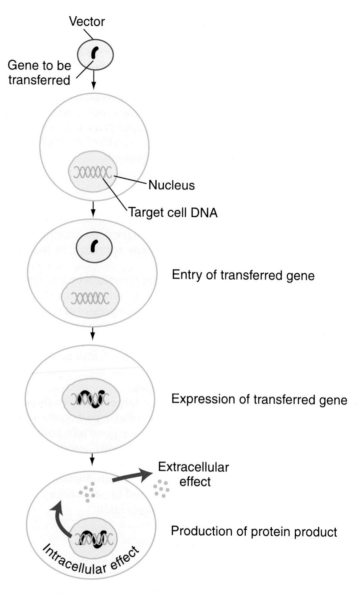

Figure 1.12 Simplified schematic representation of the basis of gene therapy (see text for details)

Vector

Gene to be transferred

Nucleus

Target cell DNA

Entry of transferred gene

Expression of transferred gene

Extracellular effect

Production of protein product

Intracellular effect

- entry of the genetic material (often still associated with its vector) into the cell cytoplasm;
- transfer of the nucleic acid into the nucleus of the recipient cell;
- this is often, but not always, followed by integration of the foreign genetic material into the cellular genetic material, known as deoxyribonucleic acid (DNA);
- the foreign gene (whether integrated or not) is expressed, resulting in the synthesis of the desired protein product. The protein product may be retained within the cell, or it is excreted from the cell.

In common with the peptide and protein-based "new biotherapeutics" described above, successful *delivery* is one of the major practical problems in gene therapy. To be effective, the genetic material must:

- reach the appropriate cellular target;
- penetrate into the target cells;
- (usually) integrate with the cell's DNA;
- avoid destruction by the body's immune system.

These challenges in gene delivery combine to form formidable barriers to the success of gene therapy. At a practical level, two techniques are used for gene therapy delivery:

- *ex vivo* gene therapy;
- *in vivo* gene therapy.

The *ex vivo* technique used to deliver, for example, a gene to a patient who is deficient in that gene, entails removal of target cells from the body, followed by their incubation with a nucleic acid-containing vector. After the vector delivers the nucleic acid into the human cells (assuming this is possible), they are placed back into the body, where they hopefully produce the missing gene. In order for this approach to be successful, the target cells must be relatively easy to remove from the body and reintroduce into the body. Success with this protocol has been achieved using various cell types, including blood cells, epithelial cells, muscle cells and hepatocytes.

In vivo gene therapy involves the direct administration of the vector (or naked DNA) to the patient. For example, vectors can be directly injected into a tumor mass; a further example involves the investigation of aerosolized vectors for the delivery of the cystic fibrosis gene to respiratory tract epithelial cells. However, direct injection of a vector or naked DNA is not always feasible, because the target cells are not always localized to one specific area of the body (for example, blood cells). Furthermore, the efficiency of integration (transduction) of the naked DNA into the host DNA is low. The foreign gene is not integrated into the target cell chromosome, so expression levels are limited. Thus this technique, while adequate for vaccine strategies, appears to give insufficient protein yields for many other applications.

An alternative *in vivo* approach is to use vectors capable of recognizing and binding only to specific cell types, so that the genetic material is delivered only to specific target cells. The simplicity of this *in vivo* approach renders it the ideal method of choice. However to date, no such bio-specific vectors have been developed for routine therapeutic use, although intensive research in this area is ongoing.

1.6.2.3   *Vectors for gene therapy*

The various vectors used to introduce genes into recipient cells are generally divided into viral, particularly retroviral, and non-viral carriers, such as cationic-liposomes. Viral strategies exploit the unique ability of viruses to seek out and fuse with target cells, and incorporate their genetic material into the cell so that it becomes integrated with the cell's DNA. The use of appropriate viruses as vectors for therapeutic genes requires inserting the therapuetic gene into the virus. Safety issues are a large concern here as the virus must also be selectively disabled so that it cannot pursue its normal life-cycle once inside its human host and cause a viral infection.

Most of the research on viral vectors has concentrated on retroviruses. The problems associated with retroviruses as vectors, which illustrate some of the problems associated with the use of viruses as a whole, include:

- Most retroviruses can only integrate into actively replicating cells, which clearly restricts their use.
- Retroviruses do not infect all dividing cell types as cellular entry requires an appropriate viral receptor on the surface of the target cell. As the identity of most retroviral receptors remains unknown, it is difficult to predict the range of cell types the virus will infect during treatment. Physiological complications may arise if integration and transfection occur in non-target cells.
- Using retroviral vectors, the transferred gene demonstrates a propensity to integrate randomly into the chromosomes of recipient cells. Integration of transferred DNA in the middle of a gene whose product plays a critical role in the cell could damage cellular function which may result in cell death.
- Viral particles are relatively labile and although easy to propagate, they are often damaged by subsequent purification and concentration processes.

The alternative approach is to use non-viral vectors, such lipid-based, peptide-based and polymer-based delivery systems, as described in detail in Chapter 14. Liposomes are relatively easy to manufacture, are generally non-toxic and are devoid of the capability to cause an infection (see Section 5.3.1). However, a number of limitations are associated with their use. For example, it is difficult to direct liposomes to a particular type of cell. Liposome/DNA complexes which may be internalized by the target cells are susceptible to degradation within secondary lysosomes or within the cytoplasm. In addition, liposomes do not (or minimally) integrate the transferred DNA into host cell chromosomes, which necessitates repeated administration protocols. Thus the efficiency of this approach is very low.

The various initial studies that have been carried out using gene therapy have highlighted the technical innovations required to achieve successful gene transfer and expression. These, in turn, should render future ("second-generation") gene therapy protocols more successful. Research into improving gene delivery is ongoing and is discussed in Chapter 14.

1.7 CONCLUSIONS

The purpose of any delivery system is to enhance or facilitate the action of therapeutic compounds. It should now be apparent that conventional drug delivery systems are associated with a number of limitations which can reduce drug efficacy. These limitations include an *inability* to:

- facilitate adequate absorption of the drug;
- facilitate adequate access to the target site;
- prevent non-specific distribution throughout the body (resulting in possible toxic side-effects and drug wastage);
- prevent premature metabolism;
- prevent premature excretion;
- match drug input with the required timing (zero-order or variable input) requirements

Limitations of conventional drug delivery systems are particularly acute for the new biotherapeutics, such as peptide and protein drugs and nucleic acid therapies.

Advanced drug delivery and targeting systems are thus being developed in order to optimize drug therapy and overcome these limitations. Further chapters will describe these new and emerging technologies, with reference to the various routes of delivery under investigation.

1.8 FURTHER READING

Aulton, M. E. (ed). (1988) *Pharmaceutics: The science of dosage form design*. Churchill Livingstone, Edinburgh.

Burkitt, H. G. and Young, B. (1993) *Wheater's Functional Histology: A text and colour atlas*, 3rd edn. Churchill Livingstone.

Evers, P. (1997) *Developments in drug delivery: technology & markets*, 2nd edn. Financial Times Pharmaceutical and Healthcare Publishing.

Walsh, G. (1998) *Biopharmaceuticals: biochemistry and biotechnology*. John Wiley and Sons, Chichester.

Brody, T.M., Larner, J. and Minneman, K.P. (eds) (1988) *Human Pharmacology: Molecular to Clinical*, 3rd edn. Mosby St Louis.

Gibaldi, M. (1991) *Biopharmaceutics and Clinical Pharmacokinetics*, 4th edn. Lea & Febiger, Philadelphia.

Robinson, J.R. and Lee, V.L. (eds) (1987) *Controlled drug delivery: fundamentals and applications*, 2nd edn. Marcel Dekker Inc., New York.

Lee, V.H.L (ed.) (1991) *Peptide and protein drug delivery*. Marcel Dekker, New York.

Waller, D. and Renwick, A. (eds) (1994) *Principles of Medical Pharmacology*. Bailliere Tindall, London.

Chien, Y.W. (ed.) (1991) *Novel drug delivery systems*, 2nd edn. Marcel Dekker.

Florence, A.T. and Attwood D. (1998) *Physicochemical Principles of Pharmacy*, 3rd edn. Macmillan London.

Lee, V.H.L. and Yamamoto, A. (1990) Penetration and enzymatic barriers to peptide and protein absorption. *Advanced Drug Delivery Reviews*, 4:171–207.

Smith, P.L., Wall, D.A., Gochoco, C.H. and Wilson, G. (1992) Routes of Delivery: Case Studies: Oral absorption of peptides and proteins. *Advanced Drug Delivery Reviews*, 8:253–290.

Brayden, D.J. and O'Mahony, D.J. (1998) Novel oral drug delivery gateways for biotechnology products: polypeptides and vaccines. *Pharmaceutical Science and Technology Today*, 1:291–299.

1.9 SELF-ASSESSMENT QUESTIONS

1. Define the term bioavailability and describe the differences between (a) relative bioavailability and (b) absolute bioavailability.
2. What are the different types of epithelium found at different sites in the body?
3. List the epithelial barriers to drug absorption.
4. Describe the most likely pathway of drug absorption for (i) a large therapeutic peptide, (ii) a small hydrophilic molecule and (iii) a small hydrophobic molecule.
5. List the different routes of drug transport across epithelial membranes.
6. Describe Fick's Law and show how it can be represented mathematically.
7. List the physicochemical properties of a drug that influence absorption. How can the physicochemical properties be improved to increase drug absorption?
8. Explain the differences between log P and log D.
9. Use the Henderson-Hasselbach Equation to demonstrate that a weak base (pKa = 7.5) should have better absorption from the small intestine (pH = 6.5) than from the stomach (pH = 1).*
10. Explain how the solubility of a poorly soluble drug may be improved.
11. Give two examples where the timing of drug administration is important.
12. List the drug delivery challenges presented by the 'new biotherapeutics'.

---

* See Appendix for answer

2 Drug Delivery: Market Perspectives

Paul Evers

OBJECTIVES

On completion of this chapter the reader should be able to:

- Describe the commercial reasons for developing advanced drug delivery systems
- Describe the breakdown of the advanced drug delivery market by region
- Provide an analysis of the advanced drug delivery market in terms of therapeutic areas
- Understand the differences between the developed and developing worlds as markets for advanced drug delivery systems

2.1 INTRODUCTION

The clinical benefit offered by novel drug delivery systems over traditional routes of delivery for existing drugs is often outweighed by their
associated increased costs. The rationale for developing novel drug
delivery systems therefore lies primarily in the potential commercial
benefits of developing more effective means of delivering the new bio-
therapeutic agents. This chapter gives a market perspective to the
rationale for the development of novel drug delivery systems.

As introduced in the previous chapter, drug delivery technology, as
a separate sector within the pharmaceutical sphere, is of quite recent
origin. It had its origins in the 1950s and 1960s, when the first sustained-release oral forms appeared; the best known was probably the
Spansule capsule formulation developed by Smith Kline & French
Laboratories. That company merged with Beecham early in the 1990s
to form SmithKline Beecham and, more recently, with Glaxo-
Wellcome to form "GlaxoSmithKline".

At first, drug delivery technology was relatively crude by today's
standards and its main objective was to prolong the effect of oral doses
of medication in order, for example, to provide usefully prolonged
relief of symptoms. Because the technology was simplistic, it could not
be relied on to address any more difficult clinical needs, such as
improving the absorption of insoluble drugs. It was not until the late
1970s that advanced drug delivery technology began to evolve into a
serious branch of pharmaceutical science, capable of being used to
tackle more fundamental problems associated with pharmacotherapy.
By the mid-1990s, it was possible to identify at least six commercial
reasons for the continued research and development of advanced drug
delivery and targeting systems. These are detailed below.

2.2 COMMERCIAL IMPORTANCE OF ADVANCED DRUG DELIVERY TECHNOLOGIES

2.2.1 Convenience and compliance

Making drug treatment more convenient was the objective of the early
sustained-release oral drug delivery formulations. Convenience meant
that patients would find the medicine easier to take; they would therefore be more likely to purchase it in preference to rival products with
less convenient dosage regimes. Thus a sustained-release dosage form
gave the product an additional benefit, or in contemporary marketing
jargon it conferred "added value".

Although the consumers of medicines primarily perceived convenience as a benefit, it soon became a clinical issue as well, because it was
linked with improved compliance; that is, better adherence to prescribed dosage regimes. Poor compliance has always been a major
problem in drug therapy, especially when the treatment is for an asymp-
tomatic condition such as essential hypertension. For an active working
man or woman to have to remember to take a tablet three or four times
a day is a nuisance; it can also be embarrassing. Missed doses are

common in this kind of situation. Good compliance is also a problem for the elderly, for whom forgetfulness is often the main problem. An article published in 1997[1] estimated that some 50% of prescribed medications are taken incorrectly. Any measure which improves compliance will result in drug therapy that is closer to the intention of the prescribing physician. Thus, to the prescriber, improved compliance represents added value, just as convenience does to the consumer.

The treatment of hypertension is a classic example of the importance of user-friendly dosage forms in giving products commercial advantage. When beta-blocking drugs came to be widely used as antihypertensives, the available drugs had relatively short half-lives and dosing three or four times a day was required. Those manufacturers who added long-acting formulations to their product range gained commercial advantage thereby; Inderal LA (propranolol sustained-release, from ICI, which is now AstraZeneca) was a case in point. Later beta-blockers such as atenolol (Tenormin, also ICI/AstraZeneca) tended to have an intrinsically longer duration of action.

2.2.2   Efficiency

One of the fastest-growing groups of prescription drugs in the 1960s was the non-steroidal anti-inflammatory drugs, known generally by the acronym NSAIDs. These drugs (exemplified by ibuprofen and indomethacin) gave effective relief of pain and stiffness in arthritis. The first generation of NSAIDs consisted exclusively of short-acting drugs; each dose gave relief of symptoms for around four to six hours. This brevity of action was not just inconvenient for the patient; it also meant that the effect of a dose taken at bedtime had dissipated by the time the patient awoke in the morning. He or she then had to face the prospect of an hour or more of pain and stiffness while waiting for the first dose of the day to take effect. As NSAIDs have a tendency to cause gastric irritation, they have to be taken with or after food, so that it was not possible for the patient simply to swallow a tablet on waking.

One solution to this problem – and one that is still valid, judging by the continued commercial success of the relevant products – was to develop sustained-release formulations of the most effective NSAIDs. Voltarol (Voltaren-XR in the USA) Retard (diclofenac) was one of the most successful of all prescription pharmaceuticals during its first years and is still among the leading NSAID products today. The reason is not simply that the long-acting product was more convenient for the patient to take; it also, and more importantly, made the treatment more effective by matching the timing of pharmacological effect to the patient's clinical need. This is a separate issue from convenience and compliance.

Another example of specialized delivery systems providing more efficient drug therapy is the use of transdermal patches (see Section 8.6) to deliver drugs in a manner that maintains a fairly constant blood-level, without the peaks and troughs, and their concomitant disadvantages (see Section 1.5.1), typical of most oral dosage forms. Most of the

---

[1] Sam A.P. and Fokkens J.G. (1997) The Drug Delivery System: Adding therapeutic and economic value to pharmacotherapy. *Pharmaceutical Technology Europe*, 9:36–40

products available in transdermal forms are drugs of this type; they include Transiderm-Nitro (glyceryl trinitrate) used for prophylaxis of angina pectoris, and Estraderm TTS (estradiol) used for hormone replacement therapy and to prevent postmenopausal osteoporosis. The efficiency of these products has made them commercially successful.

Efficiency and convenience have not always been compatible in the history of advanced drug delivery systems. Attempts to produce more convenient dosage forms using the technology available in the 1960s and 1970s sometimes led to products with greatly reduced therapeutic efficiency because, in delaying absorption of drug, the formulation also reduced absorption efficiency and bioavailability. This was a major spur to the growth of specialist advanced drug delivery companies such as Alza and Elan, which focused their attention, in different ways, on developing prolonged-release dosage forms which would also optimize efficiency of absorption.

2.2.3 Protecting franchises

The example of Voltarol Retard, cited in the preceding section, is one of a company which has developed an innovative drug, acting to protect its franchise in that product when patent expiry draws near. Every proprietary product eventually loses its patent exclusivity (usually 20 years after the patent was applied for or granted) and it is then open to any other manufacturer to manufacture and sell the same drug, perhaps under its own brand name. It is, of course, necessary to obtain a license to manufacture and market the product, but the procedures for doing this are much simpler and more abbreviated than those which the pioneer company had to follow when the drug was new.

The consequence is that copies of the original product appear on the market, always at much lower prices than the original, and the company which developed the drug in the first place almost invariably sees its market share plummet – unless it has taken steps to prevent this from happening.

Drug delivery technology is one of the resources open to a company seeking to preserve its market share in this kind of circumstance. For example, if the original product was relatively short-acting, the originator company may launch a new, prolonged-action form shortly before expiry of the original patent. Prescribers are encouraged to switch their "brand loyalty" to the new form, which usually has the same name as the product which they have been prescribing for many years, with the addition of a suffix to indicate prolonged action (thus Voltarol Retard; Inderal LA). Naturally, this approach works best when the drug has some physicochemical features, familiar to the company's pharmaceutical scientists, which make it technically difficult for a rival company to develop its own long-acting formulation.

Examples of the successful use of advanced drug delivery technology to prolong the commercial viability of original brands continue to be claimed throughout the industry. A prime example is the calcium channel blocker nifedipine used in the treatment of hypertension and angina, which was developed by Bayer and marketed as Adalat. It was licensed to Pfizer for the US market, where it was sold as Procardia. Sophisticated prolonged-release formulations developed by the specialist advanced drug delivery company Alza have been used by both Pfizer and Bayer, to market long-acting nifedipine as Procardia XL and Adalat CR, respectively.

2.2.4 Adding value to generics

A generic pharmaceutical product is one on which the original patent has expired, and which may now be sold by companies other than the originator; in some countries they must use the generic, or short chemical, name – the INN – while in others they may introduce their own brand names. As described in the preceding section, generics are always sold at prices significantly lower than the original brand, and low price is the generic product's traditional *raison d'être*. However, generic manufacturers, just like originator companies, may use advanced drug delivery technology to give their products added value, and distinguish them from the original brand and also from rival generics.

This is an indication of the evolving maturity of the generic sector of the pharmaceutical market. For many years generic manufacturers were simply cut-price manufacturing concerns, exploiting market opportunities in the wake of patent expires. However, the proliferation of generic companies in some countries has led to fierce price wars between them, and the cut-price benefit is no longer sufficient to ensure success in this sector. So generic companies have begun to develop other attributes to add value to their products, and one avenue, ripe for exploration, is the possibility of applying special delivery technology to appropriate generic products.

2.2.5 Market expansion

Drug delivery technology can be used to expand the pharmaceutical market by providing a means for convenient administration of drugs which previously had to be given by injection. By making it possible for the patient to self-administer the drug, such technology makes the drug more widely available for general use, especially in the primary care environment.

Ongoing development work in this context has focused on large molecular weight drugs such as calcitonin and insulin, which cannot be given by the oral route because they are destroyed by gastric acid and/or enzymes in the small intestine (see Sections 1.6.1 and 6.3.3). Calcitonin is widely used in the treatment of osteoporosis but until very recently has had to be given by injection. The inconvenience for both doctor (or nurse) and patient has tended to reduce the usefulness of calcitonin in the routine management of osteoporosis. One alternative is to give calcitonin by nasal inhalation; the drug is absorbed into the bloodstream via the nasal mucosa. The major pharmaceutical company Rhone-Poulenc Rorer (now Aventis) has developed a nasal calcitonin product called Calcimar Intranasal, which awaits approval in the US. Attempts are also being made to develop formulations which protect the large mole-cule from gastrointestinal degradation.

2.2.6 Creating new markets

This is another "leading edge" role for advanced drug delivery technology, where the market opportunity has not yet been matched by proven and practicable technical solutions. The main candidate is gene therapy (see Section 1.6.2 and Chapter 14). This is an experimental – some would say speculative – area; potential markets are vast but the technology is still in development, and pressure from investors is creating some confusion. Candidates for gene therapy, as described in Chapter 14, include diseases due to single genetic defects, where the treatment would involve delivering intact genes into those body cells that need it; and diseases where genetic defects (often multiple) have been recognized as one of many causative factors. The problem here is identifying and producing the missing genes, and then delivering them to the target cells.

As described in Section 1.6.2, common to both types of gene therapy is the need to develop means of safely delivering genes into target cells within the patient's body. One current experimental technique involves removing some of those cells from the body, inserting the genes into them, and then returning them to the patient. Clearly, this technique is not practicable for general therapeutic use. Most attention is currently concentrated on the use of appropriate viruses as carriers for the therapeutic genes. There are serious problems, especially regarding the dangers of viral replication in the patient, and of immune responses – as introduced in Section 1.6.2.

The challenge of developing successful delivery technologies for gene therapy is a world removed from the simple, sustained-release oral formulations which were the achievements of the first pharmaceutical scientists to specialize in advanced drug delivery technology. The potential, in commercial terms and in terms of human well-being, is too vast to estimate.

2.3 MARKET ANALYSIS

Market assessment in the pharmaceutical sphere is not an exact science; it has an element of educated guesswork overlaid on hard market statistics. This is partly because of the wide variations between market conditions in different regions of the world and individual countries within those regions. This is also partly due to the many different ways by which pharmaceutical products travel from manufacturer to consumer, so that it is almost impossible to keep close watch over all the channels of distribution.

Within the pharmaceutical sphere, the market for advanced drug delivery systems presents its own problems; not least the fact that it is not easily delimited, like the market for NSAIDs, or antibiotics, or asthma therapies. In any therapeutic category where advanced drug delivery products are used, they form only a part of total drug consumption. In order to measure the size of the total advanced drug delivery market, one must begin by calculating the sizes of the various therapy-area markets in which these products are used, then estimating the proportion of each market which is accounted for by advanced drug delivery products. That proportion will differ from one category to the next.

The market figures that follow are estimates, based on available published data and estimates, based, *inter alia*, on epidemiological and demographic records.

2.3.1 Market size

The annual value of the total world market for all advanced drug delivery products was around $16 billion in 1997. This is in line with market estimates for recent years, assuming an overall growth rate around 20% per annum. This would be an exceptional rate of market increase for any conventional pharmaceutical sector. Its validity in the context of advanced drug delivery products rests on a number of factors. First, the continuing pace of innovation in drug delivery technologies, leading to improved performance and increasing reliance on advanced drug delivery formulations. Then, the exploitation of new delivery routes and targeting technologies, bringing advanced drug delivery technology to a wider range of therapeutic applications. In addition, there is a continuing trend towards optimizing existing pharmaceuticals because of a reduction in the rate at which new drugs are introduced. Finally, the introduction of advanced drug delivery formulations by generics manufacturers as a means of achieving product differentiation and advantage lends its own impetus to market growth.

Over the next 5–10 years, additional growth drivers are also expected to become important, including the first successful outcomes to research into delivery systems for gene therapy, new targeting systems for anticancer therapies, and additional sectors including mucosal formulations.

For these reasons, it is expected that the advanced drug delivery market will grow at more than 20% per annum to the millennium and beyond.

2.3.2 Division of the market by region

For all of its existence (that is, since the late 1950s) the modern pharmaceutical industry has been concentrated in the developed regions of the world. Only inexpensive kinds of drugs (e.g. unbranded antibiotics, and vaccines) have been as widely available in the developing countries as in more prosperous ones. This split between richer and less prosperous markets has been especially noticeable in the regional distribution of the advanced drug delivery market, which was originally characterized by relatively high-priced products, so that its distribution among the main pharmaceutical market regions of the world tended to show disproportionately higher shares among the more prosperous regions – North America, Western Europe and Japan. Established advanced drug delivery products are now often no more expensive than other established pharmaceuticals; for example, sustained-release forms of non-steroidal anti-inflammatory drugs (NSAIDs) used in arthritis are priced comparably with unmodified forms. However, other factors, in particular demographic and epidemiological ones, tend to maintain the differential. For example, osteoarthritis, the commonest form of arthritis, is more prevalent in elderly individuals, and this segment of the population is increasing in developed countries, leading to growth in the NSAID market.

New developments in advanced drug delivery always result, at first, in high-priced products which are more affordable in developed economies. This will apply particularly to gene therapy delivery systems and targeted anticancer therapies, because these are expected to command very high prices. At the same time, delivery systems which were revolutionary and high-priced on their first introduction (e.g. dry powder inhalers for asthma therapy) are gradually becoming comparable in price to conventional dosage forms. The increasing use of advanced drug delivery technology by generic companies is bringing it more into the realm of everyday medicine.

Table 2.1 gives an estimate of the regional division of the advanced drug delivery market for 1997 and 2001.

Table 2.1 Regional division of the advanced drug delivery market for 1997 and 2001

	North America		Europe		Japan		Rest of world	
	Value $ billion	*Share %*	*Value $ billion*	*Share %*	*Value $ billion*	*Share %*	*Value $ billion*	*Share %*
1997	5.0	31	4.75	30	3.25	20	3.0	19
2001	14.0	33	11.75	28	7.50	18	8.75	21

Source: author's estimates
Figures have been rounded.

2.3.3 Analysis by therapeutic area

Cardiovascular drugs

The global cardiovascular market was estimated to be worth over $30 billion per annum in 1998. Antihypertensive drugs form the largest product category within this market, accounting for sales of some $20 billion. Some antihypertensives are also used for long-term maintenance in angina, while there is a separate group of drugs used for short-term angina relief.

Annual sales of antihypertensive and anti-anginal products using advanced drug delivery technology are estimated to be around $5 billion worldwide at 1995 levels, representing one-sixth or more of all cardiovascular sales. This share will increase in the near term, as sales of older drugs in conventional dosage forms decline.

Anti-inflammatory drugs

The market for prescription drugs used in the treatment of major inflammatory diseases, including arthritis and rheumatism, is currently valued at $7 billion worldwide. Non-steroidal anti-inflammatory drugs (NSAIDs) account for over 85% of this market. Early NSAIDs, which tended to be inherently short-acting, were overshadowed by longer-acting new products during the 1970s and 1980s, and there were also widespread introductions of long-acting dosage forms, giving a new lease of life to products such as Ciba's Voltarol, AHP's Lodine, Aventis's Orudis, Boots' Brufen and Froben, Hoechst's Surgam and Merck's Indocid. In fact Voltarol is the leading product in this market, with sales around $1 billion, largely contributed by the long-acting version.

This market is expected to remain static in the short-term future, because research has failed hitherto to yield a safe and effective drug which fundamentally alters the inflammatory disease process. NSAIDs are essentially palliative, and revenues from these drugs will decline in response to pressure to reduce prices. Products incorporating advanced drug delivery technology are estimated to represent up to 40% of the total NSAID market.

Anti-cancer drugs

The global cancer market is valued at around $8 billion. Most usage is still in the area of cytotoxic drugs, with hormonal therapy growing dramatically in recent years due to the increasing use of drugs such as tamoxifen. The anti-cancer market now also embraces novel adjunctive therapies such as Amgen's Neupogen (G-CSF), used to protect against anaemia following chemotherapy and radiotherapy, and GlaxoSmithKline's Zofran (ondansetron), given to combat nausea and vomiting. Because of their high price, these new products represent an unusually large share of the market; most cytotoxic and hormonal products are mature and relatively low-priced.

The main opportunity for advanced drug delivery systems in this market is in the area of targeted drug delivery. Current research is focused on the development of carriers such as liposomes and on the use of monoclonal antibodies as targeting agents (see Sections 5.2 and 5.3). The eventual market opportunity is considerable – cancer is still one of the commonest fatal diseases, and some of the most deadly forms are resistant to available therapies. The potential market for effective targeting delivery systems may eventually exceed $5 billion. Whether, and how soon, it achieves this figure will depend on the speed with which successful products come to market.

Anti-asthma therapies

The asthma market is thought to be worth some $6 billion worldwide, and consists mainly of inhaled products – bronchodilators and corticosteroids. It is a growing market because the incidence of asthma is increasing, especially in developed countries. It has been postulated that this increase is partly related to overuse of inhaled bronchodilators, which can mask progression of the underlying inflammatory disease process. Current recommendations specify the routine use of anti-inflammatory therapy (e.g. inhaled steroids) for mild asthma, with bronchodilators used to relieve acute attacks in more serious cases.

The asthma market will almost certainly continue to grow, with increasing use of inhaled therapy, favoring stronger growth of steroids over bronchodilators in the current climate of opinion.

The conventional metered-dose inhaler (MDI) cannot be classified as a product of advanced drug delivery technology; it is essentially a low-technology device and the drug delivered is not formulated or modified in any way to enhance targeting. However, inhalation products now available go a considerable way towards compensating for the drawbacks of early metered-dose aerosols. The major suppliers (including AstraZeneca, 3M and GlaxoSmithKline) have developed improved delivery devices, as well as dry powder formulations and control of medication particle size to optimize penetration into the lung (see Chapter 10). However, it seems likely that the main factor driving this market upwards in the near term will be the rising prevalence of asthma, fuelling annual market growth in the region of 8–10%.

Diabetes

Insulin is the only currently effective treatment for the millions of diabetics who suffer from Type I diabetes (also known as insulin-dependent and juvenile onset diabetes). There are also a significant number of people with Type II diabetes (also known as maturity-onset diabetes) who need insulin. Insulin is a peptide, and if given orally it is broken down by enzymes in the gut (see Section 1.6.1). Thus it has always been given by injection. Although manufacturers have introduced user-friendly devices such as insulin pens, an effective, less invasive alternative would be instantly popular. This is an area in which active research is under way, including a project at Inhale Therapeutic systems to develop an inhalation dosage form (see Chapter 10).

Worldwide sales of insulin are currently in the region of $2 billion. It is estimated that if an effective pulmonary formulation is developed and receives approval, there would be a 20% switch from the injectable products within a year. The same would apply in the case of an effective oral product. Assuming an initial high price (perhaps 30% above that of injectable insulin), this represents potential sales of $400 million for the new product a year after launch.

2.3.4 Analysis by mode of administration

Oral

The market for oral advanced drug delivery products probably accounts for almost half of all drug-delivery formulations, which means that it is now worth more than $8 billion (Table 2.2). There is a continuing demand for oral delivery systems, not only to preserve the commercial viability of major drug products as they come off-patent but also to solve specific problems such as delivery of large molecular weight drugs including calcitonin and insulin. Thus, although this sector of the market may have a smaller share of the total in 5–10 years time, it will continue to be a major opportunity for growth.

Table 2.2 Division of
advanced drug
delivery market by
route of administration,
1997

Route	1997	
	Share %	*Value* $ billion
Oral	50	8.0
Parenteral	19	3.0
Inhalation	19	3.0
Transdermal	6	1.0
Mucosal	6	1.0

Source: author's estimates
Figures have been rounded

Inhalation

Drug delivery by the pulmonary route is already very important in commercial terms, with the widespread and increasing incidence of asthma in the developed world. Significant improvements in inhaler technology have already been made, and increasing use of these more sophisticated devices is already driving market growth; so will advances in absorption efficiency being sought by companies such as Inhale Therapeutic Systems.

Separately, there is active research into the possibility of delivering, by the inhalation route, drugs which previously had to be given by injection. The newly-emerging gene therapy of cystic fibrosis is a special development. Although this condition is rare, and therefore does not represent a large market opportunity, the successful treatment of cystic fibrosis by means of inhaled gene therapy would encourage research into other therapeutic possibilities using the lung as an absorption site.

The pulmonary segment of the advanced drug delivery market is thought to be worth $3 billion worldwide, and may triple in size over the next five years.

Transdermal

The transdermal market experienced a period of dramatic growth in the early 1990s, led by the popularity of nicotine patches as an aid to smoking cessation, and the growing use of hormone replacement therapy by this route. Growth has since slowed down, as some of the enthusiasm for nicotine patches waned. Anti-smoking campaigns are continuing to fuel this sector, however. Another potent market driver in the transdermal sector is the growing numbers of elderly in the populations of developed countries. This will lead to increasing use of hormone replacement therapy, not only as a short-term treatment for menopausal symptoms but for the long-term prophylaxis of osteoporosis.

Thus the transdermal market sector is expected to rise from its present value around $3 billion towards $5 billion or more in the next five years.

Mucosal

Mucosal absorption has been a rather neglected opportunity in the advanced drug delivery market; the mucous surfaces of the body – including the mouth, nose, rectum and vagina – offer less of a barrier than the skin to the systemic absorption of drugs, so it is surprising that more attention has not been paid to mucosal delivery systems. Practical difficulties include the fact that rectal dosage forms have never been widely acceptable in some countries, and the mouth and nose are not suitable for dosage forms which must remain in place for a prolonged period. However, they are ideal for rapid absorption of drugs when prompt effect is important, for example anti-anginals.

Products formulated for mucosal delivery are now thought to contribute less than 5% of the total advanced drug delivery market, but wider utilisation of the mucosal route, now being researched by companies such as Theratech, 3M and Nomen, may eventually create a market worth over $300 billion.

Parenteral

The parenteral category includes such areas of major potential as the development of novel long-acting (implant) dosage forms (see Section 4.2), injection of drugs targeted to specific sites using monoclonal antibodies (see Section 5.2.1) and liposomal carriers (see Section 5.3.1), and administration of drugs modified to cross the blood-brain barrier (see Section 13.5). Thus, although parenteral advanced drug delivery systems now account for a very small share of the total advanced drug delivery market, they are likely to make a more significant impact when current research yields marketable products. Because much of this research is at an early stage, the parenteral sector may not achieve its full potential until well into the 21st century, with sales projected to rise to $2.5 billion or more by 2005.

2.4 INDUSTRY EVOLUTION AND STRUCTURE

The first modern advanced drug delivery systems were developed by major pharmaceutical manufacturers such as Smith Kline & French Laboratories, and with the growing recognition of the importance of advanced drug delivery technology there was a trend in these companies towards the establishment of special formulation units in their R&D divisions. This sector soon attracted the attention of pharmaceutical entrepreneurs who saw opportunities for specialist formulation companies. By the late 1970s there were a number of such companies in operation, including Alza, Elan, Eurand and Pharmatec International.

For the most part, these companies were based on core proprietary technologies, mainly involving oral dosage forms, which they offered to pharmaceutical clients as off-the-shelf solutions to absorption problems; they also undertook specially designed R&D projects aimed at solving specific problems in this area. Typically, there would be a development fee for such work, paid in stages as the project reached successive goals; finally, the client would either pay the developer royalties on the sales of the successful formulation, or subcontract production of the finished product to the advanced drug delivery company. These types of arrangements are still the basis for most development work in the advanced drug delivery sector carried out on behalf of pharmaceutical clients by specialist companies.

Some of the early entrants into this field have expanded their activities into delivery routes other than their original core technology, so that they can offer solutions in the transdermal, inhalation and other fields as well as oral formulations. This is true of Alza, Elan and 3M, the latter being something of a hybrid since it is also a pharmaceutical company in the conventional sense. By contrast, some companies in this field are linked to specific routes of administration; Inhale Therapeutic systems, as its name implies, focuses on inhalation technology, while Pharmatec International, one of the oldest-established advanced drug delivery concerns, remains committed to the oral route.

Drug delivery technology demands continual innovation in order to meet increasingly complex clinical demands and accommodate the needs of sophisticated new drugs. This places a heavy burden on existing specialist companies in terms of R&D commitment; it has led to the birth of a considerable number of small, research-driven concerns, often built around pharmaceutical specialists and teams from academia or the formulation departments of major pharmaceutical companies. Like companies in the biotechnology sector, these new ventures are set up to develop and exploit specific technologies, but their path to financial self-sufficiency is often shorter than that of a typical new biotech venture, because the regulatory hurdles are fewer when a new chemical entity is not involved.

One area in which this does not apply is gene therapy. Here, the underlying technology is so new that it cannot even be described as "pharmaceutical" in any conventional sense. Likewise, the delivery technology is pushing back the boundaries of human knowledge, exploring the use of viruses as carriers for the genetic material, as well as other vehicles including liposomes. Since this applied research is, unusually, going hand-in-hand with fundamental research into the nature of the biological mechanisms involved, the development timetable is an extended one.

In summary, the current structure of the advanced drug delivery industry is a complex one, embracing specialist companies which offer off-the-shelf and custom-developed delivery systems, some involved in a range of delivery routes, others concentrating on a single route of administration. There are leading-edge research teams in areas such as gene therapy, while some pharmaceutical concerns still maintain their own specialist advanced drug delivery formulation units developing essentially pharmaceutical solutions to formulation problems.

2.5   FURTHER READING

Evers, P. (1997) *Developments in Drug Delivery: Technology & Markets*, 2nd edn. Financial Times Pharmaceutical and Healthcare Publishing, London.

Bassett, P.D and DM Reports (1999) *Drug Delivery Systems: Trends, Technologies and Market Opportunities*, 2nd edn. Drug & Market Development, Southborough MA USA.

Burd, G. (1999) *Innovation in Drug Delivery Systems: A Strategic Insight into the Global Drug Delivery Industry.* Smi Publishing, London.

Scussa, F. (1999) Therapeutic categories gain strength. *MedAdNews*, 18(5):20–26.

2.6 SELF-ASSESSMENT QUESTIONS

1. Name 4 of the commercial reasons for developing advanced drug delivery systems.

2. What major contribution have advanced drug delivery systems made to anti-inflammatory drug therapy?

3. Discuss the importance of the developing world as a market for advanced drug delivery systems.

3 Advanced Drug Delivery and Targeting: An Introduction

Anya M. Hillery

OBJECTIVES

On completion of this chapter the reader should be able to:

- Use the appropriate terminology to describe drug delivery and targeting systems
- Describe the different mechanisms of rate-controlled release used in drug delivery and targeting
- Outline the different types of drug targeting systems used in advanced drug delivery and targeting
- Describe the properties of an "ideal" dosage form and an "ideal" route of delivery
- Outline some of the different strategies to increase drug absorption

The purpose of this chapter is to provide a general overview and describe some of the fundamentals of advanced drug delivery and targeting, prior to going into specific detail on advanced drug delivery and targeting technologies, and specific routes of delivery, in the subsequent chapters.

3.1   TERMINOLOGY OF DRUG DELIVERY AND TARGETING

The terminology describing drug delivery and targeting is extensive and ever-growing. Systems are diversely referred to as "controlled release", "sustained release", "zero-order", "reservoir", "monolithic", "membrane-controlled", "smart", "stealth" etc. Unfortunately, these terms are not always used consistently and, in some cases, may even be used inaccurately. For clarity and consistency, some common terms used in this book are defined as follows:

- *Prolonged/sustained release*: the delivery system prolongs therapeutic blood or tissue levels of the drug for an extended period of time.
- *Zero-order release*: the drug release does not vary with time; thus the delivery system maintains a (relatively) constant effective drug level in the body for prolonged periods (see Section 1.5.1).
- *Variable release*: the delivery system provides drug input at a variable rate, to match, for example, endogenous circadian rhythms, or to mimic natural biorhythms.
- *Bio-responsive release*: the system modulates drug release in response to a biological stimulus (e.g. blood glucose levels triggering the release of insulin from a drug delivery device).
- *Modulated/self-regulated release*: the system delivers the necessary amount of drug under the control of the patient.
- *Rate-controlled release*: the system delivers the drug at some predetermined rate, either systemically or locally, for a specific period of time.
- *Targeted-drug delivery*: the delivery system achieves site-specific drug delivery.
- *Temporal-drug delivery*: the control of delivery to produce an effect in a desired time-related manner.
- *Spatial-drug delivery*: the delivery of a drug to a specific region of the body (thus this term encompasses both route of administration and drug distribution).
- *Bioavailability*: the rate and extent at which a drug is taken up into the body (see Section 1.2).

In this book, the term "drug delivery system" (DDS) is used as a general term to denote any type of advanced delivery system. Conventional drug delivery systems are simple oral, topical or injection formulations. A DDS, as used here, represents a more sophisticated system which may incorporate one, or a combination, of advanced technologies such as rate-control, pulsatile release or bio-responsive release to achieve spatial and/or temporal delivery. A drug delivery and targeting system (DDTS) specifically describes an advanced delivery system that incorporates some type of specific targeting technology (such as, for example, monoclonal antibodies); such systems are currently most advanced for use in the parenteral administration of drugs. Also, rate-control and drug targeting are treated as two separate issues in this book and are dealt with in detail in Chapters 4 and 5 respectively.

3.2 RATE-CONTROLLED RELEASE IN DRUG DELIVERY AND TARGETING

Drug release from a delivery system can be zero-order, variable or bio-responsive. Although there are literally hundreds of commercial products based on controlling drug release rate from delivery systems, there are in fact only a small number of mechanisms by which drug release rate is controlled:

- Diffusion-controlled release mechanisms
- Dissolution-controlled release mechanisms
- Osmosis-controlled release mechanisms
- Mechanical-controlled release mechanisms
- Bio-responsive controlled release mechanisms

Rate-control is briefly described below and is further described in considerable detail in Chapter 4 and also Chapter 16.

3.2.1 Diffusion-controlled release

In this case, the drug must diffuse through either a polymeric membrane or polymeric or lipid matrix, in order to be released. Diffusion-controlled devices can be divided into (Figure 3.1):

Figure 3.1 Diffusion-controlled reservoir (a) and matrix (b) systems

- *reservoir devices*: in which the drug is surrounded by a rate-controlling polymer membrane (which can be non-porous, or microporous);

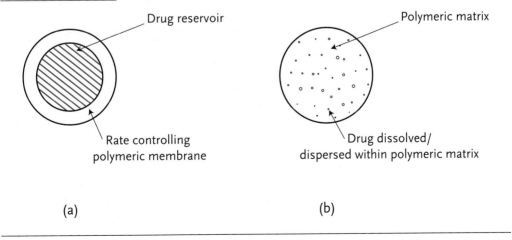

Drug reservoir

Polymeric matrix

Rate controlling polymeric membrane

Drug dissolved/ dispersed within polymeric matrix

(a)

(b)

- *matrix (also described as monolith) devices*: in which the drug is distributed throughout a continuous phase composed of polymer or lipid.

3.2.1.1 Diffusion-controlled reservoir devices

The rate of diffusion of drug molecules through the membrane follows Fick's Law (see Section 1.3.3.2) and is thus dependent on the partition and diffusion coefficient of the drug in the membrane, the available surface area, the membrane thickness and the drug concentration gradient. If the drug concentration gradient remains constant, for example where solid drug particles are present and constant dissolution maintains the concentration of the drug in solution, the rate of drug release does not vary with time and zero-order controlled release is attained (see Chapter 4 and Figure 4.4).

Diffusion-controlled reservoir devices are used in a wide variety of routes including those shown in Table 3.1.

3.2.1.2 Diffusion-controlled matrix devices

A drug dissolved in a matrix system is also known as a monolithic solution, whereas a drug dispersed in a matrix system is referred to as a monolithic dispersion. Regardless of a drug's physical state in the polymeric matrix, such devices do not usually provide zero-order drug release properties. This is because as the drug molecules at the surface of the device are released, those in the centre of the device have to migrate longer distances to be released, which takes a longer time. This increased diffusion time results in a decrease in the release rate from the device with time. Generally the rate of release is found to decrease in proportion to the square root of time ("$M \propto t^{1/2}$" kinetics; see Chapter 4 and Figure 4.8). However, the decrease in drug release rate can be compensated for by designing systems of special geometry, which provide an increasing surface area over time. Examples of diffusion-controlled matrix devices in drug delivery are shown in Table 3.1.

3.2.2 Dissolution-controlled release

In dissolution-controlled drug release devices, drug release is controlled by controlling the dissolution rate of an employed polymer. As

Table 3.1 Examples of commercial diffusion-controlled reservoir and matrix devices

Device type	Route	Commercial examples
Reservoir devices	*Parenteral*	Norplant subdermal implant
	Ocular	Ocusert implant
		Vitrasert intravitreal implant
	Transdermal	Transderm-Scop transdermal patch system
		Catapres-TTS transdermal system
	Vaginal	Cernidil vaginal insert
		Estring vaginal ring
Matrix devices	*Parenteral*	Compudose cattle growth implant
	Transdermal	Deponit transdermal patch

for diffusion-controlled release, dissolution-controlled devices can be divided into:

- *reservoir devices*: in which the drug is surrounded by a polymeric membrane which retains the drug. After a certain period of time the polymeric membrane dissolves, thereby releasing the drug;
- *matrix devices*: in which the drug is distributed throughout a polymeric matrix, which dissolves with time, thereby releasing the drug.

Since the dissolution of polymeric materials is the key to this mechanism, the polymers used must be water-soluble and/or degradable in water. The choice of a particular polymer for a particular controlled release dosage form depends on various factors such as the dissolution mechanism, delivery period, delivery route, the drug etc. In general, synthetic water-soluble polymers tend to be widely used for oral-controlled release dosage forms. Biodegradable polymers tend to be used for injectable, or implantable, drug delivery systems.

3.2.2.1 *Dissolution-controlled reservoir devices*

In dissolution-controlled reservoir devices, the drug release is controlled by the thickness and/or the dissolution rate of the polymer membrane surrounding the drug core. Once the coating polymer dissolves, the drug is available for dissolution and absorption. Such systems are often used for sustained release oral drug delivery. Drug cores can be coated with polymers of different coating thickness, so that drug release can be delayed for certain periods, for example 1, 3, 6 and 12 h after administration. The coated drug particles can be placed in a capsule, or compressed into tablets. By using a dosage form incorporating a spectrum of different coating thicknesses, the overall drug release from the dosage form (as a whole, rather than from the individual microparticles) can adjust to give zero-order drug release. Spansule, Sequel and SODAS capsules are examples of dissolution-controlled reservoir devices for oral drug delivery of various drugs.

3.2.2.2 *Dissolution-controlled matrix devices*

In this case, drug release is controlled by dissolution of the matrix. Since the size of the matrix decreases as the dissolution process continues, the amount of drug released also decreases with time. The decrease in drug release can be compensated in part by constructing a non-linear concentration profile in the polymer matrix. This strategy is used in the oral dosage form, Adalat, where the core of the dissolution matrix contains more drug than the outer layer.

Matrix dissolution devices are widely used in parenteral therapy. For example, Zoladex subcutaneous implant comprises a bulk-eroding, poly(lactide-co-glycolide) (PLGA) matrix system for the delivery of goserelin (gonadorelin analog). PLGA polymers are also widely used in the fabrication of dissolution-controlled microspheres for parenteral administration, e.g. Lupron Depot for the delivery of goserelin. Microparticulates made of proteins, in particular albumin, are also widely used in the preparation of injectable drug carriers. These, and other systems, are discussed in detail in Chapter 4.

3.2.3   Osmosis-controlled drug release

Osmosis is defined as the movement of water through a semi-permeable membrane into a solution (see Section 4.6.1). The movement of water results in an increase in pressure in the solution and the excess pressure is known as the osmotic pressure. Osmotic pressure can used to pump out a drug at a constant rate from the delivery system. Device and formulation parameters can be controlled so that drug release is zero-order. An important consideration is that osmotic-controlled devices require only osmotic pressure to be effective, thus such devices operate essentially independently of the environment. Hence, *in vitro* drug release rate is often consistent with the *in vivo* release profile. Also, for oral delivery, changes in pH or ionic strength in the gastrointestinal tract will not affect the drug release rate.

In parenteral therapy, the subcutaneously implantable, osmotic mini-pumps developed by the Alza Corp. are used widely in experimental animal studies. The DUROS implant pump is a modified version of the Alzet pumps and was developed specifically for the controlled delivery of peptides and proteins (see Section 4.6.1.2). Osmotic mini-pumps, such as the Oros osmotic pump, are also available for controlled release via the oral route (see Section 6.7.5.1); commercial products include, Procardia XL (nifedipine) and Efidac 24 (pseudoephedrine for congestion; chlorpheniramine for allergy).

3.2.4   Mechanical-controlled drug release

Mechanically driven pumps are common tools for the intravenous administration of drugs in the hospital setting. They allow physicians and patients to precisely control the infusion rate of a drug. Externally programmable pumps can facilitate:

- zero-order controlled drug release;
- intermittent drug release.

Ideally, a pump should deliver the drug at the prescribed rate(s) for extended periods of time and thus should incorporate a wide range of delivery rates, ensure accurate, precise and stable delivery, contain reliable pump and electrical components and finally, provide a simple means to monitor pump status and performance. A pump should also be convenient for the patient and thus should ideally be reasonably small in size and inconspicuous, have a long reservoir life and be easy to program. The biocompatibility of the device surface is also an important issue for consideration. Other safety concerns include danger of over-dosage, drug leakage and pump blockage.

3.2.5   Bio-responsive controlled drug release

Bio-responsive controlled drug delivery systems modulate drug release in response to changes in the external environment (see Section 16.3). For example, drug release may be controlled by the way in which pH or ionic strength affects the swellability of a polymeric delivery system. More sophisticated systems incorporate specific enzymes which causes changes in localized pH or increases in localized concentrations of specific substrates such as glucose. The change in pH caused by the biotransformation of the substrate by the enzyme thereby causes a change in permeability of a pH-sensitive polymeric system in response to the specific biomolecule. Such systems may be used to modulate the release of drug through a controlled feedback mechanism.

3.3 DRUG TARGETING SYSTEMS

An important point to remember is that while rate-controlled systems can deliver the drug at a predetermined rate, they are generally unable to control the *fate* of the drug, once it enters the body. Drug targeting systems are used to achieve site-specific drug delivery. Site-specific drug delivery is desirable in therapeutics, in order to improve:

- *drug safety*, as toxic side-effects caused by drug action at non-target sites are minimized;
- *drug efficacy*, as the drug is concentrated at the site of action rather than being dispersed throughout the body;
- *patient compliance*, as increased safety and efficacy should make therapy more acceptable and thus improve compliance.

In its simplest form, drug targeting can be achieved by the local administration of the therapeutic compound; this strategy is feasible even with conventional dosage forms. For example, if the site for desired drug action is the skin, the medication may be applied in ointment, lotion, or cream form, directly on the desired site. Direct injection of an anti-inflammatory agent into a joint is another example of site-specific delivery which is achievable without having recourse to a highly specialized drug delivery and targeting system.

Sophisticated drug targeting technology is also available, particularly for oral and parenteral delivery. However, technology is not yet advanced sufficiently for the design of "magic bullet" drug delivery systems, proposed by Paul Ehrlich at the turn of the 20th century (see Section 1.4.1), in which the drug is precisely targeted to its exact site of action. For oral delivery, systems are available to achieve site-specific delivery within the gastrointestinal tract; for example, targeting the drug to the small intestine, colon, or gut lymphatics. Drug delivery systems available for targeted oral delivery include those that use enteric coatings, prodrugs, osmotic pumps, colloidal carriers and hydrogels; these technologies are discussed in Chapter 6.

Technologies for targeted drug delivery are most advanced for parenteral administration. Such technologies are concerned with delivering drugs to specific targets in the body and also to protect drugs from degradation and premature elimination. They include the use of:

- *soluble carriers*, such as monoclonal antibodies, dextrans, soluble synthetic polymers;

- *particulate carriers*, such as liposomes, micro- and nano-particles, microspheres;
- *target-specific recognition moieties*, such as monoclonal antibodies, carbohydrates and lectins.

These technologies, and the various anatomical, physiological and pathological issues that pertain to their use, are discussed in detail in Chapter 5.

Recent advances in biological and chemical sciences have led to the development of various "Smart" technologies to ensure more effective drug delivery and targeting of drugs to specific sites within the body. Such approaches include the use of:

- antibody-directed enzyme/prodrug therapy (ADEPT);
- virus-directed prodrug/enzyme therapy (VDEPT);
- chemical drug delivery systems.

The advantages and limitations of these systems are discussed in detail in Chapter 16.

3.4 DOSAGE FORMS FOR ADVANCED DRUG DELIVERY AND TARGETING

3.4.1 Types of dosage forms for drug delivery and targeting systems

A wide variety of types of drug delivery and targeting systems are available, in a wide range of sizes, from the molecular level right up to large devices.

Molecular

Drugs can be covalently attached to water-soluble carriers, such as monoclonal antibodies, carbohydrates, lectins and immuno-toxins. Such systems are used to achieve site-specific drug delivery following parenteral administration. Release of the attached drug molecules at the target site can be achieved by enzymatic or hydrolytic cleavage. Larger complexes, some undergoing clinical trials, include drug conjugates with soluble natural, or synthetic, polymers.

Nano- and microparticles

Nanoparticles are solid colloidal particles, generally less than 200 nm. Such systems include poly(alkyl-cyanoacrylate) nanoparticles used for parenteral drug delivery and targeting.

Microparticles are colloidal particles in the micrometer scale, typically in the size range 0.2–100 μm. Synthetic polymers, such as poly(lactide-co-glycolide), are widely used in the preparation of microparticulate drug delivery systems and also as biodegradable implantable devices. Natural polymers, such as albumin, gelatin and starch, are also used as microparticulate drug carriers. Liposomes, vesicular structures based on one or more lipid bilayer(s) encapsulating an aqueous core, represent highly versatile carriers. Liposomes can be prepared using a variety of techniques to give a wide range of sizes (approximately 30 nm–10 μm), structures and physicochemical properties, to facilitate the encapsulation of both water-soluble and lipid-soluble drugs (see Section 5.3.1). Commercial products based on liposome technology are available and many more products are in clinical trials, for a variety of indications.

Macrodevices

Macrodevices are widely used in many applications, including:

- *parenteral drug delivery*: mechanical pumps, implantable devices;
- *oral drug delivery*: solid dosage forms such as tablets and capsules which incorporate controlled release/targeting technologies;
- *buccal drug delivery*: buccal adhesive patches and films;
- *transdermal drug delivery*: transdermal patches, iontophoretic devices;
- *nasal drug delivery*: nasal sprays and drops;
- *pulmonary drug delivery*: metered-dose inhalers, dry-powder inhalers, nebulizers;
- *vaginal drug delivery*: vaginal rings, creams, sponges;
- *ophthalmic drug delivery*: ophthalmic drops and sprays.

3.4.2 Properties of an "ideal" dosage form

Although available in a wide variety of shapes, sizes and mechanisms of rate-controlled release, desirable attributes of *all* drug delivery systems include:

Patient acceptability and compliance

Parenteral delivery systems involve the use of needles. This is painful for the patient, as well as generally requiring the intervention of medical professionals. The oral route, which involves merely swallowing a tablet, liquid or capsule, thus represents a much more convenient and attractive route for drug delivery. Transdermal patches are also well accepted by patients and convenient. Some other dosage forms, for example nebulizers, pessaries and suppositories, may meet with more limited patient compliance.

Reproducibility

The dosage form should allow accurate and reproducible drug delivery, a particularly important consideration for drugs with a narrow therapeutic index.

Ease of termination

The dosage form should be easily removed either at the end of an application period, or in the case where continued drug delivery is contra-indicated. A transdermal adhesive system is easily removed if necessary, as is a buccal patch. However, non-biodegradable poly-meric implants and osmotic pumps must be surgically retrieved at the end of treatment. Although a biodegradable polymeric implant does not require surgical retrieval, its continuing biodegradation makes it difficult to terminate drug delivery, or to maintain the correct dose at the end of its lifetime.

Biocompatibility and absence of adverse effects

The drug delivery system should be non-toxic and non-immunogenic. For example, concerns over the body's responses to a foreign material often raise the issues of biocompatibility and safety of implantable devices. The use of dosage forms containing penetration enhancers, which potentiate drug absorption via a variety of mechanisms and are used in oral, buccal, transdermal, nasal, ophthalmic, pulmonary and vaginal drug delivery, has raised serious questions about the potential deleterious effects they exert on epithelial tissue. As well as the possi-bility of direct damage to the epithelium, the increased epithelial per-meability may allow the ingress of potentially toxic agents.

Large effective area of contact

For drugs absorbed via passive mechanisms (see Section 1.3.3), increasing the area of contact of the drug with the absorbing surface will increase the amount absorbed. The dosage form can influence the size of the area over which the drug is deposited. For example, the use of nasal drops offers a larger solution/membrane surface area for immediate absorption than if the drug solution is delivered in the form of a nasal spray (see Section 9.4.3). Increasing the size of a transdermal patch increases transdermal bioavailability.

Prolonged contact time

Drug delivery to epithelial sites is often limited by a variety of physio-logical clearance mechanisms at the site of administration. Clearance mechanisms include mucociliary clearance and intestinal motility. Ideally, the dosage form should facilitate a prolonged contact time between the drug and the absorbing surface, thereby facilitating absorption. Bioadhesive materials (sometimes also termed mucocad-hesive) adhere to biological substrates such as mucus or tissue and are often included in dosage forms in order to increase the effective contact time.

3.5 ROUTES OF ADMINISTRATION

3.5.1 Properties of an "ideal" route of administration

Routes of drug administration that can be utilized in order to achieve systemic delivery of a drug include: parenteral, oral, buccal, transder-mal, nasal and pulmonary. Although the oral route is the preferred route of administration, many drugs are unsuitable for oral delivery and must be given parenterally. However, alternative routes (in particular the transdermal and pulmonary routes) are assuming greater importance as alternative non-injectable routes of systemic delivery. In order to maximize the amount of drug entering the systemic circulation from the site of administration, the delivery site should possess certain properties, as discussed below. No single route matches all the physiological requirements of an "ideal" absorption site; the relative extent to whether these criteria can be fulfilled for each particular route are summarized in Table 3.2 and discussed in more detail in the relevant chapters.

Large surface area

A large surface area obviously facilitates absorption. For example, due to the presence of the Folds of Kerckring, the villi and the microvilli, the available surface area of the small intestine of the gastrointestinal tract is very large, making this region an extremely important one for oral drug delivery. The surface area of the lungs, which has evolved physiologically for the highly efficient exchange of gases, is also very extensive, making this region a promising alternative route to the parenteral and oral routes for systemic drug delivery.

Low metabolic activity

Degradative enzymes may deactivate the drug, prior to absorption. Poor drug bioavailability may thus be expected from an absorption site in which enzyme activity is high, such as the gastrointestinal tract. Furthermore, drugs which are orally absorbed must first pass through the intestinal wall and the liver, prior to reaching the systemic circulation. These "first-pass" effects can result in a significant loss of drug activity. Drug delivery via other routes (nasal, buccal etc.) avoid intestinal first-pass effects, and as metabolic activity at these sites is often lower than in the gastrointestinal tract, these routes are highly attractive alternatives for the systemic delivery of enzymatically labile drugs.

Contact time

As described above, the length of time the drug is in contact with the absorbing tissue will influence the amount of drug which crosses the mucosa. Materials administered to different sites of the body are removed from the site of administration by a variety of natural clearance mechanisms.

For example, intestinal motility moves material in the stomach or small intestine distally towards the large intestine; it has been estimated that in some cases residence of a drug in the small intestine can be in the order of minutes. In the buccal cavity, the administered dosage form is washed daily with 0.5–2 litres of saliva.

In the nasal cavity and the upper and central lungs, an efficient self-cleansing mechanism referred to as the "mucociliary escalator" is in place to remove any foreign material, including undissolved drug particles. Particulates entering the airways are entrapped within a mucus blanket and ciliary action propels the mucus along the airways, to the

Feature	Parenteral	Oral	Dermal	Buccal	Pulmonary	Nasal	Vaginal
Accessible	+++	+++	+++	++	+	++	+
Patient acceptability	-	+++	+++	++	++	++	+
Rate of uptake	+++	++	+	+	+++	+++	+
Surface area	+++	+++	+++	++	+++	++	++
Blood supply	+++	+++	+	++	+++	+++	+++
Enzyme activity	++	+++	+	+	+	+	+
First-pass effects	-	+++	-	-	-	-	-
Permeability	+++	+++	+	++	+++	+++	+++
Reproducibility	+++	+	+++	++	+	+	+
Clearance mechanisms	+	+++	+	+	+/++/+++*	+++	+

+++ = high, ++ = medium, + = low, - absent *Depends on location

Table 3.2 Comparison of the features associated with various routes of systemic drug delivery

throat, where the mucus and any entrapped particulates are swallowed.

Typical vaginal delivery systems such as foams, gels and tablets are removed in a relatively short period of time by the self-cleansing action of the vaginal tract. In the eye, materials are diluted by tears and removed via the lachrymal drainage system.

Blood supply

Adequate blood flow from the absorption site is required to carry the drug to the site of action post-absorption and also to ensure that "sink" conditions are maintained (see Section 1.3.3.2).

Accessibility

Certain absorption sites, for example the alveolar region of the lungs, are not readily accessible and thus may require quite complex delivery devices to ensure the drug reaches the absorption site. Delivery efficiency to such sites may also therefore be low. In contrast, other sites, such as the skin, are highly accessible.

Lack of variability

Lack of variability is essential to ensure reproducible drug delivery. This is a particularly important criterion for the delivery of highly potent drugs with a narrow therapeutic window. Due to such factors as extremes of pH, enzyme activity, intestinal motility, presence of food/fluid etc., the gastrointestinal tract can be a highly variable absorption site. Similarly, diseases such as the common cold and hayfever are recognized to alter the physiological conditions of the nose, contributing to the variability of this site. The presence of disease can also severely compromise the reproducibility of drug delivery in the lungs. Cyclic changes in the female menstrual cycle mean that large fluctuations in vaginal bioavailability can occur.

Permeability

A more permeable epithelium obviously facilitates greater absorption. Some epithelia are relatively more permeable than others. For example, the skin is an extremely impermeable barrier, whereas the permeability of the lung membranes towards many compounds is much higher than the skin and is also higher than that of the small intestine and other mucosal routes. The vaginal epithelium is relatively permeable, particularly at certain stages of the menstrual cycle.

3.5.2 Overview of the routes of drug delivery

The various routes of drug delivery are discussed in detail in subsequent chapters; the description below constitutes a brief introductory outline.

Parenteral drug delivery

The main clinical role of parenteral therapy is to administer drugs that cannot be given by the oral route, either because of their poor absorption properties, or propensity to degrade in the gastrointestinal tract. Injection by the iv route is also used when an immediate drug effect is required.

Injections are unpleasant and patient acceptance and compliance via this route are low. Intravenous injections may only be given by qualified medical professionals, making this route expensive and inconvenient. Intramuscular and subcutaneous preparations are self-injectable; however, patients dislike them. In addition, elderly, infirm and pediatric patients cannot administer their own injections and require assistance, thereby increasing inconvenience to these patients and the cost of their therapy. Increased medical complications can result from the poor compliance associated with the parenteral route.

Furthermore, the parenteral route is normally associated with short-term effects. There has always been a need for injectable formulations that could offer a prolongation of action similar to that achievable by the oral route. Novel sophisticated implant devices have been developed which can adequately control drug dosage and provide a prolonged duration of effect. Implants are available as biodegradable and non-biodegradable polymeric devices and as mini-pumps, and are described in detail in Chapter 4; new-generation implantable technologies, such as bioresponsive implants, are discussed in Chapter 16. The other major thrust of research in the parenteral field involves the delivery of drugs to specific targets in the body. Parenteral drug delivery and targeting systems are discussed in detail in Chapter 5.

Oral drug delivery

It is estimated that 90% of all medicines usage is in oral forms and oral products consistently comprise more than half the annual drug delivery market. It is the preferred route of administration, being convenient, controlled by the patient and needs no skilled medical intervention. Considerable success has been achieved with various types of controlled-release systems for peroral delivery, which are used to prolong drug effects.

However, there are also many disadvantages associated with this route. For example, the oral route is highly variable, so that there is considerable potential for bio-inequivalence amongst orally administered drugs. The route is also characterized by adverse environmental conditions, including extremes of pH, intestinal motility, mucus barriers, the presence of p-glycoprotein efflux systems, high metabolic activity and a relatively impermeable epithelium. Such factors mean that many drugs are unsuitable for delivery via this route, particularly the "new biotherapeutics", which demonstrate poor GI membrane permeability and enzymatic instability.

Research is currently focusing on 3 main areas to improve oral drug delivery: (i) improving the retention of devices in the GI tract and therefore contact time with the absorbing surface, via the use of mucoadhesives; (ii) increasing the absorption of poorly absorbed moieties, via the use of penetration enhancers and other mechanisms; (iii) improving targeting to areas of the GI tract, via the use of osmotic pumps, target-specific ligands, colloidal carriers and other mechanisms. These and other technologies are described in Chapter 6.

Buccal and sub-lingual drug delivery

Although currently a minor route for drug delivery, the oral cavity is associated with many advantages as site for drug delivery (Table 3.2), suggesting that this route will grow in importance over the coming years. The sub-lingual route is characterized by a relatively permeable epithelium, and is suited to the delivery of low molecular-weight lipophilic drugs, when a rapid onset of action is required. Dosage forms include sub-lingual sprays and fast-dissolving tablets. The buccal route, in contrast, is highly suited to retentive systems. Advanced drug delivery systems such as buccal adhesive patches are now being developed in order to provide prolonged mucosal adhesion and sustained delivery of drugs. Oral transmucosal drug delivery is discussed in detail in Chapter 7.

Transdermal drug delivery

The transdermal route, discussed in Chapter 8, has emerged as a viable alternative route to the parenteral and oral routes, in order to achieve the systemic delivery of drug molecules. Although the skin provides a highly effective barrier against external damage and desiccation, transdermal technology has been developed to overcome this resistance and now several systemically active drugs are delivered transdermally.

Advanced delivery systems include transdermal patches, which are now well established and accepted by patients. Technologies under development include, for example, iontophoresis, which uses a small electric current to propel the drug through the skin. Drug delivery via iontophoresis occurs at enhanced rates and amounts in comparison to patch technology, which uses simple passive diffusion. The development of safe, non-toxic absorption enhancers to facilitate transdermal absorption is a further focus of current research.

Nasal drug delivery

Nasal sprays are commercially available for the systemic delivery of various peptide drugs, including buserelin, desmopressin, oxytocin and calcitonin. Although currently a relatively small market, the nasal route possesses many properties of an "ideal" delivery site (Table 3.2) and it can be expected that the already demonstrated success of this route will be built on further, so that this route should increase in importance in the future. New technologies in nasal delivery are primarily concerned with strategies to increase the rate of systemic drug absorption, in particular, in developing absorption promoters with minimal toxicity. Nasal drug delivery is discussed in detail in Chapter 9.

Pulmonary drug delivery

Drug delivery by inhalation has a long history and is an obvious way of administering agents that act on the respiratory system. A more recent advance has been the investigation of this route for systemic drug delivery, although the morphology of the lungs makes drug access to the airways difficult. Furthermore, particles that gain access to the upper airways may subsequently be cleared by mucociliary clearance mechanisms. Pulmonary drug delivery research is addressing factors such as the use of optimized drug delivery devices and novel drug delivery systems, such as liposomes. Systemic drug delivery via the lungs has largely focused on nebulization procedures, which are the most efficient at delivering the emitted dose to the peripheral lung. Such issues are discussed in detail in Chapter 10.

Vaginal drug delivery

The vaginal route, discussed in Chapter 11, constitutes another mucosal route of emerging importance for systemic drug delivery. As with other mucosal routes, a major challenge lies in the development of safe, non-toxic absorption enhancers, to potentiate drug absorption. Although associated with many advantages for drug delivery (see Table 3.2), the route is also seriously limited by a lack of reproducibility, primarily due to cyclic changes in the vaginal epithelium. Furthermore, the route is only applicable to approximately 50% of the population, so that it may be that the future of this route lies in the treatment of diseases specific or more common to the female population.

Ophthalmic drug delivery

In contrast to the other routes described above, ophthalmic drug delivery systems are designed to deliver drugs locally to the ocular tissue, to avoid systemic uptake and associated side-effects. Research has focused on the development of systems which will improve the retention of drug at the corneal surface in order to overcome the problems associated with tear film drainage. Ophthalmic drug delivery is discussed in Chapter 12.

CNS drug delivery

Similar to the ocular route, CNS delivery is concerned with localized drug delivery, in this case to the central nervous system, rather than achieving the systemic delivery of a drug. The primary challenge here is to penetrate the permeability barrier comprising the brain capillary endothelium, known as the Blood-Brain-Barrier (BBB). Various methods are under investigation, as described in Chapter 13.

3.6 STRATEGIES TO INCREASE DRUG ABSORPTION

A wide variety of strategies have been developed in an attempt of increase drug absorption. These strategies are discussed in detail in the relevant chapters; the following discussion comprises a general summary of some of the common approaches available.

3.6.1 Manipulation of the drug

As discussed in Chapter 1 (Section 1.3.4), physicochemical properties of a drug which influence drug absorption include such properties as:

- lipid solubility and partition coefficient;
- pKa;
- molecular weight and volume;
- aqueous solubility;
- chemical stability;

These properties can be manipulated to achieve more favorable absorption characteristics for a drug but will also create new drug entities. For example, various lipidization strategies can be employed (see Section 1.3.4.1) to increase the lipophilicity of the absorbing moiety and thereby increase its membrane-penetrating ability and absorption via transcellular passive diffusion. The hydrogen-bonding propensity of a drug molecule can be minimized by substitution, esterification or alkylation of existing groups on the molecules, which will decrease the drug's aqueous solubility, again favoring partitioning of the drug into lipidic membranes. The degree of ionization of a drug may be suppressed by the judicious use of buffering agents. Drug solubility may be enhanced by the use of amorphous or anhydrous forms, or the use of the corresponding salt form of a lipophilic drug. Low molecular weight analogues of an active moiety can be developed, to facilitate trans-membrane transport. Alternatively, derivatives may be prepared which are substrates of natural transport carriers.

Considerable effort has been directed towards the stabilization of therapeutic peptides and proteins both *in vitro* and *in vivo*. Several methods of modifying peptide structure to improve metabolic stability have been investigated, as outlined in Section 1.6.1.

Traditionally drug design has focused on optimizing the pharmacological properties of a drug with less concern for potential drug bioavailability, toxicity and metabolism, which all form part of the later pharmaceutical development process. However, with the increasing numbers of compounds entering pharmaceutical development there is a need to limit resource wastage in developing compounds with poor biopharmaceutical profiles. This has led to the development of more rationalized approaches to drug design in order to optimize the bioavailability of potential drug substances in the early stage of drug discovery process to ensure that new drugs can be effectively delivered to their site of action. The process of rational drug design and delivery is discussed in more detail in Chapter 16.

Although the pharmaceutical industry strives to develop drugs with appropriate pharmacokinetic and pharmacodynamic properties to ensure effective drug delivery, it is often difficult to obtain effective potency, low toxicity and acceptable bioavailability. In such cases the optimization of the dosage form becomes particularly important. Methods to improve delivery by manipulating the dosage form are described below and in the relevant chapters.

3.6.2 Manipulation of the formulation

Various formulation additives may be included in the dosage form in order to maximize drug absorption.

3.6.2.1 Penetration enhancers

Penetration enhancers are substances that facilitate absorption of solutes across biological membranes. There are currently five major types of penetration enhancers under investigation:

- *chelators*, such as EDTA, citric acid, salicylates, N-acyl derivatives of collagen and enamines;
- *synthetic surfactants*, such as sodium lauryl sulfate and polyoxyethylene-9-lauryl ether;
- *naturally occurring surfactants*, such as bile salts, phospholipids and bile salt analogues such as sodium taurodihydrofusidate;
- *fatty acids*, such as oleic acid, caprylic acid and caproic acid, and their derivatives such as acylcarnitines, acetylcholines and mono- and di-glycerides;
- *nonsurfactants*, such as unsaturated cyclic ureas and 1-alkyl and 1-alkenylazacycloalkanone derivatives.

The mechanisms of absorption promotion proposed for the different compounds are numerous and it is likely that more than one mechanism is involved (see Section 8.6.1).

The use of penetration enhancers to improve drug absorption by variety of delivery routes is presently under investigation; for example, various studies have recently been carried out to identify penetration enhancers to facilitate the absorption of peptides and proteins by various routes (Table 3.3).

However, as mentioned previously, a serious drawback associated with the use of penetration enhancers is their potential deleterious effect to the epithelial tissue, either directly, by damaging vital cell structures and/or functions, or indirectly, by increasing the permeability of the epithelium and thus paving the way for inward penetration of toxic agents and organisms. Some routes of drug delivery, such as the transdermal and buccal, allow the spatial containment of absorption enhancers within an adhesive patch, thereby limiting the adverse effects to a specific area.

Route of administration	Drugs	Absorption enhancers
Nasal	insulin	bile salts, surfactants
Buccal	human calcitonin	bile salts, surfactants
Small intestine	somatostatin analogue	palmitoyl-dl-carnitine
Large intestine	[asu1,7]-eel calcitonin	Na-salicylate
		Na$_2$EDTA
Rectal	pentagastrin, gastrin	5-methoxysalicylate
Vaginal	leuprolide	organic acids
Ocular	insulin	bile salts, surfactants
Transdermal	vasopressin	azone, DMSO

Table 3.3 The use of penetration enhancers to improve the absorption of peptides and proteins across epithelial interfaces

The design and search for safe and effective penetration enhancers is an ongoing area of research associated with all epithelial routes of delivery.

3.6.2.2 Mucoadhesives

As described in Chapter 1 (Section 1.3.2), the majority of the epithelia discussed in this book are covered by a layer of mucus. Mucoadhesives, which are generally hydrophilic polymers, may be included in a dosage form to increase drug bioavailability. These agents are believed to act by:

• increasing the contact time of the drug at the absorbing surface;
• increasing the local drug concentration at the site of adhesion/absorption;
• protecting the drug from dilution and possible degradation.

Several mechanisms by which mucoadhesives adhere to biological surface have been suggested, including the electronic, adsorption, wetting, diffusion, and fracture theories. It is likely that water movement from the mucosa to the polymer and physical entanglement of the adhesive polymer in the mucus glycoprotein chains are important in obtaining adherence.

3.6.2.3 Enzyme inhibitors

The inclusion of enzyme inhibitors in a formulation may help to overcome the enzymatic activity of the epithelial barrier. Work in this field has concentrated on the use of protease inhibitors to facilitate the absorption of therapeutic peptides and proteins. Protease inhibitors demonstrating potential to increase absorptioninclude the use of phosphoamidon, soyabean trypsin inhibitor, aprotinin and the chymotrypsin inhibitor FK-448.

3.6.2.4 Other formulation strategies

As described in Sections 1.3.4.4 and 6.4.2, the type of dosage form also profoundly influences the bioavailability of a drug. For example, because it does not have a dissolution step, the bioavailability from an aqueous solution will be greater than from a tablet, etc. Increasing the drug concentration increases the rate of drug absorption via passive diffusion mechanisms. Examples include the use of eutectic mixtures and supersaturated systems to enhance the transdermal penetration of drugs (see Chapter 8). Other formulation strategies include altering the formulation pH and tonicity to effect favorable absorption. Various further strategies are specific for the route in question, for example the use of iontophoresis to enhance the transdermal delivery of drugs.

3.7 CONCLUSIONS

This chapter has provided a broad overview of advanced drug delivery and targeting, and has introduced various key concepts pertinent to this subject.

The following chapters provide a more in-depth discussion of each of the major routes of drug delivery and discuss both advantages and disadvantages of these routes. The existing technologies employed to maximize delivery using the various routes is discussed along with the perceived challenges and opportunities for the future.

3.8 FURTHER READING

1. Evers, P. (1997) *Developments in Drug Delivery: Technology & Markets*, 2nd edn. Financial Times Pharmaceutical and Healthcare Publishing, London.
2. Robinson, J.R. and Lee, V.L. (eds) (1987) *Controlled Drug Delivery: Fundamentals and Applications*, 2nd edn. Marcel Dekker, New York.
3. Lee, V.H.L. (ed.) (1991) *Peptide and protein drug delivery*. Marcel Dekker Inc., New York.
4. Chien, Y.W. (ed.) (1991) *Novel Drug Delivery Systems*, 2nd edn. Marcel Dekker, New York.

3.9 SELF-ASSESSMENT QUESTIONS

1. Explain the following terms: (a) sustained release, (b) zero-order release, (c) bio-responsive release, (d) rate-controlled release and (e) targeted drug delivery.
2. List the different mechanisms by which rate-controlled release may be achieved.
3. Outline the differences between a reservoir device and a matrix device.
4. List the reasons why site-specific drug delivery is desirable in therapeutics.
5. List the various technologies presently being evaluated for drug targeting.
6. List the properties of an "ideal" dosage form.

7. List the properties of an "ideal" route of administration.

8. Outline the advantages and disadvantages of the following routes of administration: (a) parenteral, (b) oral and (c) pulmonary.

9. Outline how the physicochemical properties of a dosage form can be modulated to improve drug absorption.

10. Outline how a drug formulation may be improved to enhance drug absorption.

Rate Control in Drug Delivery and Targeting: Fundamentals and Applications to Implantable Systems

Hongkee Sah and Yie W. Chien

OBJECTIVES

On completion of this chapter the reader should be able to:

- Understand the advantages and disadvantages of implant therapy
- Describe the different types of non-degradable polymeric implants
- Describe the different types of biodegradable polymeric implants
- Describe rate control in drug delivery and targeting
- Give some examples of implant systems presently used in drug delivery
- Give examples of osmotic implant systems

4.1 INTRODUCTION

An implant is a single-unit drug delivery system that has been designed to deliver a drug moiety at a therapeutically desired rate, over a prolonged period of time. Such systems are most commonly used for sustained parenteral administration, including ocular and subcutaneous drug delivery. This chapter focuses on such implant systems and the mechanisms of rate control which form an intrinsic component of implantable systems. As these rate control mechanisms are applicable to many other drug delivery systems, this chapter also serves as a general introduction to the methods of rate control which are achievable using advanced drug delivery and targeting strategies.

Implants are available in many forms, including:

- *polymers*, which can be biodegradable or non-degradable and are available in various shapes (rod, cylinder, ring, film, etc.), sizes and mechanisms of drug release;
- *mini-pumps*, which can be powered by osmotic or mechanical mechanisms.

An implant requires specialized administration to initiate therapy. They are commonly implanted subcutaneously, either into the loose interstitial tissues of the outer surface of the upper arm, the anterior surface of the thigh or the lower portion of the abdomen. However, implants may also be surgically placed in, for example, the vitreous cavity of the eye (intravitreal implant), or intraperitoneally.

4.1.1 Historical development of implants

In the late 1930s, a pellet comprising compressed finely-powdered estradiol particles was implanted subcutaneously in animals, which caused animals to gain weight at a rate much faster than animals without an implant. Scientists further fabricated pellet-type implants comprising other steroidal hormones including testosterone, progesterone, deoxycorticosterone and dromostanolone propionate.

Release from such pellet-type implants is governed by the dissolution of the particular drug moiety in the body fluids and thus is not amenable to external control. A pellet-type implant also lacks pellet-to-pellet reproducibility in the rate of drug release. Thus attempts were made to optimize the approach. In the early 1960s, it was reported that hydrophobic small molecular weight compounds permeated through a silicone rubber capsule at relatively low rates. When implanted in animals, the system released drugs at reasonably constant rates and also elicited little inflammation at the site of implantation. The use of a silicone elastomer as a diffusion barrier to control the release of compounds such as steroidal hormones, insecticides, anesthetics and antibiotics was later demonstrated. The rate of drug release was subject to external control by manipulating the thickness, surface area, geometry and chemical composition of the silicone elastomers.

As a silicone rubber membrane is not permeable to hydrophilic or high molecular weight compounds, concerted efforts were made to develop other biocompatible polymers for use in implantable devices. Such polymers include poly(ethylene-co-vinyl acetate), poly (ethylene), poly(propylene), poly(hydroxymethyl methacrylate), poly(lactide-co-glycolide), poly(anhydrides) and poly(ortho esters). The characteristics and applications of each important polymer family will be discussed later in this chapter.

4.2 ADVANTAGES AND DISADVANTAGES OF IMPLANTATION THERAPY

Implants possess several advantages, but also disadvantages, as drug delivery systems depending on the nature of the drug being delivered. A brief overview of both the advantages and disadvantages of implantable drug delivery is given below.

4.2.1 Advantages

The advantages of implantation therapy include:

- *Convenience*: effective drug concentrations in the bloodstream can be maintained for long periods by methods such as continuous intravenous infusion or frequent injections. However, under these regimens, patients are often required to stay in hospital during administration for continuous medical monitoring. A short-acting drug exacerbates the situation, as the number of injections or the infusion rate must be increased, in order to maintain a therapeutically effective level of the drug. In contrast, implantation therapy permits patients to receive medication outside the hospital setting, with minimal medical surveillance. Implantation therapy is also characterized by a lower incidence of infection-related complications in comparison to an indwelling catheter-based infusion system.
- *Compliance*: by allowing a reduction, or complete elimination, of patient-involved dosing, compliance is increased immensely. A person can forget to take a tablet, but drug delivery from an implant is largely independent of patient input. Some implantable systems involve periodical refilling, but despite this factor the patient has less involvement in delivering the required medication.
- *Potential for controlled release*: implants are available which deliver drugs by zero-order controlled release kinetics. As discussed in Chapter 1 (Section 1.5.1), zero-order controlled release offers the advantages of:
  (i)   avoiding the peaks (risk of toxicity) and troughs (risk of ineffectiveness) of conventional therapy;
  (ii) reducing the dosing frequency;
  (iii) increasing patient compliance.

- *Potential for intermittent release*: externally programmable pumps (discussed later in this chapter) can facilitate intermittent release. As discussed in Chapter 1 (Section 1.5.2), intermittent release can facilitate drug release in response to such factors as:

  (i)   circadian rhythms;
  (ii)   fluctuating metabolic needs;
  (iii) the pulsatile release of many peptides and proteins.

- *Potential for bio-responsive release*: bio-responsive release from implants is an area of ongoing research and is discussed in Chapter 16.
- *Improved drug delivery*: using an implant system the drug is delivered locally or to the systemic circulation with minimal interference by biological or metabolic barriers. For example, the drug moiety bypasses the gastrointestinal tract and the liver. This bypassing effect is particularly of benefit to drugs which are either absorbed poorly or easily inactivated in the gastrointestinal tract and/or the liver before systemic distribution.
- *Flexibility*: considerable flexibility is possible with these systems, in the choice of materials, methods of manufacture, degree of drug-loading, drug release rate, etc.
- *Commercial*: an implantable dosage form diversifies the product portfolio of a given drug (see Section 2.2). From a regulatory perspective, it is regarded as a new drug product and can extend the market protection of the drug for an additional 5 years (for a new drug entity) or 3 years (for existing drugs).

4.2.2 Disadvantages

The disadvantages of implantation therapy include such factors as:

- *Invasive*: as described in Section 3.5.2, either a minor or a major surgical procedure is required to initiate therapy. This requires the appropriate surgical personnel, and may be traumatic, time-consuming, cause some scar formation at the site of implantation and, in a very small portion of patients, may result in surgery-related complications. The patient may also feel uncomfortable wearing the device.
- *Termination*: non-biodegradable polymeric implants and osmotic pumps must also be surgically retrieved at the end of treatment. Although a biodegradable polymeric implant does not require surgical retrieval, its continuing biodegradation makes it difficult to terminate drug delivery, or to maintain the correct dose at the end of its lifetime.
- *Danger of device failure*: there is a concomitant danger with this therapy that the device may for some reason fail to operate, which again requires surgical intervention to correct.
- *Limited to potent drugs*: the size of an implant is usually small, in order to minimize patients' discomfort. Therefore, most systems have a limited loading capacity, so that often only quite potent drugs, such as hormones, may be suitable for delivery by implantable devices.

- *Possibility of adverse reactions*: the site of implantation receives a high concentration of the drug delivered by an implant. This local high drug concentration may trigger adverse reactions.
- *Biocompatibility issues*: concerns over body responses to a foreign material often raise the issues of biocompatibility and safety of an implant (discussed in the next section).
- *Commercial disadvantages*: developing an implantable drug delivery system requires an enormous amount of R&D investment in terms of cost, effort, and time. If a new biomaterial is proposed to fabricate an implant, its safety and biocompatibility must be thoroughly evaluated to secure the approval of regulatory authorities. These issues can attribute to significant delay in the development, marketing and cost of a new implant.

4.3   BIOCOMPATIBILITY ISSUES

Implants may cause short- and long-term toxicity, as well as acute and chronic inflammatory responses.

Adverse effects may be caused by:

- *The intact polymer*: this may be due to the chemical reactivity of end or side groups in a polymer, organometallics used as polymerization initiators, or extractable polymeric fragments.
- *Residual contaminants*: such as residual organic solvents, unreacted monomers and additives used as fillers.
- *Toxic degradation products*: this effect is applicable to biodegradable polymers; for example, degradation of poly(alkylcyanoacrylate) leads to the formation of formaldehyde which is considered toxic in humans. In the case of a bioerodible poly(vinylpyrrolidone), the accumulation of the dissolved polymer in the liver raises a long-term toxicity issue.
- *Polymer/tissue interfacial properties*: the implant interface is a unique site where different chemicals co-exist and interact. If the surface of an implant has an affinity towards specific chemicals, an abnormal boundary layer will develop. The subsequent intra-layer rearrangement or reactions with other species then trigger tissue reactions. The defence reactions of the host tissue often lead to encapsulation of an implant by layers of fibrous tissues. Since the encapsulation frequently impedes drug release, *in vitro* drug release data may not permit the prediction of *in vivo* drug release patterns. High local drug concentrations at the site of implantation over extended periods of time can also cause severe local irritation or adverse tissue reactions.

The performance and response of the host toward an implanted material is indicated in terms of biocompatibility. Major initial evaluation tests used to assess the biocompatibility of an implant are listed in Table 4.1. These tests include:

- observation of the implant/tissue interactions at the site of implantation;

Biological Effect	Prolonged Contact[a]		Permanent Contact[b]	
	Tissue/Bone[c]	Blood	Tissue/Bone	Blood
Cytotoxicity	x	x	x	x
Sensitization	x	x	x	x
Irritation or intracutaneous reactivity	Δ	x	Δ	x
Systemic toxicity (acute toxicity)	Δ	x	Δ	x
Subchronic toxicity (subacute toxicity)	Δ	x	Δ	x
Chronic toxicity			x	x
Genotoxicity	x	x	Δ	x
Implantation	x	x	x	x
Haemocompatibility		x	x	x
Carcinogenicity			x	x

Table 4.1 Examples of major initial tests for assessing the biocompatibility of an implant

Source: FDA General Program Memorandum #G95-1 [a]Contact duration ranges from 24 hours to 30 days. [b]Contact duration is longer than 30 days. [c]Tissue includes tissue fluids and subcutaneous spaces. x: ISO (International Standards Organizations) evaluation tests for consideration. Δ: Additional tests which may be applicable

- assessment of the intensity and duration of each inflammatory response;
- histopathological evaluation of the tissues adjacent to the implant.

4.4 NON-DEGRADABLE POLYMERIC IMPLANTS

Non-degradable polymeric implants are divided into two main types (see also section 3.2):

- *reservoir devices*, in which the drug is surrounded by a rate-controlling polymer membrane (which can be non-porous, or microporous);
- *matrix devices*, in which the drug is distributed throughout the polymer matrix.

In both cases, drug release is governed by *diffusion*, i.e. the drug moiety must diffuse through the polymer membrane (for a reservoir device) or the polymeric matrix (for a matrix device), in order to be released.

The choice of whether to select a reservoir-type, or a matrix-type, implantable system depends on a number of factors, including:

- the drug's physicochemical properties;
- the desired drug release rate;
- desired delivery duration;
- availability of a manufacturing facility.

For example, it is generally easier to fabricate a matrix-type implant than a reservoir system, so this may determine the selection of a matrix system. However, if drug release is the overriding concern, a reservoir system may be chosen in preference to a matrix system. This is because reservoir systems can provide zero-order controlled release, whereas drug release generally decreases with time if a matrix system is used.

4.4.1 Reservoir-type non-degradable polymeric implants

4.4.1.1 Solution diffusion

For solution diffusion, a drug reservoir is bound by a polymeric membrane which has a compact, non-porous structure and functions as a rate-controlling barrier (Figure 4.1).

Silicones are used extensively as nondegradable non-porous membranes. They are polymerized from siloxanes and have repeating $OSi(R_1R_2)$ units. They vary in molecular weight, filler content, R_1 and R_2, and the type of reactive silicone ligands for cross-linking. Variations in these parameters permit the synthesis of a wide range of material types such as fluids, foams, soft and solid elastomers (Figure 4.2).

Poly(ethylene-co-vinyl acetate) (EVA copolymer) is also widely used as a non-degradable polymeric implant. These copolymers have the advantages of:

- *Ease of fabrication*: the copolymers are thermoplastic in nature, thus an implantable device is easily fabricated by extrusion, film casting or injection molding.
- *Versatility*: the copolymers are available in a wide range of molecular weights and ethylene/vinyl acetate ratios. As the ethylene domain is crystalline, an increase in the content of ethylene unit affects the crystallinity and the solubility parameter of the copolymer. Thus the release rate of a drug from the device can be tailored as required.

Other polymeric materials commonly used as non-porous, rate-controlling membranes are given in Table 4.2.

The penetration of a solvent, usually water, into a polymeric implant initiates drug release via a diffusion process. Diffusion of drug molecules through non-porous polymer membranes depends on the size of

Figure 4.1 Reservoir-type polymeric implant

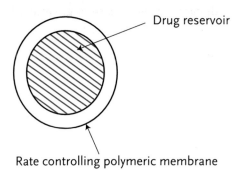

Drug reservoir

Rate controlling polymeric membrane

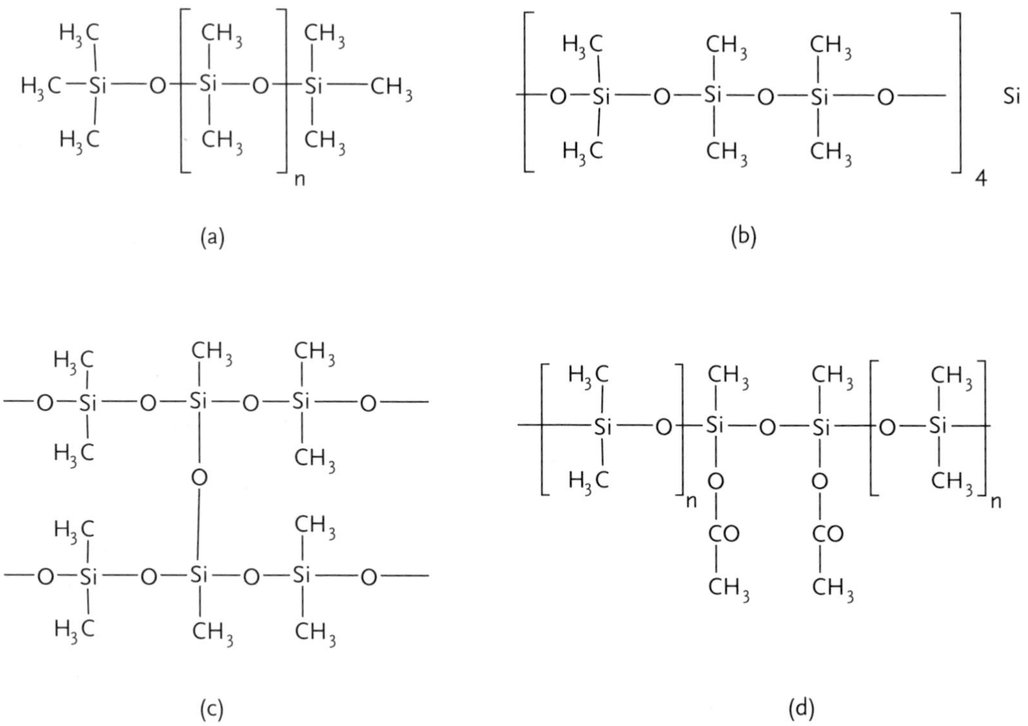

(a)

(b)

(c)

(d)

Figure 4.2 Structure of silicones (a) silicone fluid (Dow Corning 360 Medical Fluid); (b) silicone foam elastomer; (c) silicone elastomer (vulcanized Silastic 382 Medical-grade Elastomer); and (d) silicone elastomer (vulcanized Silastic Medical Adhesive Type A)

the drug molecules and the spaces available between the polymeric chains. Even through the space between the polymer chains may be smaller than the size of the drug molecules, drug can still diffuse through the polymer chains due to the continuous movement of polymer chains by Brownian motion.

For transport through the membrane, there are three barriers to be circumvented (Figure 4.3):

Table 4.2 Polymers used for fabrication of reservoir systems

Polymers providing solution-diffusion mechanism
Silicone rubber, especially polydimethyl siloxane (Silastic)
Silicone-carbonate copolymers, Surface-treated silicone rubbers
Poly(ethylene-vinyl acetate), Polyethylene, Polyurethane (Walopur)
Polyisopropene, Polyisobutylene, Polybutadiene
Polyamide, Polyvinyl chloride, Plasticized soft nylon
Highly cross-linked hydrogels of polyhydroxyethyl methacrylate,
Polyethylene oxide, Polyvinyl alcohol, or Polyvinyl pyrrolidone

Polymers providing pore-diffusion mechanism
Cellulose esters, Cellulose triacetate, Cellulose nitrate
Modified insoluble collagen
Polycarbonates, Polyamides, Polysulfonates
Polychloroethers, Acetal polymers, Halogenated polyvinylidene fluoride
Loosely cross-linked hydrogels of polyhydroxyethyl methacrylate,
Polyethylene oxide, Polyvinyl alcohol or Polyvinyl pyrrolidone

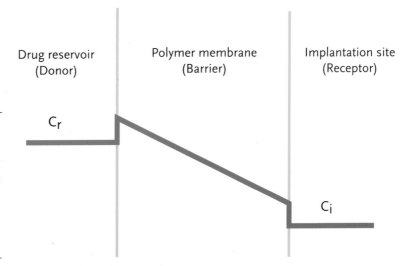

Drug reservoir
(Donor)

Polymer membrane
(Barrier)

Implantation site
(Receptor)

C_r

C_i

Figure 4.3 The steady-state concentration profile of a drug in a reservoir-type polymeric implant C_r = concentration of drug in the reservoir, C_i = concentration of drug at the site of implantation

- the reservoir–membrane interface;
- the rate-controlling membrane;
- the membrane–implantation site interface.

The drug molecules in the reservoir compartment initially partition into the membrane, then diffuse through it, and finally partition into the implantation site. The rate of drug diffusion follows Fick's Law (see Section 1.3.3.2):

$$dm/dt = (Dk/h) . A . \Delta C \qquad \text{(Equation 4.1)}$$

where dm/dt = the rate of drug diffusion
  D = the diffusion coefficient of the drug in the membrane
  k = the partition coefficient of the drug into the membrane
  h = the membrane thickness
  A = the available surface area
  ΔC = the concentration gradient, i.e. $C_r - C_i$ where C_r and C_i denote the drug concentrations in the reservoir and at the site of implantation respectively.

As sink conditions apply;

$$\Delta C \approx C_r$$

hence

$$dm/dt = (Dk/h) . A . C_r \qquad \text{(Equation 4.2)}$$

Substituting further:

$$dm/dt = P . A . C_r \qquad \text{(Equation 4.3)}$$

where P, the permeability constant, is defined as Dk/h and has the units cm/s. The release rate of a drug from different polymeric membranes can be compared from the corresponding P values.

Substituting again:

$$dm/dt = K_1 C_r \qquad \text{(Equation 4.4)}$$

where K_1 is a pseudo-rate constant and is dependent on the factors D, A, k and h. This is the familiar form of a first-order rate equation and indicates that the rate of diffusion is proportional to drug concentration.

However, in this system, the drug reservoir consists of either:

• solid drug particles, or
• a suspension of solid drug particles in a dispersion medium

so that the concentration of drug (C_r) in the system always remains *constant*, so that Equation 4.4 simplifies to:

$$dm/dt = K_2 \qquad \text{(Equation 4.5)}$$

where K_2 is a constant and is dependent on C_r.

Equation 4.5 is the familiar form of a zero-order rate equation and indicates that the drug release rate does not vary with time (Figure 4.4). Thus the release rate of a drug from this type of implantable device is constant during the entire time that the implant remains in the body.

Figure 4.4 "M ∝ t" Zero-order controlled release profile of a reservoir-type non-degradable polymeric implant (porous or compact membrane)

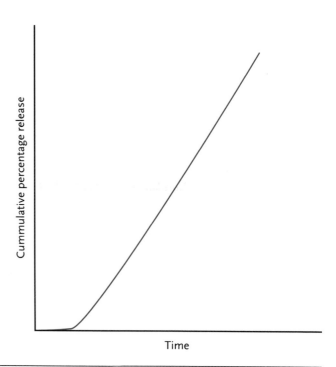

Cummulative percentage release

Time

4.4.1.2 Pore-diffusion

In some cases, the rate-controlling polymeric membrane is not compact but porous. Microporous membranes can be prepared by making hydrophobic polymer membranes in the presence of water-soluble materials such as poly(ethylene glycol), which can be subsequently removed from the polymer matrix by dissolving in aqueous solution. Cellulose esters, loosely cross-linked hydrogels and other polymers given in Table 4.2 also give rise to porous membranes.

In microporous reservoir systems, drug molecules are released by diffusion through the micropores, which are usually filled with either water or oil (e.g. silicone, castor and olive oil). Solvent-loading of a porous membrane device is achieved simply by immersing the device in the solvent. When this technique presents some difficulty, the implantable device is placed inside a pressure vessel and pressure is then applied to facilitate the filling of the solvent into pores. The transport of drug molecules across such porous membranes is termed pore-diffusion. The selection of a solvent is obviously of paramount importance, since it affects drug permeability and solubility.

In this system, the pathway of drug transport is no longer straight, but tortuous. The porosity ε of the membrane and the tortuosity τ of the pathway must therefore also be considered. Thus for a porous polymeric membrane, Equation 4.4 is modified as follows:

$$dm/dt = D_s . A . C_s . \varepsilon/\tau h \qquad \text{(Equation 4.6)}$$

where C_s, the drug solubility in a solvent, is the product of K and C_r and D_s is the drug diffusion coefficient in the solvent.

As for the non-porous reservoir device, in the microporous system, both:

- the surface area of the membrane and
- the drug concentration in the reservoir compartment

remain unchanged, thus "M ∝ t" kinetics is again demonstrated and zero-order controlled release is attained (Figure 4.4).

4.4.1.3 Examples of non-degradable reservoir devices

Norplant subdermal implant

The Norplant contraceptive implant is a set of six flexible, closed capsules made of a dimethylsiloxane/methylvinylsiloxane copolymer containing levonorgestrel. The silicone rubber copolymer serves as rate-controlling membrane. The capsules are surgically implanted subdermally, in a fan-like pattern, in the mid-portion of the upper arm. The implant releases levonorgestrel continuously at the rate of 30 μg/day (the same daily dose provided by the oral uptake of the progestin-only minipill) over a 5-year period. After the capsules are removed, patients are promptly returned to normal fertility.

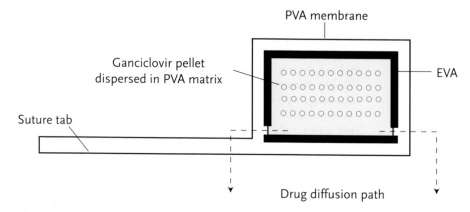

PVA membrane

Ganciclovir pellet
dispersed in PVA matrix

EVA

Suture tab

Drug diffusion path

Figure 4.5 Structure
of Vitrasert implant

Vitrasert intravitreal implant

The Vitrasert implant has been developed to deliver therapeutic levels
of ganciclovir locally to the eye, for the treatment of retinitis infected
by Cytomegalovirus (CMV) (see Section 12.4.2). Localized delivery to
the eye minimizes the systemic side effects of the drug. The implant is
surgically placed in the vitreous cavity of the eye and delivers therapeutic levels of ganciclovir for up to 32 weeks.

The implant consists of a tablet-shaped ganciclovir reservoir. The
drug is initially completely coated with poly(vinyl alcohol) (PVA) and
then coated with a discontinuous film of hydrophobic, dense poly(ethylene-co-vinyl acetate) (EVA). Both polymers are nonerodible and
hydrophobic (the PVA used in the implant is cross-linked and/or high
molecular weight, to ensure it does not dissolve when exposed to
water). The entire assembly is coated again with PVA to which a
suture tab made of PVA is attached (Figure 4.5).

The first step for drug release involves the dissolution of ganciclovir
by ocular fluids permeating through the PVA and EVA membranes. The
drug molecules permeate through the PVA membrane, then through the
pores of the discontinuous film of EVA and finally through the outer
PVA membrane into the vitreous cavity, at the rate of approximately
1 μg/hr over a 7- to 8-month period. The release rate can be further
tailored by varying the membrane characteristics of PVA and EVA.

4.4.2 Matrix-type non-degradable polymeric implants

In a matrix-type implant the drug is distributed throughout a polymeric matrix (Figure 4.6).

Matrix-type implants are fabricated by physically mixing the drug
with a polymer powder and shaping the mixture into various geome-
tries (e.g. rod, cylinder, or film) by solvent casting, compression/injec-
tion molding or screw extrusion.

The total payload of a drug determines the drug's physical state in a
polymer:

- *Dissolved*: the drug is soluble in the polymer matrix. A dissolved
  matrix device (also known as a monolithic solution) appears at a
  low payload.

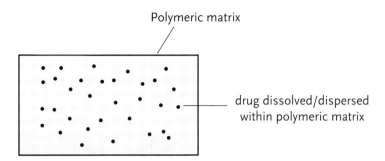

Polymeric matrix

drug dissolved/dispersed within polymeric matrix

Figure 4.6 Matrix-type polymeric implant

- *Dispersed*: the drug is present above the saturation level, additional drug exists as dispersed particles in the polymer matrix (also known as a monolithic dispersion).
- *Porous*: with further increase in total drug payload, the undissolved drug particles keep in contact with one another. When the drug content occupies more than 30% volume of the polymer matrix, the leaching of drug particles results in the formation of pores or microchannels that are interconnected.

Figure 4.7 A matrix-type implant in which a drug is dissolved. The initial diffusion of drug molecules leaves a drug-depleted polymeric zone with a length h, which increases with time. This event leads to an increase in diffusional distance over time

Regardless of a drug's physical state in the polymeric matrix, the release rate of the drug decreases over time. Initially, drug molecules closest to the surface are released from the implant. As release continues, molecules must travel a greater distance to reach the exterior of the implant and thus increase the time required for release (Figure 4.7). This increased diffusion time results in a decrease in the release rate from the device with time (Figure 4.8). Numerous equations have been developed to describe drug release kinetics obtainable with dissolved,

Time

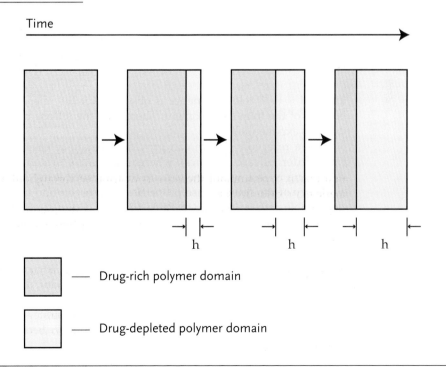

h   h   h

Drug-rich polymer domain

Drug-depleted polymer domain

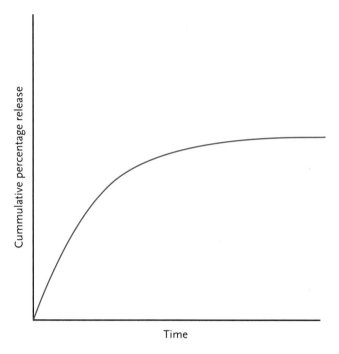

Figure 4.8 Drug release by diffusion through a non-degradable polymeric matrix. There is a decrease in the release rate from the device with time

dispersed, and porous-type matrix implants, in different shapes, including spheres, slabs and cylinders. Suffice to say here that in all cases, the release rate initially decreases proportionally to the square root of time:

$$dm/dt = k_d/t^{1/2} \qquad \text{(Equation 4.7)}$$

where k_d is a proportionality constant dependent on the properties of the implant, thus:

$$M \propto t^{1/2} \qquad \text{(Equation 4.8)}$$

This "$M \propto t^{1/2}$" release kinetics is observed for the release of up to 50–60% of the total drug content. Thereafter, the release rate usually declines exponentially.

Thus a reservoir system can provide constant release with time (zero-order release kinetics) whereas a matrix system provides decreasing release with time (square root of time-release kinetics). A summary of the drug release properties of reservoir and matrix non-degradable devices in given in Table 4.3.

The decreasing drug release rate with time of a matrix system can be partially offset either by:

- designing a special geometry that provides increasing surface over time (this strategy is used in the Compudose implant, described in Section 4.4.2.1 below), or
- using reservoir/matrix hybrid-type systems (this strategy is used in the Synchro-Mate-C and Implanon implants, described in Section 4.4.3).

Table 4.3 A summary of the drug release properties of reservoir and matrix non-degradable implant devices	System	Release Mechanism	Release Properties	Release Kinetics
	Reservoir	Diffusion through a polymeric membrane (which can be compact or microporous)	Constant drug release with time	Zero-order release "$M \propto t$"
	Matrix	Diffusion through a polymeric matrix	Drug release decreases with time	Square root of time release "$M \propto t^{1/2}$"

4.4.2.1 Examples of matrix-type implants

Compudose cattle growth implant

In the Compudose implant microcrystalline estradiol is dispersed in a silicone rubber matrix, which is then used to coat a biocompatible inert core of silicone rubber, that does not contain any drug particles (Figure 4.9). This particular design, consisting of a thin layer of the drug-containing matrix and a relatively thick drug-free inert core, minimizes tailing in the drug release profile.

When this implant is placed under the skin of an animal, estradiol is released and enters into systemic circulation. This stimulates the animal's pituitary gland to produce more growth hormone and causes the animal to gain weight at a greater rate. At the end of the growing period, the implant can be easily removed to allow a withdrawal period before slaughter.

The Compudose implant is available with a thick silicone rubber coating (Compudose-400) and releases estradiol over 400 days, whereas one with a thinner coating (Compudose-200) releases the drug for up to 200 days.

Syncro-Mate-B implant

The implant consists of a water-swellable Hydron (cross-linked ethylene glycomethacrylate) polymer matrix in which estradiol valerate (Norgestomet) crystals are dispersed. It is used for the synchronization of estrus/ovulation in cycling heifers. Once implanted in the animal's ear, the implant delivers estradiol valerate at the rate of 504 μg cm^{-2} day$^{-1/2}$ over a period of 16 days.

Figure 4.9 Structure of Compudose cattle growth implant

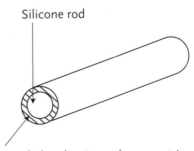

Silicone rod

Estradiol - releasing polymer matrix

4.4.3 Reservoir/matrix hybrid-type polymeric implants

Reservoir/matrix hybrid-type non-degradable polymeric implants are also available. Such systems are designed in an attempt to improve the "$M \propto t^{1/2}$" release kinetics of a matrix system, so that release approximates the zero-order release rate of a reservoir device. Examples of these types of systems include:

Syncro-Mate-C subdermal implant

To make this implant, an aqueous solution of PEG is first loaded with estradiol valerate (Norgestomet) at a saturation level. This suspension is then dispersed in a silicone elastomer by vigorous stirring. The mixture is blended with a cross-linking agent, which results in the formation of millions of individually sealed microreservoirs. The mixture is then placed in a silicone polymer tube for *in situ* polymerization and molding. The tube is then sectioned to make tiny cylindrical implants (Figure 4.10a). Drug molecules initially diffuse through the microreservoir membrane and then through the silicone polymer coating membrane. This implant provides zero-order release kinetics, rather than square root of time-release kinetics. The two open ends of the implant do not affect the observed zero-order release pattern because their surface area is insignificant compared to the implant's total surface area.

Implanon (Organon)

Implanon is fabricated by dispersing the drug, 3-ketodesogestrel, in an EVA copolymer matrix. This polymer matrix is then coated with another EVA copolymer, which serves as a rate-controlling membrane (Figure 4.10b). The drug permeation through the polymer membrane occurs at a rate that is 20 times slower than that through the polymer matrix, thus diffusion through the *membrane* is rate-limiting, which again improves the matrix-type square root of time-release kinetics, so that the release is like the zero-order release rate of a reservoir device. Following implantation in the upper arm, a single rod of Implanon releases 3-ketodesogestrel at the rate of > 30 μg/day for up to 3 years.

EVA copolymers are also used in fabricating Progestasert and Ocusert which are an intrauterine and an ocular drug delivery device for pilocarpine and progesterone, respectively. These are discussed in Chapters 11 and 12.

Figure 4.10 Hybrid-type polymeric implants (a) Syncro-Mate-C: matrix containing microreservoirs of drug, (b) Implanon: membrane coating a drug containing matrix

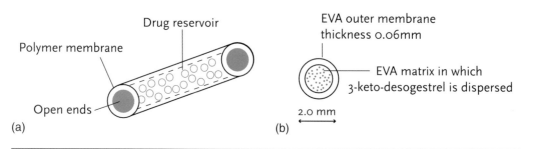

Polymer membrane

Drug reservoir

Open ends

(a)

EVA outer membrane thickness o.o6mm

EVA matrix in which 3-keto-desogestrel is dispersed

2.0 mm

(b)

4.5 BIODEGRADABLE POLYMERIC IMPLANTS

Since the 1950s, most implants have been fabricated from non-biodegradable, inert polymers such as silicone rubber, polyacrylamide and poly(ethylene-vinyl acetate) copolymers. However, some fundamental limitations of such implants include:

- The implants must be surgically removed after they are depleted of drug.
- Water-soluble or highly-ionized drugs and macromolecules, such as peptides and proteins, have negligible diffusivities through dense hydrophobic membranes.
- It is difficult to achieve versatile release rates – drug release rate is determined largely by the intrinsic properties of the polymers.

Such limitations prompted scientists to develop biodegradable polymeric implants. Degradation can take place via:

- *bioerosion* – the gradual dissolution of a polymer matrix;
- *biodegradation* – degradation of the polymer structure caused by chemical or enzymatic processes.

Degradation can take place by one or both mechanisms. For example, natural polymers such as albumin may be used; such proteins are not only water-soluble, but are readily degraded by specific enzymes. The terms degradation, dissolution and erosion are used interchangeably in this chapter, and the general process is referred to as polymer degradation.

Thus polymers used in biodegradable implants must be water-soluble and/or degradable in water. Table 4.4 lists some of the water soluble and biodegradable polymers that can be used for the fabrication of biodegradable implants.

Polymer degradation is classified into two patterns (Figure 4.11):

- bulk erosion;
- surface erosion.

In bulk erosion, the entire area of polymer matrix is subject to chemical or enzymatic reactions, thus erosion occurs homogeneously throughout the entire matrix Accordingly, the degradation pattern is sometimes termed homogeneous erosion.

In surface erosion, polymer degradation is limited to the surface of an implant exposed to a reaction medium. Erosion therefore starts at the exposed surface and works downwards, layer by layer. Due to the

Table 4.4 Synthetic polymers used in the fabrication of biodegradable implants

Water-soluble polymers	Degradable polymers
Poly(acrylic acid)	Poly(hydroxybutyrate)
Poly(ethylene glycol)	Poly(lactide-co-glycolide)
Poly(vinylpyrrolidone)	Polyanhydrides

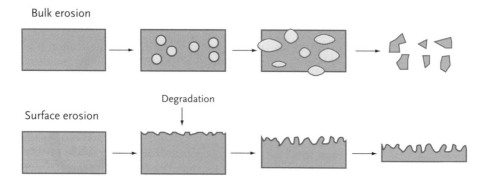

Bulk erosion

Surface erosion

Degradation

Figure 4.11 Bulk and surface dissolution of biodegradable polymers

difference in degradation rates between the surface and the center of the polymer matrix, the process is alternatively termed heterogeneous erosion. A drug distributed homogeneously in a surface-eroding matrix implant, of which the surface area is invariant with time, shows constant release with time over the period of implantation.

Polymer characteristics (type of monomer, degree of cross-linking, etc.) play a crucial role in determining whether the polymer is bulk- or surface-eroding. If water is readily able to penetrate the polymer, the entire domain of polymer matrix is easily hydrated and the polymer undergoes bulk erosion. On the contrary, if water penetration into its center is limited, the erosion front is restricted to the surface of the polymer matrix and the implant undergoes surface erosion. In practice, the polymer degradation occurs through a combination of the two processes.

As for non-degradable polymeric implants, biodegradable polymeric implants are divided into two main types:

- *reservoir devices* in which the drug is surrounded by a rate-controlling polymer membrane (such devices are particularly used for oral-controlled release – see Section 6.6.3);
- *matrix devices* in which the drug is distributed throughout the polymer matrix.

The drug release for biodegradable polymeric implants is governed not by diffusion through a membrane, but by *degradation* of the polymer membrane or matrix.

If the rate of polymer degradation is slow compared to the rate of drug diffusion, drug release mechanisms and kinetics obtained with a biodegradable implant are analogous to those provided by a non-biodegradable implant (therefore a reservoir system gives a zero-order release profile and a matrix system gives a square root of time release profile). After drug depletion, the implant subsequently degrades at the site of implantation and eventually disappears.

However, in many cases, drug release takes place *in parallel* with polymer degradation. In such cases the mechanism of drug release is complicated as drug release occurs by drug diffusion, polymer degradation and/or polymer dissolution. The permeability of the drug through the polymer increases with time as the polymer matrix is gradually opened up by enzymatic/chemical cleavage. The references cited at the end of this chapter deal with the relevant mathematical treatments of this topic.

4.5.1 Poly-lactide and poly-lactide-co-glycolide polymers

Polyesters, such as poly(lactic acid) (PLA) and poly(lactic-co-glycolic acid) (PLGA), are examples of biomaterials that are degraded by homogeneous bulk erosion.

The polymers are prepared from lactide and glycolide, which are cyclic esters of lactic and glycolic acids. The lactic acid can be in either the L(+) or D(–) form, or the DL-lactic acid mixture can be used. Low molecular weight polymers (< 20,000 g/mol) are directly synthesized from lactic and glycolic acid via polycondensation. High molecular polymers (> 20,000 g/mol) are prepared via ring-opening polymeriza-tion (Figure 4.12). Variations in lactic acid:gycolic acid ratios, as well as molecular weights, affect the degree of crystallinity, hydrophobic-ity/hydrophilicity, and water uptake. Lactic acid-rich copolymers are more stable against hydrolysis than glycolic acid-rich copolymers.

Polymer degradation generally takes place in four major stages:

- Polymer hydration causes disruption of primary and secondary structures.
- Strength loss is caused by the rupture of ester linkages in the polymers.
- Loss of mass integrity results in initiation of absorption of poly-meric fragments.
- Finally smaller polymeric fragments are phagocytosed, or complete dissolution into glycolic and lactic acids occurs (Figure 4.12).

4.5.1.1 *Zoladex*

Zoladex is a commercially available PLA/PLGA implant, designed to deliver goserelin (a GnRH agonist analog) over a 1- or 3-month period. As described in Chapter 1 (Section 1.5.2), chronic administration of GnRH agonists evokes an initial agonist phase, which subsequently causes *antagonistic* effects and a suppression of gonadotrophin secre-tion. Thus implants of GnRH analogues can be used clinically in the treatment of sex-hormone responsive tumors and endometriosis.

Zoladex implants are indicated for use in the palliative treatment of advanced breast cancer in pre- and peri-menopausal women, in the palliative treatment of advanced carcinoma of the prostate and in the management of endometriosis, including pain relief and the reduction of endometriotic lesions. The implant is fabricated by dispersing goserelin in a PLGA matrix and molding it into a cylindrical shape, which can be injected subcutaneously.

The release profile of goserelin from the implants has been well char-acterized during product development. For example, in a study of a Zoladex implant loaded with 10.8 mg of drug, the goserelin present at the surface of the implant was released rapidly, so that mean concen-trations increased and reached peak levels within the first 24 hours. The initial release was then followed by a lag period up to 4 days, in which there was a rapid decline in the plasma concentration of the drug.

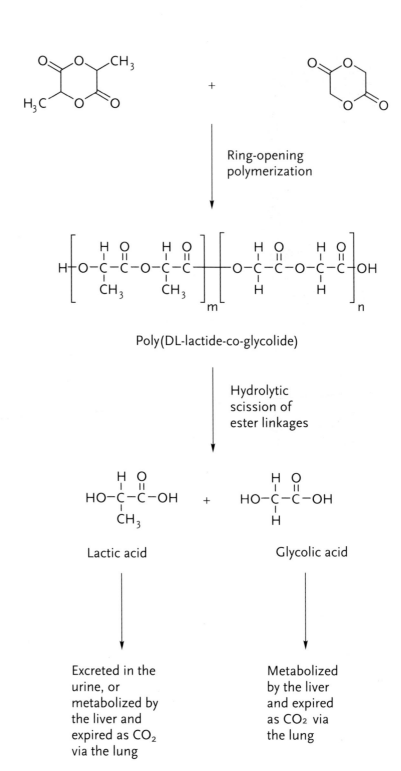

Poly(DL-lactide-co-glycolide)

Ring-opening
polymerization

Hydrolytic
scission of
ester linkages

Lactic acid

Glycolic acid

Excreted in the
urine, or
metabolized by
the liver and
expired as CO_2
via the lung

Metabolized
by the liver
and expired
as CO_2 via
the lung

Figure 4.12 Synthesis
and *in vivo* degradation
of PLGA polymers

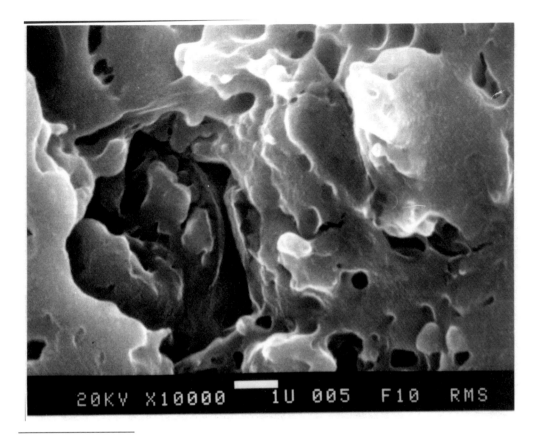

```
20KV  X10000    1U  005    F10    RMS
```

Figure 4.13 Scanning electron micrograph of a PLGA matrix incubated in distilled water at (37°C for 21 days). Pores and channels produced by extensive polymer degradation are visualized in the micrograph. The bar size is 1 μm. (Reproduced from *Journal of Applied Polymer Science*, 58: 197–206, 1995)

The lag period represents the time required to initiate polymer degradation. As water penetrates the polymer matrix and hydrolyzes the ester linkages, the essentially hydrophobic polymer becomes more hydrophilic. Extensive polymer degradation is followed by the development of pores or microchannels in the polymer matrix, which are visible by scanning electron microscopy (Figure 4.13). After the initial induction period required to initiate polymer degradation, drug release is accelerated thereafter by polymer degradation. In the above study this maintained the mean goserelin concentrations in the range of about 0.3 to 1 ng/ml until the end of the treatment period.

The discontinuous two phases drug release can be controlled and avoided by manipulating the degradation properties of the polymer so that it is possible for the Zoladex implant to provide continuous release over a 28-day period.

4.5.1.2 *Lupron depot*

The Lupron Depot comprises a PLA/PLGA microsphere delivery system for the delivery of the GnRH analog, leuprolide, over a 1-, 3-, or 4-month period. The release rate is determined by the polymer composition and molecular weight (Table 4.5).

The Lupron Depot microspheres are indicated for the treatment of male patients with prostate cancer and female patients suffering from endometriosis and anemia due to fibroids. Each depot formulation is

Table 4.5 Lupron Depot characteristics	Release Rate	Polymer Composition	Polymer MW
	1 month	PLGA (75:25)[a]	12,000 to 14,000
	3 or 4 months	PLA	12,000 to 18,000

[a]lactic acid:glycolic acid monomer ratio.

supplied in a single dose vial containing lyophilized microspheres and an ampoule containing a diluent. Just prior to intramuscular injection, the diluent is withdrawn by a syringe and injected into the single-dose vial to homogeneously disperse the microspheres.

An initial burst release of leuprolide from the microsphere depot occurs *in vivo*, followed by quasi-linear release for the rest of the time period. The efficacy of leuprolide depot formulations was found to be the same as the efficacy achieved with daily subcutaneous injections of 1 mg leuprolide formulation.

4.5.2 Polyanhydrides

Polyanhydrides, such as poly[bis(p-carboxyphenoxy)propane:sebacic acid] copolymers (Figure 4.14), are also used for the fabrication of biodegradable implants. Polymer degradation occurs via hydrolysis,

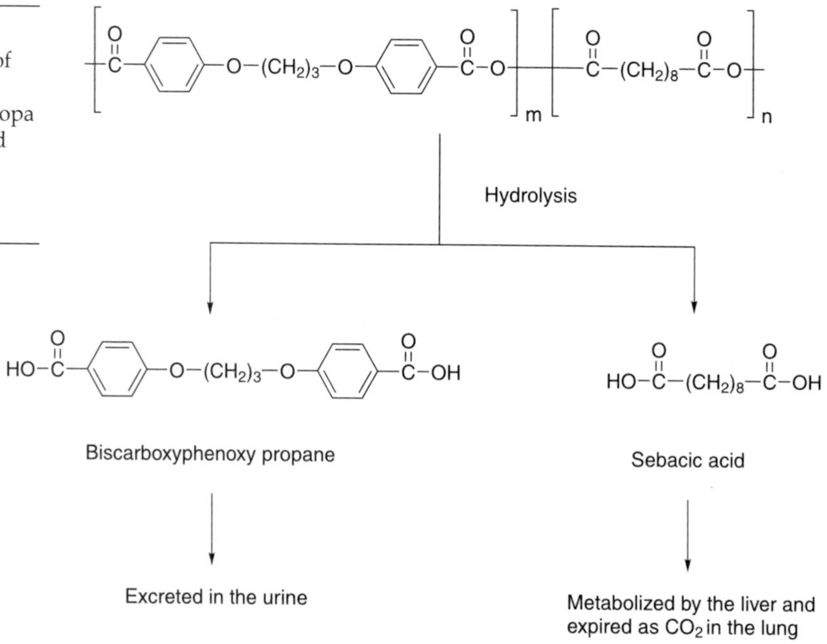

Figure 4.14 The chemical structure of poly[bis(p-carboxyphenoxy)propane: sebacic acid] and the pathway and products of its metabolism

the biscarboxyphenoxypropane monomer is excreted in the urine and the sebacic acid monomer is metabolized by the liver and is expired as carbon dioxide via the lung (Figure 4.14).

Erosion rates of poly (anhydride) copolymers are controlled by adjusting their molecular weight and biscarboxyphenoxy propane:sebacic acid ratio. Sebacic acid-rich copolymers display much faster degradation rates than biscarboxyphenoxy propane-rich copolymers. Changes in the ratio of the monomers are reported to provide various degradation rates ranging from 1 day to 3 years.

4.5.2.1 *Gliadel*

Gliadel is a biodegradable polyanhydride implant composed of poly[bis(p-carboxyphenoxy) propane:sebacic acid] in a 20:80 monomer ratio, for the delivery of carmustine. The implant is indicated in the treatment of recurrent glioblastoma multiforme (GBM) which is the most common and fatal type of brain cancer.

To fabricate the implant, the polyanhydride and the drug moiety are dissolved in dichloromethane. The solution is spray dried to produce microspherical powders in which the drug is homogeneously dispersed. The powders are then compressed into a disk-shaped wafer, approximately 14 mm in diameter and 1 mm thick.

Up to eight Gliadel wafers are implanted in the cavity created when a neurosurgeon removes the brain tumor. The wafers gradually degrade in the cavity and allows the delivery of high, localized doses of the anti-cancer agent for a long period, thereby minimizing systemic side-effects. Preliminary clinical reports with this system are highly encouraging.

In contrast to bulk-eroding PLA/PLGA polymers, the polyanhydride undergoes surface erosion. The thin-disk type morphology of the wafer confers a high surface-to-volume ratio on the implant, so that the total surface area of the implant is kept almost constant over the time of polymer degradation, which facilitates a constant release of carmustine with time.

4.5.3   Other biodegradable polymers

4.5.3.1 *Poly(ortho esters)*

Poly(ortho esters) offer the advantage of controlling the rate of hydrolysis of acid-labile linkages in the backbone by means of acidic or basic excipients physically incorporated in the matrix. This results in polymer degradation proceeding purely by surface erosion, which results in zero-order drug release from disk-shaped devices.

4.5.3.2 *Poly(caprolactones)*

Poly(ϵ-caprolactone) (PCL) is synthesized by anionic, cationic or co-ordination polymerization of ε-caprolactone. Degradable block copolymers with polyethylene glycol, diglycolide, substituted caprolactones and *l*-valerolactone can also be synthesized. Like the lactide polymers, PCL and its copolymers degrade both *in vitro* and *in vivo* by bulk hydrolysis, with the degradation rate affected by the size and shape of the device and additives.

4.5.3.3 Poly(hydroxybutyrate)

Poly(hydroxybutyrate) may be synthesized by fermentation from *Alcaligenes eutrophus*. The polymers have been shown to be useful for the controlled release of buserelin (a GnRH agonist analog) in both rats and humans.

4.5.4 Natural biodegradable polymeric implants

In addition to synthetic biodegradable polymers discussed so far, naturally occurring biopolymers have also been used for fabricating implantable drug delivery systems. Examples of natural biopolymers are proteins (e.g. albumin, casein, collagen, and gelatin) and polysaccharides (e.g. cellulose derivatives, chitin derivatives, dextran, hyaluronic acids, inulin, and starch).

Collagen, a major structural component of animal tissues, is being used increasingly in various biomedical and cosmetic applications. After implantation, collagen provokes minimal host inflammatory response or tissue reaction and its initial low antigenicity is practically abolished by the host's enzymatic digestion.

A collagen-based therapeutic implantable gel technology has recently been developed, in which the drug moiety (a chemotherapeutic agent) is incorporated within the meshwork of rod-shaped collagen molecules. The collagen matrix is then converted to an injectable gel by a chemical modifier. Changes in the composition and structure of the gel can adjust its solubility, strength and resorption properties.

Figure 4.15 Schematic illustration of the delivery of a drug to local tissues via the collagen implant injectable gel technology (courtesy of Matrix Pharmaceuticals Inc., Fremont, CA, USA)

Direct injection of the gel into solid tumors and skin lesions provides high local concentrations of a drug specifically where needed (Figure 4.15). The gel is injected intradermally in a fanning or tracking manner to disperse the gel formulation throughout the tumor. Drug retention at the site of implantation is further enhanced by the addition of chemical modifiers such as the vasoconstrictor, epinephrine (adrenaline). This adjunct reduces blood flow and acts as a chemical tourniquet to hold the therapeutic agent in place.

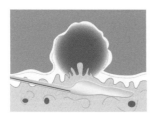

The chemotherapeutic gel is injected intradermally at the base of the wart

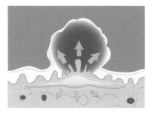

Active therapeutic drug disperses from the gel providing high local concentration of drug in and around diseased tissue. Vasoconstrictor reduces local blood frow, slowing clearance of drug from the site. Slow dispersion limits normal tissue exposure to active therapeutic drug.

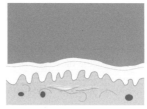

After release of active drug, the gel biodegrades.

The most advanced products based on the implantable gel technology include the Intradose (cisplatin/epinephrine) injectable gel for treatment of solid tumors and the Advasite (fluorouracil/epinephrine) injectable gel for treatment of cutaneous diseases, including external warts, basal cell carcinoma, squamous cell carcinoma and psoriasis.

4.6 IMPLANTABLE PUMPS

The driving force for drug release from a pump is a *pressure* difference that causes the bulk flow of a drug, or drug solution, from the device at a controlled rate. This is in contrast to the polymeric controlled release systems described above, where the driving force is due to the *concentration* difference of the drug between the formulation and the surrounding environment. Pressure differences in an implantable pump can be created by osmotic or mechanical action, as described below.

4.6.1 Osmotic implantable pumps

Osmosis is defined as the movement of water through a semi-permeable membrane into a solution. The semi-permeable membrane is such that only water molecules can move through it; the movement of solutes, including drugs, is restricted (although the extent of this restriction depends on the characteristics of the membrane, see below).

If a solution containing an osmotic agent (e.g. NaCl) is separated from water by a semipermeable membrane, the water will flow across the semipermeable membrane, into the solution containing the osmotic agent (Figure 4.16). Osmosis results in an increase in pressure in the solution and the excess pressure is known as the osmotic pressure.

The volume flow rate arising from the influx of water into the solution is determined by a number of factors:

- The *osmotic pressure*: $\Delta\pi$ is the difference in the osmotic pressure between osmotic agent-containing, and osmotic agent-free, compartments.
- The *back pressure*: water influx into the osmotic compartment generates a back pressure which retards the volume flow rate of water. ΔP is the difference in the hydrostatic pressure between the two

Figure 4.16 Process of osmosis: the influx of water across a semi-permeable membrane

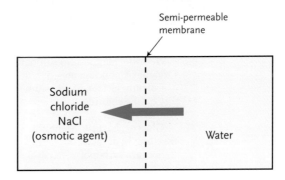

compartments and represents the degree of back pressure generated.

- The *effective surface area*, *A*, of the membrane.
- The *thickness* of the membrane, *h*.
- The *membrane selectivity* toward an osmotic agent and water, described by the osmotic reflection coefficient σ. An ideal semipermeable membrane has the σ value of 1, which means that it allows the passage of only water molecules. In contrast, a leaky semipermeable membrane with σ value approaching zero does not exhibit such selectivity and permits the transport of not only water, but also an osmotic agent.
- the *permeability coefficient* of the membrane, L_p.

These parameters affecting the volume influx of water can be expressed by:

$$\frac{dV}{dt} = \frac{A\,L_p\,(\sigma\Delta\pi - \Delta P)}{h} \qquad \text{(Equation 4.9)}$$

Common semipermeable membranes and osmotic agents used in osmotic pumps are summarized in Table 4.6.

Osmotic pressure can be used for controlled drug release. The osmostic pressure can pump out drug at a constant rate, as described below. An important consideration is that because the pumping principle is based on osmosis, pumping rate is unaffected by changes in experimental conditions. Hence, *in vitro* drug release rate is often consistent with the *in vivo* release profile.

Table 4.6 Semipermeable membranes and osmotic agents commonly used in osmotic pressure-activated implantable pumps

Semi-permeable membrane

Cellulose acetate derivatives
    Cellulose acetate, Plasticized cellulose triacetate, Cellulose acetate methyl carbamate, Cellulose acetate Ethyl carbamate, Cellulose acetate phthalate, Cellulose acetate succinate
Other polymers
    Poly(ethylene-vinyl acetate), Highly plasticized polyvinyl chloride, Polyesters of acrylic acid and methacrylic acid, Polyvinylalkyl ethers, Polymeric epoxide, Polystyrenes

Osmotic agents

Inorganic osmotic agents
    Sodium chloride, Sodium carbonate, Sodium sulphate, Calcium sulphate, Mono- and Di-basic potassium phosphate, Magnesium chloride, Magnesium sulphate, Lithium chloride
Organic osmotic agents
    Calcium lactate, Magnesium succinate, Tartaric acid, Acetamide, Choline chloride
Carbohydrates
    Glucose, Lactose, Mannitol, Sorbitol, Sucrose
Swelling hydrogels
    Sodium carbopol

4.6.1.1 Alzet miniosmotic pumps

The Alzet miniosmotic pump consists of (Figure 4.17):

- *Semipermeable membrane*: serves as the housing for the entire pump and allows only water molecules to migrate into the osmotic sleeve.
- *Osmotic chamber*: contains sufficient contents of an osmotic agent.
- *Reservoir wall*: a cylindrical cavity molded from a synthetic elastomer, which is easily deformable by gentle squeeze. The fexible reservoir wall is impermeable to water molecules.
- *Drug reservoir*: contains the drug in solution/suspension.
- *Flow moderator*: a stainless steel, open-ended tube with a plastic end-cap, which serves as a pathway for the exit of drug solution/suspension.

In this process, water crosses the outer semi-permeable membrane of the pump. The characteristics of the semipermeable membrane including permeability, pore size, and thickness are key factors determining the rate at which water molecules enter the osmotic sleeve. The water that is drawn across the semipermeable membrane causes the osmotic chamber to expand. This force compresses the flexible drug reservoir, discharging the drug solution through the flow moderator.

Figure 4.17 Cross-sectional view of the Alzet osmotic pump, showing the various structural components

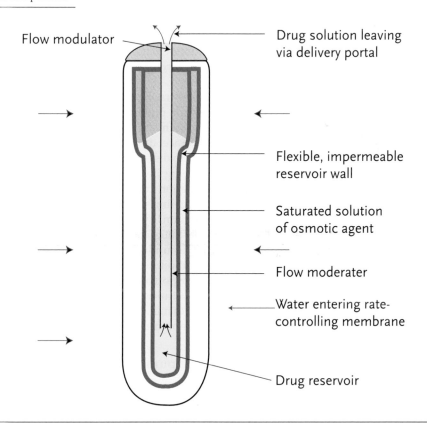

Flow modulator

Drug solution leaving via delivery portal

Flexible, impermeable reservoir wall

Saturated solution of osmotic agent

Flow moderater

Water entering rate-controlling membrane

Drug reservoir

The osmotic pump can deliver a drug at a constant rate, if:

- the osmotic sleeve contains a sufficient amount of an osmotic agent so that the osmotic pressure remains unchanged for the duration of implantation, and
- the drug reservoir contains a saturated solution of the drug (this ensures that the concentration of drug is constant).

The selection of a semipermeable membrane is equally important since its properties, including A, h and σ, affect drug permeation (see Equation 4.9).

Alzet miniosmotic pumps permit easy manipulation of drug release rate ($0.25 \sim 10$ $\mu l/hr$) over a wide range of periods (1 day to 4 weeks). Also, as stated above, *in vitro* drug release rate from the osmotic pumps is often consistent with the *in vivo* release profile. These advantages mean that the miniosmotic pumps are used widely in experimental animal studies, to investigate, for example, the effects of drug administration regimen upon dose-response curve, as well as pharmacokinetic and pharmacodynamic profiles and drug toxicity. Alzet osmotic kits are also available, which allow the localized administration of drugs to the central nervous system of animals.

4.6.1.2   *Duros implant pump*

The Duros implant pump is a modified version of the Alzet miniosmotic pump which additionally contains a piston to control drug flow, between the osmotic engine and the drug resorvoir (Figure 4.18).

Water is drawn in across the semipermeable membrane and results in the expansion of the osmotic chamber. This force is delivered via the piston to the drug reservoir, forcing the contents of the drug reservoir to exit through the orifice.

Duros technology is demonstrating considerable promise for the controlled delivery of peptides and proteins. For example, a single implantation of the Duros pump in animals resulted in constant-rate release of biologically active leuprolide acetate (a GnRH analog) for one year. The use of non-aqueous vehicles to disperse peptides/proteins in the reservoir compartment is also being investigated. Although peptides and proteins are prone to degradation in aqueous solutions, adverse physicochemical reactions are sometimes avoided by dispersing them in a nonaqueous dispersion medium. Typical nonaqueous vehicles used in the drug reservoir compartment of the Duros implantable pump include waxes that soften around body temperature, hydrogenated vegetable oils such as peanut oil, sesame oil and olive oil, silicone oil, fatty acid monoglycerides or polyols. In addition, suspending agents, such as hydroxypropyl cellulose, poly(vinyl pyrrolidone) and poly(acrylic acid) are added to minimize the sedimentation rate of proteins inside the reservoir compartment.

4.6.2   Mechanical implantable pumps

The advance in microelectronics in the 1970s provided the momentum to develop externally programmable implantable pump systems. Such

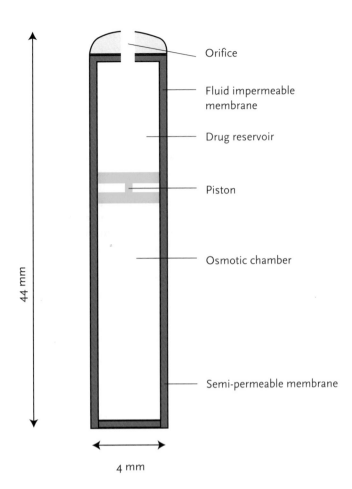

44 mm

4 mm

Figure 4.18 Cross-sectional view of the Duros implant, showing the various structural components

Orifice

Fluid impermeable membrane

Drug reservoir

Piston

Osmotic chamber

Semi-permeable membrane

pumps were finally developed in the early 1980s and they allow physicians and patients to *precisely control* the infusion rate of a drug. Thus externally programmable pumps can facilitate:

- zero-order drug release
- intermittent drug release.

Most implantable pumps are made of titanium which has proven records of excellent biocompatibility and long life. They are usually implanted intraperitoneally, in a pocket created in the abdominal wall of patients, under the subcutaneous fat layers, but above the muscular fascias. They are secured to the muscular fascia by suturing, which prevents pumps from flipping over or migrating in the pump pocket, thereby allowing patients to resume routine physical activities. Intraperitoneal insulin pump therapy is advantageous over a subcutaneous injection, as insulin infused into the peritoneal membrane surrounding abdominal organs is absorbed faster and more completely than via subcutaneous injection. Arterial or intraspinal delivery is also possible with a proper surgical procedure. A silicone rubber catheter is attached to the pumps, through which infusate is delivered to various body sites. The catheter is replaced if it becomes blocked, for example, by the deposition of infusate inside the lumen, fibrous tissue encapsulation or clotting at the tip.

4.6.2.1 SynchroMed implantable pump

The SynchroMed implantable pump was the first externally programmable implant pump to be introduced in the United States (in 1988). The major components are a miniature peristaltic pump, a drug reservoir (18 ml), a battery, an antenna, a microprocessor and a catheter through which infusate is delivered to a specific site.

The infusion rate of a drug solution can be programmed by a portable computer with specialized software which transmits instructions by radiotelemetry to the pump. The pump is driven by a step motor, controlled by signals from the micropocessor and is capable of delivering infusate at varying rates (0.004–0.9 ml/hr). The programmer provides the implantable pump with versatile delivery patterns, including a straight continuous-flow pattern or a more complex pattern that allows a varying dose at different times of the day to meet the patient's changing metabolic requirements.

The SynchroMed pump is approved for use in:

- chemotherapy (using floxuridine, doxorubicin, cisplatin, or methotrexate);
- the treatment of chronic, intractable cancer pain (using morphine sulfate);
- osteomyelitis treatment (using clindamycin);
- spasticity therapy (using the muscle relaxant, baclofen).

However, the SynchroMed pump is not suitable for the delivery of insulin. The pressure of the roller heads on the tubing in the peristaltic pump causes intensive shear stresses which lead to stability problems for labile peptides and proteins.

4.6.2.2 MiniMed implantable pump

In the MiniMed implantable pump, a piston pump drives insulin through the delivery catheter. A patented solenoid motor controls the piston movement, to aspirate insulin from the reservoir chamber into the piston chamber and then push it through the insulin delivery catheter.

A hand-held programmer can change the pumping rate to administer the desired insulin dose to the diabetic patient. Thus the pump can be responsive to the diabetic's fluctuating insulin needs. Many conventional insulin preparations are prone to denaturation when exposed to body fluids and temperature, or when agitated (see Section 1.6.1). The ensuing aggregation and precipitation may cause blockage of the catheter attached to the pump. However, the Minimed pump uses an insulin formulation, developed by Hoechst, which includes a small amount of Genapol (polyethylene glycol and polypropylene glycol), to increase the stability of the polypeptide.

4.6.2.3 Arrow implantable pump

The Arrow implantable pump is non-programmable and delivers infusate (2-deoxy-5-fluorouridine, morphine sulfate, baclofen, or heparinized saline) at 3 pre-set flow rates. The pump is divided into two chambers by accordion-like movable bellows. Infusate is placed in the inner drug reservoir chamber and Freon propellant in the outer chamber (Figure 4.19).

Drug delivery from this pump is powered by the Freon propellant. When the Arrow pump is implanted subcutaneously, it is warmed by the patient's body temperature so that the propellant-containing chamber expands and exerts pressure on the movable bellows. Infusate is thus forced out of the reservoir chamber to an attached catheter through a filter and flow restrictor. This mechanism allows the delivery of infusate at a fairly constant rate to surrounding tissues or blood vessels. It should be noted, however, that the vapour pressure exerted by the outer chamber can be affected by changes in altitude/elevation or body temperature.

The Infusaid pump is another fixed-rate implantable pump that shares many similar features, including the Freon pumping principle, with the Arrow pump.

4.7 CONCLUSIONS

Implantable devices possess many advantages for drug delivery. Many different types of system are available and technology is expanding rapidly. Indeed, there now exists bio-responsive implantable systems, and implants for gene therapy; such advances are described in Chapter 16 (New Generation Technologies). However, despite the striking advances in this field, implantable systems will always be limited by the invasive nature of this therapy.

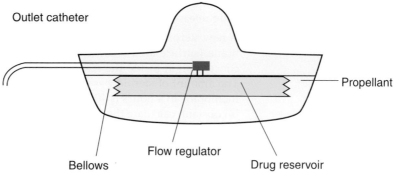

Figure 4.19 The cross-sectional view of the Arrow model 3000 implantable pump, showing the pumping mechanism

Outlet catheter

Propellant

Bellows

Flow regulator

Drug reservoir

4.8 FURTHER READING

Ogata, N., Kim, S.W., Feijen, J. and Okano T. (eds) (1996) *Advanced Biomaterials in Biomedical Engineering and Drug Delivery Systems.* Springer.

Chasin, M. and Langer, R. (eds) (1990) *Biodegradable Polymers as Drug Delivery Systems.* Marcel Dekker, New York.

Tsirita, T., Hayashi, T., Ishihara, K., Kataoka, K. and Kimura, Y. (eds) (1993) *Biomedical Applications of Polymeric Materials.* CRC Press, Boca Raton, Florida.

Chemical & Engineering News, June 9, 26–37 (1997).

Baker, R. (ed.) (1987) *Controlled Release of Biologically Active Agents.* John Wiley, New York.

Controlled Release of Polymeric Formulations, ACS Symposium Series 33 (1976).

Chien, Y.W. (ed.) (1992) *Novel Drug Delivery Systems,* 2nd edn. Marcel Dekker, New York.

Polymer-Based Drug Delivery to the Brain, *Science and Medicine,* 3:2–11 (1996).

Kost, J. (ed.) (1990) *Pulsed and Self-Regulated Drug Delivery.* CRC Press, Boca Raton, Florida.

Anderson, J.M. and Kim, S.W. (eds) (1984) *Recent Advances in Drug Delivery Systems.* Plenum Publishing, New York.

Hrushesky, W.J.M., Langer, R. and Theeuwes, F. (eds) (1991) Temporal Control of Drug Delivery. *Annals of the New York Science Academy,* Volume 618.

Kydonieus, A. (ed.) (1991) *Treatise on Controlled Drug Delivery: Fundamentals, Optimization, Application.* Marcel Dekker, New York.

4.9 SELF-ASSESSMENT QUESTIONS

1. A company is trying to develop a reservoir-type polymeric implant for the controlled release of estradiol for 3 months. Which techniques would you recommend to the company to increase the drug release rate?

2. A new steroidal drug is allowed to pass through a siloxane membrane (surface area = 23.64 cm^2, thickness = 0.85 cm). The drug concentration inside the reservoir compartment is 0.0004 g/cm^3. The amount of steroid passing through the reservoir through the membrane in 4 hours is 40 μg. Provided that the drug release rate is constant, calculate the flux (F) that is defined as the amount of a solute flowing through a membrane per unit time.*

3. The release rate of a drug from conventional non-degradable matrix-type polymeric implant usually decreases over time. Describe a technique that can be used to overcome this problem.

4. What is the main reason for developing a reservoir/matrix hybrid-type polymeric implant?

5. Which polymer is most extensively used as non-degradable non-porous membrane to develop reservoir-type polymeric implants?

6. Which of the following is/are an example(s) of non-biodegradable matrix-type implant? (a) Norplant (b) Compudose (c) Implanon and/or (d) Zoladex.

7. Which of the following products is made of a surface-eroding polymer? (a) Lupron Depot (b) Zoladex (c) Gliadel and/or (d) Vitrasert.

8. Which one of the following polymers undergoes homogeneous bulk erosion? (a) Poly(lactide-co-glycolide) (b) Poly[bis(p-carboxyphenoxy)propane:sebacic acid) (c) Poly(ortho esters) and/or (d) Poly(ethylene-vinyl acetate).

9. What is the principle that has been utilized in the development of the Alzet and the Duros implant pumps in which a drug solution or suspension is confined in a semi-permeable membrane that allows only water molecules to move through it?

10. The release rate (dM/dt) of a drug from an osmotic pump can be described as $C_d (dV/dt)$ where C_d is the drug solubility in its reservoir compartment. The effective surface area, permeability coefficient, thickness, and osmotic reflection coefficient of the semi-permeable membrane used for the pump are 3.0 cm^2, 0.7×10^{-4} cm^2/day, 500 μm, and 0.8, respectively. Initially, the pump has a reservoir compartment with a drug having C_d of 100 mg/ml, and the observed $\Delta \pi$ is 100 atm. If we change the reservoir medium and osmotic agent to increase C_d of the drug from 100 to 300 mg/ml and to increase $\Delta \pi$ from 100 to 300 atm, by how much will the release rate of the drug increase?*

---

* See Appendix for answer

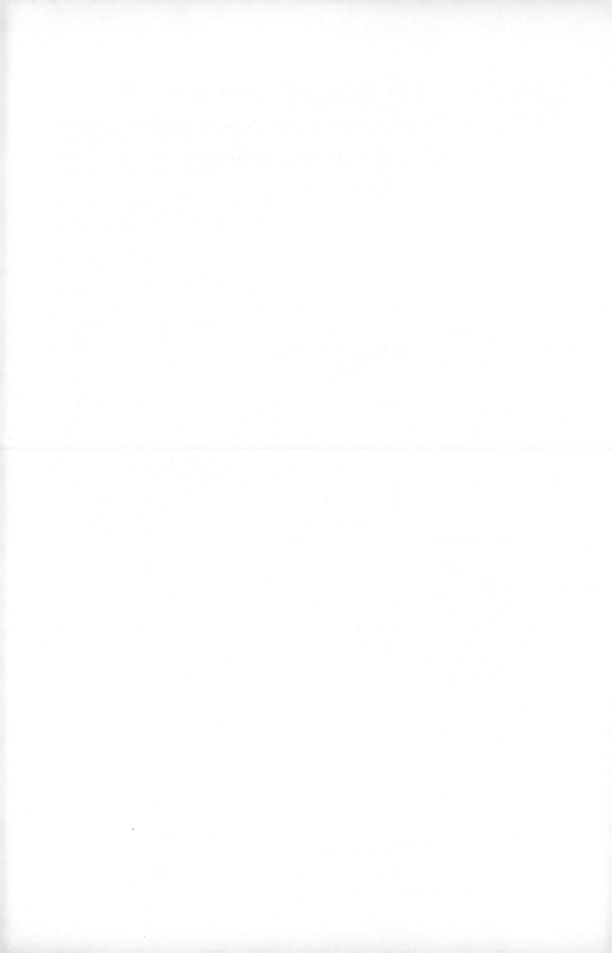

Drug Targeting Systems: Fundamentals and Applications to Parenteral Drug Delivery

Daan J.A. Crommelin, Wim E. Hennink and Gert Storm

OBJECTIVES

On completion of this chapter the reader should be able to:

- Describe different carrier systems and homing devices that are being used in drug targeting
- Describe physiological, anatomical and pathological hurdles encountered in developing drug targeting strategies
- Describe the different pharmaceutical problems encountered in the development of a targeted drug delivery system
- Discuss the pros and cons of a hypothetical carrier system/homing device/drug combination for a specific disease

5.1 INTRODUCTION

Routine parenteral administration by injection serves to deliver drugs to specific body tissues. The most important routes of injection of these sterile products are intramuscular (im), intravenous (iv) and subcutaneous (sc). Basic parenteral formulation involves the selection of appropriate bases (e.g. aqueous, oily and emulsions) to achieve the desired bioavailability following injection. The detailed description of these areas of pharmaceutics lie outside the remit of this text and the reader is refered to information provided in the further reading section of Chapter 1. This chapter focuses on advanced drug delivery and targeting systems administered via the parenteral route and serves to provide the reader with a basic understanding of the principal approaches to drug targeting.

5.1.1 Rationale for the development of parenteral drug delivery and targeting systems

As introduced in Chapter 1, there are many limitations associated with conventional drug therapy. An intravenously administered drug is subject to a number of pharmacokinetic processes *in vivo* which can decrease the drugs therapeutic index, including:

- *Distribution*: intravenously administered drugs distribute throughout the body and reach non-target organs and tissues, resulting in drug wastage and (possibly) toxic side-effects.
- *Metabolism*: the drug may be rapidly metabolized in the liver or other organs.
- *Excretion*: the drug may be cleared rapidly from the body through the kidney.

As a result of these processes, only a small fraction of the drug will reach the target tissue. Moreover, it may be cleared rapidly from this site and, therefore, not be available long enough to induce the desired effect. Reaching the target cell is often not the ultimate goal; in many cases the drug has to enter the target cell to reach an intracellular target site. Again, as discussed in Chapter 1, many drugs do not possess the required physicochemical properties to enter target cells; they may be too hydrophilic, too large or not transportable by the available active-transport systems.

Drug delivery and targeting systems (DDTS) aim to overcome the limitations of conventional drugs and thus improve drug performance. An ideal DDTS should:

- specifically target the drug to target cells or target tissue;
- keep the drug out of non-target organs, cells or tissue;
- ensure minimal drug leakage during transit to target;
- protect the associated drug from metabolism;
- protect the associated drug from premature clearance;
- retain the drug at the target site for the desired period of time;

- facilitate transport of the drug into the cell;
- deliver the drug to the appropriate intracellular target site;
- be biocompatible, biodegradable and non-antigenic.

In certain situations, some of these requirements may be inappropriate. For example, the drug may work outside the cell, thus cell penetration may not be necessary. In this chapter there are also examples mentioned of passive targeting approaches (see below), where the drug does not have to be specifically targeted to the cell or tissue.

The parenteral route of administration is associated with several major disadvantages (see Section 3.5.2). Parenteral administration is invasive and may require the intervention of trained medical professionals. Strict regulations for parenteral formulations govern their use and generally dictate that they are as simple as possible and the inclusion of excipients in the formulation is kept to an absolute minimum. Furthermore, developing a DDTS requires an enormous amount of R&D investment in terms of cost, effort and time, which can cause a significant delay in the development and marketing of a system and the final product will be relatively expensive. Parenteral DDTS must, therefore, offer real therapeutic advantages to justify their use. Table 5.1 lists a number of pharmacokinetic considerations to decide if the use of DDTS is indicated for a particular drug.

Drugs used in the treatment of diseases which are life threatening, or that dramatically affect the quality of life of the patient, are prime candidates for inclusion in a DDTS. Such drugs include those used in treatment of cancer, as well as life-threatening microbial, viral and fungal diseases. Chronic diseases such as arthritis can also be found on the priority list.

5.1.2 Generalized description of parenteral drug delivery and targeting systems (DDTS)

The technology used for targeted drug delivery with carrier systems differs from the technology to achieve prolonged release profiles for a drug. If prolonged release of a drug via the parenteral route is required, subcutaneous or intramuscular injection of a controlled-release system is the first option to consider. The relevant technology is already available and validated for many years.

Table 5.1 Pharmacokinetic considerations related to drug targeting	<ul><li>Drugs with high total clearance are good candidates for targeted delivery.</li><li>Carrier-mediated transport is suitable for response sites with a relatively small blood flow.</li><li>The higher the rate of elimination of free drug from either central or response compartments, the greater the need for targeted drug delivery; this also implies a higher input rate of the drug–carrier ccombination to maintain the therapeutic effect.</li><li>For maximizing the targeting effect, the release of drug from the carrier should be restricted to the response compartment.</li></ul>

Table 5.2
Components of a drug
delivery and targeting
system (DDTS)

DDTS Component	Purpose
The active moiety	To achieve the therapeutic effect
The carrier system, which can be either soluble or particulate	To effect a favorable distribution of the drug To protect the drug from metabolism To protect the drug from early clearance
A "homing device"*	To specifically target the drug to the target cells or target tissue

*not necessary when "passive" targeting approaches are used

Examples include:

- the long, medium and short acting insulin formulations, prepared by crystal manipulation or physical complex-formation;
- depot injections (aqueous suspensions, oily injections) of contraceptives and psychotropic drugs;
- polymeric implants, for example Zoladex (see Chapter 4);
- infusion pumps (see Chapter 4).

In contrast, a DDTS generally comprises three functionally specific units, as shown in Table 5.2.

A "homing device" is a target-specific recognition moiety. For example, galactose receptors are present on liver parenchymal cells, thus the inclusion of galactose residues on a drug carrier can target the carrier to these cells. A number of different target-specific recognition moieties are available and discussed further below. However, an important point to note here is that target-specific recognition moieties are not the idealized "magic bullets", capable of selectively directing the drug to the appropriate target and ignoring all other non-target sites. Although the homing device can increase the *specificity* of the drug for its target site, the process must rely on the (random) encounter of the homing device with its appropriate receptor, during its circulation lifetime.

The carrier systems that are presently on the market or under development can be classified in two groups on the basis of size:

- soluble macromolecular carriers;
- particulate carrier systems.

This classification is sometimes rather arbitrary, as some soluble carriers are large enough to enter the colloidal size range. Another useful distinction is that with macromolecular carrier systems the drug is *covalently attached* to the carrier and has to be released through a chemical reaction. In contrast, with colloidal carriers, the drug is generally *physically associated* and does not need a chemical reaction to be

Table 5.3 Particulate drug carrier systems	Particulate Carriers	Particulate Matrix Material	Typical Size of Particulate
	Liposomes	Phospholipids	0.03–30 μm
	Micelles	PEG/polypeptides	0.03 μm
	Nanoparticles	Poly(alkylcyano-acrylates)	0.1–1 μm
	Microspheres	Poly(lactide-co-glycolide)	
		Starch	
		Albumin	0.2–150 μm
	Lipoproteins	Lipids/proteins	0.01–0.09 μm

released. Here, diffusion barriers comprise the major hurdles to avoid premature release.

Soluble carriers include antibodies and soluble synthetic polymers such as poly(hydroxypropyl methacrylate), poly(lysine), poly(aspartic acid), poly(vinylpyrrolidone), poly(N-vinyl-2-pyrrolidone-co-vinyl-lamide) and poly (styrene co-maleic acid/anhydride).

Many particulate carriers have been designed for drug delivery and targeting purposes for intravenous administration (Table 5.3). They usually share three characteristics:

- Their size range: minimum size is approximately 0.02 μm; the maximum size relevant for drug targeting is approximately 10–30 μm.
- They are all biodegradable.
- The drug is physically associated with the carrier and, in general, drug release kinetics are controlled either by diffusional transport or matrix degradation.

A full appreciation of the respective advantages and disadvantages of soluble and particulate carriers cannot be gained without first considering the anatomical, physiological and pathological considerations described below.

5.1.3 Anatomical, physiological and pathological considerations

The body is highly compartmentalized and should not be considered as a large pool without internal barriers for transport. The degree of body-compartmentalization, or in other words, the ability of a macromolecule or particulate to move around, depends on its physicochemical properties, in particular its:

- molecular weight/size;
- charge;
- surface hydrophobicity;
- the presence of homing devices for interaction with surface receptors.

The smaller the size, the easier a molecule can passively move from one compartment to another. An important question is whether and

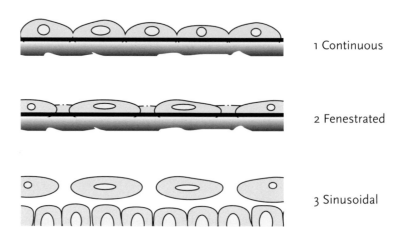

Figure 5.1 Schematic illustration of the structure of the wall of different classes of blood capillaries.
(1) Continuous capillary (as found in the general circulation). The endothelium is continuous with tight junctions between adjacent endothelial cells. The subendothelial basement membrane is also continuous.
(2) Fenestrated capillary (as found in exocrine glands and the pancreas). The endothelium exhibits a series of fenestrae which are sealed by a membranous diaphragm. The subendothelial basement membrane is continuous.
(3) Discontinuous (sinusoidal) capillary (as found in the liver, spleen and bone marrow). The overlying endothelium contains numerous gaps of varying size. The subendothelial basement is either absent (liver) or present as a fragmented interrupted structure (spleen, bone marrow)

1 Continuous

2 Fenestrated

3 Sinusoidal

where the carriers can pass through the endothelial lining of the blood circulation. Under physiological conditions, the situation exists as depicted in Figure 5.1. The endothelial lining is continuous in most parts of the body and the endothelial cells are positioned on a basal membrane. The exact characteristics of this barrier are still under investigation, but it is clear that particulate systems greater than 10 nm cannot pass this barrier through pores. Only in the sinusoidal capillaries of the liver, spleen and bone marrow can "pores" (so-called fenestrae) be found. In the lining of these capillaries the basal membrane is fragmented or even completely missing.

This anatomical information has important implications for the rational design of targeted carrier systems. If a therapeutic target is located outside the blood circulation and if normal anatomical conditions exist around the target site, a small-sized macromolecular carrier must be selected, in order to achieve sufficient "escaping tendency" from the blood circulation. Particulate carriers will generally fail to extravasate, simply because there is no possibility for endothelium penetration.

In addition to the issue of endothelial permeability, the effect of macrophages in direct contact with the blood circulation (e.g. Kupffer cells in the liver) on the disposition of carrier systems must be considered. Unless precautions are taken, particulate carrier systems are readily phagocytosed by these macrophages and tend to accumulate in these cells. Phagocytic uptake by the cells of the mononuclear phagocyte systems (MPS; also sometimes known as the reticuloendothelial system, RES) has been described in Chapter 1 (Section 1.3.3.2). The MPS comprises both:

- *fixed cells*: macrophages in liver (also known as Kuppfer cells), spleen, lung, bone marrow and lymph nodes, and
- *mobile cells*: blood monocytes and tissue macrophages

and constitutes an important part of the body's immune system; its functions include:

- the removal and destruction of bacteria;
- the removal and metabolism of denatured proteins;
- antigen processing and presentation;

- storage of inert colloids;
- assisting in cellular toxicity.

The cells of the MPS are always on the alert to phagocytose "foreign body-like material". Thus as well as being responsible for the removal of particulate antigens such as microbes, other foreign particulates, such as microspheres, liposomes and other particulate carriers, are also susceptible to MPS clearance.

Clearance kinetics by the MPS are highly dependent on the physico-chemical properties of the particulate, in particular on particulate size, charge and surface hydrophobicity:

Particle size

Particulates in the size range of 0.1–7 μm tend to be cleared by the MPS, localizing predominantly in the Kuppfer cells of the liver.

Particle charge

For liposomes, it has been shown that negatively charged vesicles tend to be removed relatively rapidly from the circulation whereas neutral vesicles tend to remain in the circulation for longer periods.

Surface hydrophobicity

Hydrophobic particles are immediately recognized as "foreign" and are generally rapidly covered by plasma proteins known to function as opsonins, which facilitate phagocytosis. The extent and pattern of opsonin adsorption depends highly on surface characteristics such as charge and hydrophilicity. Strategies to decrease MPS clearance, by increasing the hydrophilicity of the particle surface, are described below.

A further consideration is that under *pathological* conditions, endothelium exhibits modified characteristics. In general, the permeability is enhanced; this phenomenon is called the enhanced permeability and retention (EPR) effect. For example, the endothelial fenestrations in inflammation sites can be as large as 0.2 μm. Also, in tumor tissue, even larger fenestrations can be found. However, in this case, the pattern is not uniform and depends on the tumor type and stage of development. Even within one tumor, highly permeable sites can be identified in close proximity to sites of low permeability. Also, necrotic tissue affects tumor permeability. Because of the EPR effect, particles in the colloidal size range can enter tumor tissue, or sites of inflammation. This phenomenon can be exploited for drug delivery.

5.1.4 Passive and active targeting

5.1.4.1 *Passive targeting*

Passive targeting exploits the "natural" (passive) distribution pattern of a drug carrier *in vivo* and no homing device is attached to the carrier. For example, as described above, particulate carriers tend to be phago-cytosed by cells of the MPS. Consequently, the major organs of accumulation are the liver and the spleen, both in terms of total uptake and uptake per gram of tissue. An abundance of MPS macrophages and a rich blood supply are the primary reasons for the preponderance of particles in these sites. After phagocytosis, the carrier and the associated drug are transported to lysosomes and the drug is released upon disintegration of the carrier in this cellular compartment. This passive targeting to the MPS (and particularly to the liver) is advantageous in a number of situations, including:

- the treament of macrophage-associated microbial, viral or bacterial diseases (e.g. leishmaniasis);
- the treatment of certain lysosomal enzyme deficiencies;
- the immunopotentiation of vaccines;
- the activation of macrophages, by loading the carrier system with macrophage-activating agents such as interferon γ, to fight infections or tumors.

If the drug is not broken down by the lytic enzymes of the lysosomes, it may be released in its active form from the lysosomal compartment into the cytoplasm and may even escape from the phagocyte, so causing a prolonged release systemic effect. Figure 5.2 depicts this "macrophage mediated release of drugs".

Technology is available to reduce the tendency of macrophages to rapidly phagocytose colloidal drug carrier complexes. The process of "steric stabilization" involves the coating of the delivery system with synthetic or biological materials, which make it energetically unfavorable for other macromolecules to approach. A standard approach is to graft hydrophilic, flexible poly(ethylene glycol) (PEG) chains to the surface of the particulate carrier.

This repulsive steric layer reduces the adsorption of opsonins and consequently slows down phagocytosis. The net effect of PEG attach-

Figure 5.2 Schematic representation of the concept of "macrophage mediated controlled release of drugs"

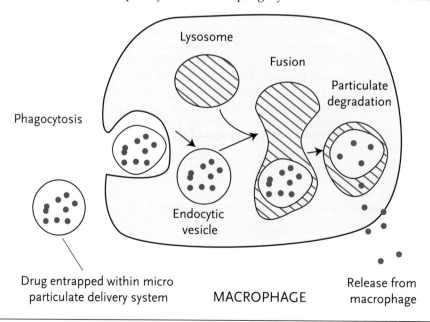

ment is that macrophage/liver uptake of the particles is delayed or reduced, thus increasing the circulation time.[1]

Another example of passive targeting is the exploitation of the EPR effect to deliver a drug to a site of inflammation, or a tumor site. This form of passive targeting, also called "selective targeting", requires two conditions to be satisfied:

- The size of the drug-carrier system should exceed the size of normal endothelial fenestrations to ensure that the carrier system only crosses inflamed endothelium; a certain size range is preferred as there is an upper limit to the endothelial fenestration dimensions under pathological conditions.
- The circulation time in the blood compartment should be long enough to allow the carrier systems to "escape" from circulation at the pathological site.

As described above, the circulation time of a particulate carrier in the blood can be prolonged using "stealth" technology to enhance particle hydrophilicity. If the circulation time is sufficiently prolonged and the particle size does not exceed, say, 0.2 μm, then accumulation at tumor and inflammation sites (EPR-effect) can be observed.

In addition to stealth strategies, other more specific approaches include the removal of undesired ligands on the DDTS which interact with specific receptors on non-target cells.

5.1.4.2 *Active targeting*

In active targeting strategies a homing device is attached to the carrier system, to effect delivery to a specific cell, tissue or organ. Thus delivery systems designed for active targeting are usually composed of three parts: the carrier, the homing device and the drug (Table 5.1). Preferably, the homing device is covalently attached to the carrier, although successful targeting attempts of non-covalently attached homing device–carrier combinations have also been described.

Target sites for active targeting strategies can differ widely. A list of cell-specific receptors and their corresponding ligands, expressed under physiological conditions, is presented in Table 5.4. Thus, for example, galactose can be used to target a drug carrier to parenchymal liver cells, etc. In the future, it is expected that the rapidly growing field of genomics will be used to identify specific receptors for targeting purposes (see Chapter 15).

Other receptors may become available under pathological conditions. Such receptors include:

- antigenic sites on pathogens (bacteria, viruses, parasites);
- infected host cells expressing specific antigenic structures;
- tumor-associated antigens (TAAs) (i.e. antigenic structures specifically occurring at the surface of tumor cells);

---

[1] Sterically stabilized liposomes are often described as "stealth" carriers (Stealth is a registered trade name of Sequus Inc.), so called because their ability to evade recognition by the MPS was deemed analogous to the ability of stealth bombers to avoid radar detection.

Table 5.4 Examples of cell-specific ligands/carriers *in vivo*	Cell	Cell-specific ligands/carriers
	Parenchymal liver cells	Galactose, polymeric IgA, cholesterol ester-VLDL*, LDL**
	Kupffer cells	Mannose-fucose, galactose (particles), (oxidized) LDL
	Liver endothelial cells	Mannose, acetylated LDL
	Leucocytes	Chemotactic peptide, complement C3b

* VLDL = very low density lipoproteins; ** LDL = low density lipoproteins

- substances such as fibrin in blood clots (i.e. potential ligands for targeting of fibrinolytics).

Sometimes it is necessary for the carrier-bound drug to reach all target cells to be clinically successful, as is the case with antitumor therapy. So-called "bystander" effects can help to achieve fully effective therapy. Bystander effects occur when the targeted drug carrier reaches its target site, and released drug molecules also act on surrounding non-target cells. In other cases not all target cells have to be reached, as is the case, for example, for targeted gene delivery for the local production of a therapeutic protein.

Antibodies raised against a selected receptor are extensively used as homing devices. Modern molecular biotechnology permits the production of large amounts of tailor-made material. The schematic structure of IgG antibodies (150 kD) is given in Figure 5.3. The antigen

Figure 5.3 Molecular structure of IgG, Fab and single chain antibody

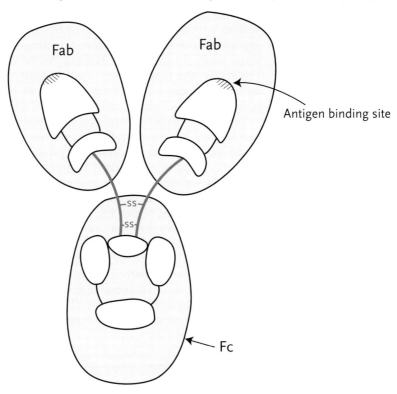

binding site of IgG molecules represents the homing part, which specifically interacts with the target (cells, pathogens, tissue). These antigen binding sites are located at both tips of the Y-shaped molecules. The sites that are responsible for the pharmacological effects of IgG, such as complement activation and macrophage interaction, are located at the stem part of the Y. The rest of the molecule forms the connection between the homing device and the pharmacologically active sites and also contributes to the long blood circulation characteristics of the IgG molecule, which has an elimination half-life much greater than 24 h.

Often, the full antibody molecule (Mw 150 kD) is not utilized for targeting, but the antigen binding domain carrying the Fab (Mw 50 kD) fragment, or even smaller fragments (single chain antibodies, Mw 25 kD) can be used. The present generation of murine monoclonal antibodies is now being replaced by humanized or human antibodies. Mouse-derived antibodies produced via the hybridoma technology can induce human anti-mouse antibodies (HAMA) in the patient. In multiple injection schemes this HAMA reaction can cause neutralization of the homing capacity of the antibody and can also cause anaphylactic reactions. However, although humanized and human antibodies do not induce HAMA, they can still raise anti-idiotypic antibodies against the binding site structure, which can also interfere with the homing performance.

Antibodies have received most attention as potential homing devices, but other potential candidates are emerging, in the cytokine and the growth hormone family and, finally, among the adhesion molecules that play a role in the homing of inflammatory cells to inflammation sites.

5.2 SOLUBLE CARRIERS FOR TARGETED DRUG DELIVERY

As described above, the major advantage of soluble carriers over particulate carriers is their greater ability to extravasate. Active targeting strategies for soluble carriers include attaching rather simple homing devices such as galactose, for targeting to liver parenchymal cells (see Table 5.4); alternatively, more complicated structures, such as antibodies, or antibody fragments (Fab or single chain antibodies) can be used as homing devices.

However, a number of disadvantages are also associated with the use of soluble carriers:

- Limited drug loading capacity: poor stoichiometry of drug to carrier limits the mass transport mediated by the drug carrier.
- The drug is covalently bound to the carrier: this can mask the active site of the drug and the conjugation reaction may damage a labile drug moiety.
- The carrier confers limited protection on the drug moiety.

A number of soluble carrier systems are described in detail below.

5.2.1 Monoclonal antibodies

Monoclonal antibodies (MAb) or MAb fragments have been described above as homing devices for soluble and particulate carriers; however, they can also be used in their own right as soluble carriers. The first marketed (1986) MAb for therapeutic use was the anti-CD3 antibody OKT3, for the prevention of rejection of kidney transplants. More recently, MAb for the treatment of post angioplasty complications (ReoPro) and for the treatment of colorectal cancers (Panorex) have been introduced.

MAb against tumor-associated antigens have been developed to assist in tumor imaging. The MAb is conjugated with a diagnostic imaging agent; commercial products include:

- Oncoscint CR/OV, for the imaging of colorectal cancer;
- Prostascint, for prostate cancer;
- CeaScan, for a number of tumors;
- Myoscint, for use in cardiac imaging.

MAb as drug delivery and targeting systems *per se* are limited because of the poor loading efficiency: only a limited number of drug molecules can bind to an antibody molecule. In order to increase the efficiency of MAb targeting, they can be used in conjunction with drug-loaded particulate carriers. In this case, a relatively high degree of drug loading can be achieved within the particulate carrier and the MAb, located on the surface of the particles, is used for targeting purposes. Further strategies include the use of antibody-directed enzyme prodrug therapy (ADEPT), which is described in Chapter 16, and the use of immunotoxins and bispecific antibodies, described below.

5.2.1.1 *Immunotoxins*

Immunotoxins comprise conjugates of:

- an MAb or MAb fragment, which acts as a targeted carrier;
- a toxin or toxin fragment, which acts as the pharmacologically active component.

The primary clinical targets of immunotoxins are tumors, based on the principle that the MAb will target the toxin to the tumor cells and the highly toxic moiety will then kill the cancer cells. Examples of toxins are ricin, diphtheria toxin and abrin, which are all glycoproteins. Their toxicity is based on their ability to block protein synthesis at the ribosomal protein assembly site. They are normally extremely toxic and not suitable for therapeutic purposes because they induce liver and vascular toxicity, even at low dose levels.

Ricin toxin consists of two protein moieties connected by a disulphide bridge. Chain A (Mw 32 kD) blocks the ribosomal activity, and chain B (Mw 34 kD) is responsible for cell entry of the A chain.

Chain A loses its toxicity when the B chain is removed. In ricin immunotoxins, the MAb replaces the B chain function and takes the responsibility for both the target cell specificity and cell entry of the A chain. Ricin immunotoxins using the anti-CD5 antibody (a marker on

T cells and some B cells) have been investigated in T and B cell lymphomas; ricin immunotoxins using the anti-CD19 antibody (a B lymphocyte marker) have been investigated in non-Hodgkin's lymphoma.

Unfortunately, studies completed so far show that the present generation of immunotoxins lack specificity and are also immunogenic; a major fraction still ends up in the liver and causes toxicity, and severe side-effects in the kidney and the GI tract have also been described. Attempts are being made to reduce liver uptake, by blocking or removing certain ligands on the ricin molecule which recognize receptors on liver parenchymal cells.

5.2.1.2 *Bispecific antibodies*

Bispecific antibodies are manufactured from two separate antibodies to create a molecule with two different binding sites. One binding site links the MAb to the target cell. The other site is chosen to bring T-lymphocytes or natural killer (NK) cells in close contact with the target site, in order to exert a pharmacological effect, for example to kill the target cell. This approach is now in early stage clinical trials.

5.2.2 Soluble polymeric carriers

Over the years, different soluble polymeric systems have been developed to improve drug performance (see Section 5.1.2). Here again, the emphasis is on the improvement in drug disposition conferred by the carrier and homing device, as well as the protection offered by the system against premature inactivation. The strategy, as shown in Figure 5.4, involves the use of a soluble macromolecule, the molecular weight of which ensures access to the target tissue. The drug moiety can be bound via either a direct linkage, or via a short chain "spacer". The spacer overcomes problems associated with the shielding of the drug moiety by the polymer backbone. The spacer allows greater exposure of the drug to the biological milieu thereby facilitating drug release. A targeting moiety, which can be either an integral part of the

Figure 5.4
Components of a soluble macromolecular site-specific delivery system

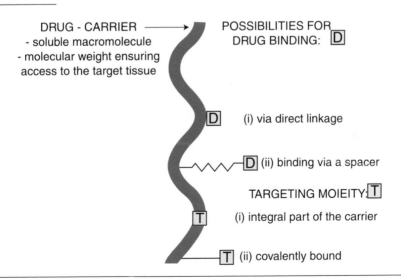

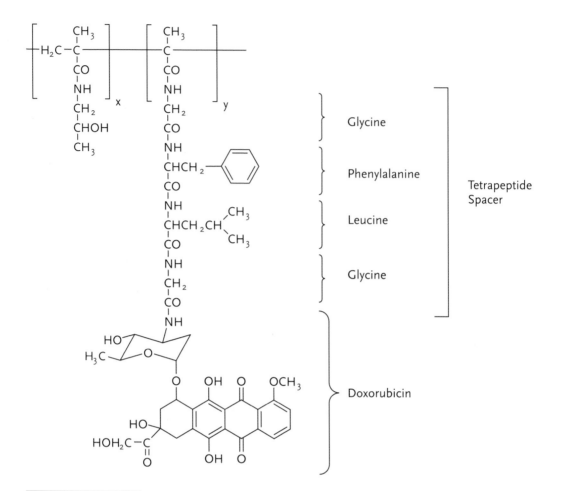

Figure 5.5 Chemical structure of a doxorubicin-N-(2-hydroxypropyl) methacrylamide (HPMA) copolymer conjugate

polymer backbone or covalently bound, may also be incorporated into the system.

A crucial feature of such carrier systems is their solubility, which enables them to be taken up into target cells by the process of pinocytosis (which has been described in Section 1.3.3.2). The intact carrier enters the target cell through pinocytotic capture. Through an endosomal sorting step, the carrier reaches the lysosomes where it is exposed to the actions of a battery of degradative enzymes. The drug-carrier linkage is designed to be cleaved by these enzymes, liberating free, active drug that can leave the lysosome by passage through its membrane, reaching the cytoplasm and other parts of the cell. Intra-lysosomal release of the drug from the carrier can also be achieved by making the drug-carrier linkage acid-labile, as the lysosomal interior has a pH of approximately 4.5–5.5.

5.2.2.1 HPMA derivatives

Poly(N-(2-hydroxypropyl)methacrylamide) (pHPMA) has been investigated as a soluble macromolecular carrier system, using doxorubicin as the active drug (Figure 5.5).

The bulk of the conjugate consists of unmodified HPMA units (x in Figure 5.5) which comprise about 90% of the carrier while the remaining units (y) are derivatized with doxorubicin. A tetrapeptide spacer (sequence Gly-Phe-Leu-Gly) connecting doxorubicin to the HPMA units proved to be cleavable by lysosomal thiol proteinases. Enzymatic cleavage breaks the peptide bond between the terminal glycogen and the daunosamine ring, liberating free doxorubicin, which can diffuse to the cytoplasm and nucleus where it (presumably) exerts its action.

Targeting moieties can also be incorporated into this delivery system. Targeting systems that have been investigated include:

- *galactose*: for targeting to parenchymal liver cells;
- *melanocyte-stimulating growth factor*: for targeting to melanocytes;
- *monoclonal antibodies*: for targeting to tumors.

Interestingly, the doxorubicin-polymer conjugate alone, without a homing device, showed an enhanced therapeutic index in animal models and considerable accumulation of the drug in tumor tissue. The EPR effect, as discussed above, is held responsible for this phenomenon. After optimizing conjugate performance in terms of doxorubicin "pay load" and desired molecular weight range of the polymer backbone, clinical grade material is now available and clinical trials are in progress to evaluate the potential of this concept.

5.2.2.2 SMANCS

The cytotoxic neocarzinostatin (NCS) is a small protein (Mw 12 kD) associated with a low molecular weight chromophore. NCS is rapidly cleared by the kidney and its cytotoxicity is non-cell specific. To modify its disposition, two poly(styrene-co-maleic acid anhydride) copolymers (Mw 1,500) have been coupled to one molecule of NCS, to give styrene-maleic-anhydride-neocarcinostatin (SMANCS) systems.

SMANCS has been shown to retain nearly all the *in vitro* activity of NCS, with much improved pharmacokinetic properties. Tumor uptake has been shown to increase in animal models, presumably by the EPR effect. Clinical successes have been reported with SMANCS in Lipiodol (a lymphographic vehicle) after intra-arterial administration in patients with unresectable hepatocellular carcinomas.

5.3 PARTICULATE CARRIERS FOR DRUG TARGETING

Advantages of particulate carriers include:

- the high drug loading that is possible with these systems;
- the drug does not have to be chemically attached to the carrier;
- a considerable degree of protection may be conferred on drug molecules encapsulated within the carrier.

However, a major limitation of these systems is their inability to cross intact endothelial barriers and leave the general circulation. In general, microparticulate carriers are phagocytosed by the macrophages of the

MPS, thereby rapidly localizing predominantly in the liver and spleen. However, sterically stabilized particulate carriers have extended circulation times and can remain in the blood, either acting as circulating drug reservoirs, or they may slowly escape from the blood pool at pathological sites with increased vascular permeability.

Intravenously administered particles with dimensions exceeding 7 μm (the diameter of the smallest capillaries) will be filtered by the first capillary bed they encounter, usually the lungs, leading to embolism. Intra-arterially administered particles with dimensions exceeding 7 μm will be trapped in the closest organ located upstream; for example, administration into the mesenteric artery leads to entrapment in the gut, into the renal artery leads to entrapment in the kidney etc. This approach is under investigation to improve the treatment of diseases in the liver.

Active targeting strategies for particulate systems are similar to those discussed for soluble macromolecular systems (see Table 5.4 and Section 5.2.1 on antibodies).

5.3.1 Liposomes

Liposomes are vesicular structures based on one or more lipid bilayer(s) encapsulating an aqueous core (Figure 5.6). The lipid molecules are usually phospholipids, amphipathic moieties with a hydrophilic head group and two hydrophobic chains ("tails"). Such moieties spontaneously orientate in water to give the most thermodynamically stable conformation, in which the hydrophilic head-group faces out into the aqueous environment and the lipidic chains orientate inwards avoiding the water phase; this gives rise to bilayer structures. In order to reduce exposure at the edges, the bilayers self-close into

Figure 5.6 Schematic illustration of a multilamellar liposome

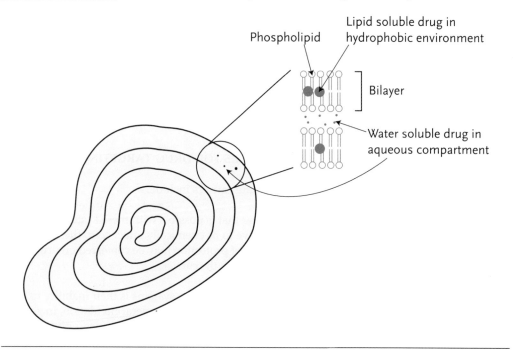

one or more concentric compartments around a central discrete aqueous phase. Dependent on the preparation protocol used, liposome diameters can vary between 0.02 and 20 μm. In general, they can be multilamellar or unilamellar; i.e. a multitude of concentrically orientated bilayers surrounds the aqueous core, or only one bilayer surrounds an aqueous core, respectively. However, other structures have also been described.

If multilamellar structures are formed, water is present in the core of the liposome, and also entrapped between the bilayers. Depending on the physico-chemical nature of the drug, it can either:

- be captured in the encapsulated aqueous phase (i.e. the aqueous core and the aqueous compartments between the bilayers (hydrophilic drugs)),
- interact with the bilayer surface (e.g. through electrostatic interactions), or
- be taken up in the bilayer structure (lipophilic drugs).

Thus liposomes can serve as carriers for both water-soluble and lipid-soluble drugs. The liposomal encapsulation of a wide variety of drugs, including antitumor and antimicrobial agents, chelating agents, peptides, proteins and genetic material have all been described.

Bilayer composition can be almost infinitely varied by choice of the constituent lipids. Phosphatidylcholine (PC), a neutral phospholipid, has emerged as the major lipid component used in the preparation of pharmaceutical liposomes. Phosphatidylglycerol and phosphatidylethanolamine are also widely used. Liposomal bilayers may also accommodate sterols, glycolipids, organic acids and bases, hydrophilic polymers, antibodies and other agents, depending on the type of vesicle required.

The rigidity and permeability of the bilayer strongly depend on the type and quality of lipids used. The alkyl-chain length and degree of unsaturation play a major role For example, a C18 saturated alkyl chain produces rigid bilayers with low permeability at room temperature. The presence of cholesterol also tends to rigidify the bilayers. Such systems are more stable and can retain the entrapped drug for relatively longer periods, whereas more "fluid" bilayer systems can be prepared if a more rapid release is required.

Liposomes can be classified on the basis of their composition and *in vivo* applications:

- *Conventional liposomes*, which are neutral or negatively charged, are generally used for passive targeting to the cells of the MPS.
- *Sterically stabilized ("stealth") liposomes*, which carry hydrophilic coatings, are used to obtain prolonged circulation times.
- *Immunoliposomes* ("antibody-targeted"), which can be either conventional or sterically stabilized, are used for active-targeting purposes.
- *Cationic liposomes*, which are positively charged, are used for the delivery of genetic material.

As phospholipid bilayers form spontaneously when water is added, the important challenge in liposome preparation is not the assembly of simple bilayers (which happens automatically), but in causing the bilayers to form stable vesicles of the desired size, structure and physicochemical properties, with a high drug encapsulation efficiency. There are many different approaches to the preparation of liposomes; however, they all have in common that they are based on the hydration of lipids:

Liposomes represent highly versatile drug carriers, offering almost infinite possibilities to alter structural and physicochemical characteristics. This feature of versatility enables the formulation scientist to modify liposomal behaviour *in vivo* and to tailor liposomal formulations to specific therapeutic needs. It has taken two decades to develop the liposome carrier concept to a pharmaceutical product level, but commercial preparations are now available in important disease areas and many more formulations are currently undergoing clinical trials. Examples of the different applications and commercial products of various types of liposomal systems are given below.

5.3.1.1 *Conventional liposomes*

These can be defined as liposomes that are typically composed of only phospholipids (neutral and/or negatively charged) and/or cholesterol. Most of the early work on liposomes as a drug-carrier system employed this liposomal type. These systems are rapidly taken up by the phagocytic cells of the MPS, localizing predominantly in the liver and spleen, and are therefore used when targeting to the MPS is the therapeutic goal (see Section 5.1.4.1). Conventional liposomes have also been used for antigen delivery and a liposomal hepatitis-A vaccine has received marketing approval in Switzerland.

A commercial product based on conventional liposomes has been introduced for the parenteral delivery of the anti-fungal drug, amphotericin B, which is poorly tolerated in conventional formulations. AmBisome, a liposomal formulation of amphotericin B, comprises SUV of diameter 50–100 nm. Two other lipid-based formulations of amphotericin B have also recently been commercially introduced:

- Abelcet consists of ribbon-like structures having a diameter in the 2–5 μm range.
- Amphocil comprises a colloidal dispersion of disk-shaped particles with a diameter of 122 nm and a thickness of 4 nm.

In spite of the large differences in structural features (a further example of "liposomal" versatility), all formulations have been shown to greatly reduce the toxicity of amphotericin B, allowing higher doses to be given and thereby improving clinical efficacy.

5.3.1.2 *Long-circulating liposomes*

At present, the most popular way to produce long-circulating liposomes is to covalently attach the hydrophilic polymer, polyethylene glycol, to the liposome bilayers. As discussed in Section 5.1.4, the highly hydrated PEG groups create a steric barrier against interactions

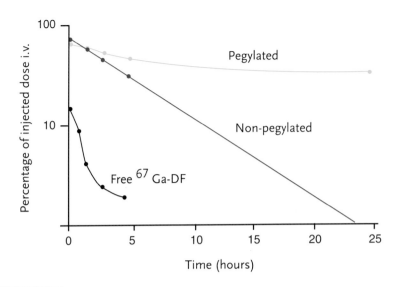

Figure 5.7
Comparison of the
blood levels of free
^{67}Ga-DF (gallium-
desferal), with ^{67}Ga-DF
encapsulated in
poly(ethylene glycol)
stabilized liposomes
and non-stabilized
liposomes upon iv
administration in rats.
From Woodle, M. *et al.*
(1990) Improved long
circulating (Stealth)
liposomes using
synthetic lipids. *Proc.
Int. Symp. Control. Rel.
Bioactive Mater.* **17**:
77–78

with molecular and cellular components in the biological environment. Figure 5.7 shows how "PEGylation" of liposomes can extend their blood circulation profile.

Long circulating liposomes can exploit the EPR effect to accumulate at sites where pathological reactions occur. For example, the commercial product Doxil (marketed as Caelyx in Europe) consists of small-sized PEGylated liposomes, encapsulating the cytostatic doxorubicin. The resulting long circulation times and small size of the vesicles facilitate their accumulation in tumor tissue via the EPR effect.

DaunoXome liposomes are also long circulating liposomes, in this case encapsulating the cytostatic daunorubicin. Although a non-stealth system, long circulation times are attained by using a particularly rigid bilayer composition, in combination with a relatively small liposome size.

The encapsulation of these anthracycline cytostatics in liposomes effects a modified biodistribution of the drug; the drug is distributed away from the heart, where it can exert considerable toxic effects, and is preferentially taken up by solid tumor tissue.

5.3.1.3 Immunoliposomes

Immunoliposomes have specific antibodies or antibody fragments on their surface to enhance target site binding. The primary focus of their use has been in the targeted delivery of anticancer agents.

Long-circulating immunoliposomes can also be prepared (see Figure 5.8). The antibody can be coupled directly to the liposomal surface, however the PEG chains may provide steric hindrance to antigen binding. Alternatively, a bi-functional PEG linker can be used, to couple liposomes to one end of PEG chains and antibodies to the other end of these chains. Steric hindrance is not a problem in the latter approach.

5.3.1.4 Cationic liposomes

Cationic liposomes are a relatively new development in liposomal therapeutics, which demonstrate considerable potential for improving

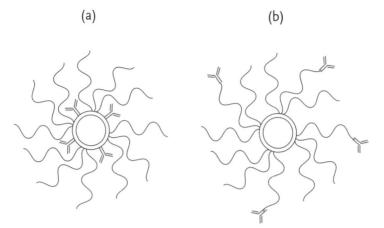

(a)   (b)

Figure 5.8
Immobilization of
antibody on PEG-
liposomes by (a) direct
coupling to the
liposome surface and
(b) coupling to the
terminal ends of the
PEG chains

the delivery of genetic material. The cationic lipid components of the
liposomes interact with, and neutralize, negatively charged DNA,
thereby condensing the DNA into a more compact structure.
Depending on the preparation method used, the complex may not be a
simple aggregate, but an intricate structure in which the condensed
DNA is surrounded by a lipid bilayer. These systems are discussed
further in Chapter 14.

5.3.2 Polymeric micelles

When amphipathic molecules (i.e. molecules with distinct hydrophilic
and hydrophobic sections) are dispersed in water, association colloids
or micelles are formed above a certain critical concentration, the critical micelle concentration (CMC). The stability of these micelles
depends on the nature of the hydrophilic and hydrophobic effects. A
high CMC value indicates rapid exchange of the constitutive components and a fast disintegration of the micelles upon dilution. A low
CMC indicates that the micelles are stable and do not disintegrate
readily.

Micelles used as DDTS must be sufficiently stable in the blood circulation and should not disintegrate upon contact with blood components. This means that their CMC should be very low. The diameter of
the micelles can be chosen so that it is in the range where the EPR effect
is observed (<0.2 μm) to allow accumulation of the drug in, for
example, tumor tissue or sites of inflammation.

Micellar systems based on amphipathic block-copolymers have
gained most attention as intravenously administered drug carrier
systems over the years. These block-copolymers are composed of a
hydrophilic PEG block and a hydrophobic block based on doxorubicin
conjugated poly(aspartic acid) or poly(β-benzyl L-aspartate).

These block-copolymers form micelles in aqueous solution with
spherical core/shell structures and diameters around 20–40 nm
(Figure 5.9). The hydrophobic core of these micelles can be loaded with
a hydrophobic drug such as doxorubicin. After intravenous administration the micelles tend to accumulate at tumor sites and release the

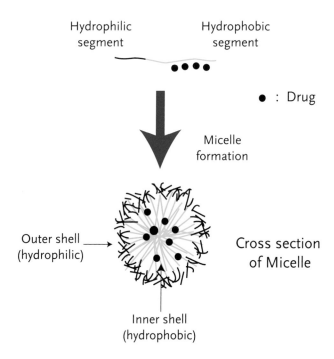

Hydrophilic segment   Hydrophobic segment

● : Drug

Micelle formation

Outer shell (hydrophilic)   Cross section of Micelle

Inner shell (hydrophobic)

Figure 5.9 Concept of micelle-forming polymeric drug

entrapped drug there. Some of the characteristics of these micellar systems are listed in Table 5.5.

Polymeric micelles loaded with doxorubicin have shown strongly increased antitumor activity in animal models. Work in progress to optimize the performance of polymeric micelles includes varying the copolymer characteristics, drug pay load, covalent binding strategies and using other types of drugs.

5.3.3 Poly(alkyl cyanoacrylate) nanoparticles

The poly(alkyl cyanoacrylates) have been used extensively as hemostatic and tissue adhesives. They can be polymerized under controlled

Table 5.5 Polymeric micelles as drug carriers

- CMC of the amphipathic copolymers is low; interaction between polymer units is so strong that blood components cannot break them up.
- Molecular weight of the polymeric unit is small enough to allow clearance through glomerular filtration.
- Diameter is large enough to prevent penetration through intact endothelium.
- Diameter can be chosen in the range where the EPR effect is observed ($< 0.2\ \mu m$).
- Release kinetics of the drug depend on the selected polymer structure (hydrophilicity/hydrophobicity balance).
- Drug is in the hydrophobic core of the micelle protected from exposure to aqueous degradation processes.
- Polymeric micellar carriers have been shown to have a high drug-carrying capacity ("pay load").

conditions to yield colloidal particles, typically in the 0.2 μm size range ("nanoparticles"), which have potential as particulate DDTS.

Drug loading efficiency varies widely between different drugs, monomers and reaction conditions. Efficient drug loading occurs with unionized and highly lipophilic drugs. Poor drug loading is therefore generally achieved for alkaline drugs because the polymerization reaction takes place under acidic conditions. Degradation proceeds via a surface erosion process (see Section 4.5) and degradation kinetics *in vivo* depend on the nature of the alkyl-chain. Poly(butyl cyanoacrylate) nanoparticles are degraded fairly rapidly (1 day), whereas poly(hexyl cyanoacrylate) nanoparticles take a number of days to degrade.

Poly(alkyl cyanoacrylate) nanoparticles accumulate in the liver (60–90% of the injected dose) and the spleen upon iv injection, with the macrophages in the liver being their major target. Nanoparticles loaded with doxorubicin have shown a markedly enhanced therapeutic index in a number of animal tumor models. This is probably due to a reduction of the peak concentration of the drug in the cardiac tissue, the organ most severely affected by doxorubicin upon injection. Release of drug from the Kupffer cells upon breakdown of the nanoparticles in the lysosomal system (see Figure 5.2) may induce a slow release pattern that is still tumoricidal, but does not evoke the cardiotoxic effects. Another application where these nanoparticles have been shown to have large therapeutic promise is the killing of pathogens that are specifically located in the Kupffer cells in the liver.

At present, attempts are being made to prolong the circulation time of poly(alkyl cyanomethacrylate) nanoparticles in the blood circulation by adsorbing PEG-coatings, for example using PEG containing non-ionic surfactants such as poloxamers or poloxamines.

5.3.4   Lipoprotein carriers

Lipoproteins are endogenous lipid carrier systems comprising a lipid core and a coat where apolipoproteins can be found. The lipid core material consists of cholesterol and other lipids (cholesterol esters, triacylglycerols and phospholipids) which are transported in plasma and other body fluids in the form of lipoproteins. The ratio of lipid to protein determines the densities of the different lipoproteins:

- chylomicrons are the least dense, composed almost entirely of lipids, size about 10–90 nm;
- VLDL, very low density lipoproteins, size about 30–90 nm;
- LDL, low density lipoproteins, size about 25 nm;
- HDL, high density lipoproteins, size about 10 nm.

These endogenous lipid carriers have been studied for the site-specific delivery of lipophilic drugs.

LDLs have a plasma half-life of 3–4 days. 90% of the LDL receptor activity is concentrated in the liver with the Kupffer cells playing a major role in the uptake process. On some tumor cells LDL receptor density is increased. This would make LDLs a highly attractive DDTS for cancer therapy. It has been suggested that one could selectively down-regulate the LDL receptor density in the liver by dietary means and in the adrenals by using corticosteroids, thereby enhancing tumor specificity. LDLs can also be actively targeted, by attaching target-specific recognition moieties. For example:

- lactosylation of LDL leads to enhanced uptake in the parenchymal liver cells instead of Kupffer cells;
- acetylation of LDL leads to enhanced uptake by endothelial cells in the liver.

HDLs tend to accumulate in the parenchymal liver cells and target specific recognition moieties such as galactose can enhance the hepatocyte uptake process. This system is being investigated for the targeting of hydrophobic antiviral prodrugs to parenchymal liver cells in viral hepatitis.

5.3.5 Other particulate carrier systems

Other particulate carrier systems which are under evaluation include:

5.3.5.1 *Albumin microspheres*

In the preparation of albumin microspheres, an aqueous solution of albumin and the drug moiety is initially emulsified in an oil, forming a water-in-oil emulsion. This can be chemically cross-linked by the addition of a cross-linking agent such as glutaraldehyde or butadione, or thermally cross-linked by applying heat. Either method produces stabilized particles for use in drug delivery. The size of the particles is based on the droplet size of the initial emulsion, and can range from 15 nm–150 μm.

5.3.5.2 *Poly(lactide-co-glycolide) (PLGA) microspheres*

PLGA microspheres can be prepared in rather narrow size ranges from 0.2 μm up to > 100 μm. The preparation, properties and degradation of these polymers have been discussed extensively in Chapter 4 (see Section 4.5.1). PLGA microspheres can now be prepared with surface oriented PEG-chains which improves *in vivo* circulation time ("stealth-effects").

5.3.5.3 *Niosomes*

Niosomes have been developed as an alternative to phospholipid-based liposomes. They are based on several different families of synthetic, non-ionic amphipatic molecules. At present, there is rather limited experience with niosomes as a parenteral delivery system and no clear advantages over liposomal systems have been established yet.

5.4 PHARMACEUTICAL ASPECTS OF CARRIER SYSTEMS

In order for parenteral DDTS to become commercial products, certain pharmaceutical issues need to be addressed, including:

- purity of the carrier material;

- reproducibility of the characteristics of the drug-carrier system;
- carrier/drug-related safety aspects, including immunological responses;
- scaling up possibilities;
- shelf life.

Historically DDTS were developed in environments where the primary goal was "proof of concept", rather than developing a commercial product. The typical pharmaceutical considerations described above were not dealt with seriously in the early days of drug carrier research, thus early drug-carrier systems were associated with long gestation periods from product development to product marketing.

The time-frame associated with the development of a drug targeting concept to a targeted drug product can be illustrated by the "liposome story". Liposomes were originally used as biochemical tools for the study of cell membrane behaviour in the 1960s; the idea to use them as drug carriers was subsequently developed in the early 1970s. It took more than twenty years to develop the system from a concept to the first commercial parenteral liposome preparation carrying a drug (amphotericin B). Although this may seem like quite a long gestational period, it must be remembered that liposomes were one of the first colloidal carrier systems designed for targeted drug delivery. Comparatively little was known about such systems and many technological and biopharmaceutical hurdles had to be overcome before marketing authorization for the first product could be obtained. Some of these hurdles encountered and solved over the years while developing liposomes as drug carriers include:

- *Poor quality of the raw material*: In the early 1980s, the quality of lipids of several suppliers could vary considerably, both in quantitative and qualitative terms. Nowadays, a few suppliers provide the global market with high-quality products. Interestingly, over the years, the price per unit has dropped considerably while the quality has improved.
- *Poor characterization of the physicochemical properties of liposomes*: Liposome behavior *in vitro* and *in vivo* is critically dependent on their physicochemical properties. Therefore a full physicochemical characterization of pharmaceutical liposomes is required in early stages of a development program (Table 5.6). In later development stages, these quality control assays can be used to obtain regulatory approval and to ensure batch-to-batch consistency.
- *Shelf life*: Shelf-life issues that need to be addressed include avoidance of pre-administration leakage of the liposome-associated drug (retention loss), size stability (occurrence of fusion or aggregation) and phospholipid degradation (occurrence of peroxidation and hydrolysis).
- *Scaling-up problems*: Several of the laboratory-scale liposome preparation methods were difficult to scale up to industrial scale.
- *Safety data*: As these carriers are novel delivery systems, there initially existed a paucity of data on their safety during chronic use. However, their existing safety record and the experience with mar-

Table 5.6 Quality control assays of liposomal formulations

Assay	Methodology/Analytical Target
Characterization	
pH	pH meter
Osmolarity	Osmometer
Phospholipid concentration	Lipid phosphorus content/HPLC
Phospholipid composition	TLC, HPLC
Cholesterol concentration	Cholesterol oxidase assay, HPLC
Drug concentration	Appropriate compendial method
Chemical stability	
pH	pH meter
Phospholipid peroxidation	Conjugated dienes, lipid peroxides, FA composition (GLC)
Phospholipid hydrolysis	HPLC, TLC, FA concentration
Cholesterol autooxidation	HPLC, TLC
Antioxidant degradation	HPLC, TLC
Physical stability	
Vesicle size distribution:	
submicron range	DLS
micron range	Coulter Counter, light microscopy, laser diffraction, GEC
Electrical surface potential, surface pH	Zeta-potential measurements, pH sensitive probes
Number of bilayers	SAXS, NMR
Percentage of free drug	GEC, IEC, protamine precipitation
Dilution-dependent drug release	Retention loss on dilution
Relevant body fluid induced leakage	GEC, IEC, protamine precipitation
Biological characterization	
Sterility	Aerobic and anaerobic cultures
Pyrogenicity	Rabbit or LAL test
Animal toxicity	Monitor survival, histology, pathology

FA = fatty acids, TLC = thin layer chromatography, HPLC = high pressure liquid chromatography, DLS = dynamic light scattering, GEC = gel exclusion chromatography, SAXS = small angle X ray scattering, IEC = ion exchange chromatography, LAL = Limulus Amebocyte Lysate

keted parenteral liposome preparations (e.g. amphotericin B, doxorubicin and daunorubicin) indicate that the safety of these systems is not a major limiting factor.

Biochemists, who worked with drug-loaded liposomes in the early days, had a completely different perception of "stability", reproducibility, upscaling and toxicity than pharmaceutical scientists, who are familiar with the development of pharmaceutical formulations. For example, for a biochemist, a shelf life of a week at –70 °C may be acceptable, whereas a pharmaceutical product would be expected to have a minimum shelf-life of two years, preferably without refrigerator cooling. It took several years and considerable "mental adaptation" to bridge this cultural gap. Currently, quality is ensured by improved purification schemes, the introduction of validated analytical techniques and a better insight into lipid degradation mechanisms leading to better shelf-life conditions (Table 5.6).

The development of liposomal systems has thus contributed greatly to the development of drug carrier systems in general and has highlighted the various pharmaceutical hurdles that must be overcome before a DDTS can reach the marketplace. In addition, liposomal development has provided fundamental knowledge on the fate of particulate systems *in vivo* and how this fate can be manipulated for therapeutic gain.

5.5 CONCLUSIONS AND PROSPECTS

In the early days of the 20th century, Paul Ehrlich developed his "magic bullet" concept: the idea that drugs reach the right site in the body, at the right time, at the right concentration. It should not exert side-effects, neither on its way to the therapeutic target, nor at the target site, nor during the clearance process. Considerable progress has been made and as discussed above, several DDTS have entered the marketplace successfully and many more are in clinical trials. These systems have in common that they are indicated for the treatment of life-threatening diseases like cancer, and severe infectious diseases and, therefore, contribute considerably to our therapeutic armamentarium.

Now in the early days of the new millennium, targeted drug delivery concepts are still in "*statu nascendi*". It has become apparent that multidisciplinary approaches, employing the combined forces of such disciplines as molecular biology, biotechnology, pathology, pharmacology, immunology, pharmaceutical sciences, engineering, clinical sciences etc. is the key to success. In particular, insights into the anatomical, physiological and pathological constraints to the targeting concept have been growing fast over the past two decades. That know-how will help to speed up new developments on a rational basis. Moreover, progress in molecular biology and biotechnology allows the engineering of protein structures and their large-scale production, and will have a great impact on drug targeting concepts and the actual production of targeted drug delivery systems.

5.6 FURTHER READING

Barenholz, Y. and Crommelin, D.J.A. (1991) Liposomes as Pharmaceutical Dosage Forms. In: *Encyclopedia of Pharmaceutical Technology* (Swarbrick, J. and Boylan, J.C., eds), Volume 9. Marcel Dekker, New York, pp. 1–39.

Crommelin, D.J.A. and Sindelar, R. (1997) *Pharmaceutical Biotechnology, An Introduction for Pharmacists and Pharmaceutical Scientists*. Harwood Academic Publishers, Amsterdam.

Crommelin, D.J.A. and Storm, G. (1990) Drug Targeting. In: *Comprehensive Medicinal Chemistry*, Volume 5, *Biopharmaceuticals* (Taylor, J.B., ed.). Pergamon Press, Oxford, pp. 661–701.

Crommelin, D.J.A. and Storm, G. (1994) Magic Bullets Revisited: From Sweet Dreams via Nightmares to Clinical Reality. In: *Innovations in Drug Delivery. Impact on Pharmacotherapy* (Sam, T. and Fokkens, J., eds). The Anselmus Foundation, Houten, pp. 122–133.

Crommelin, D.J.A. and Storm, G. (2000) Stealth Therapeutic Systems: Rationale and Strategies. In: *Targeting of Drugs: Strategies for Stealth Therapeutic Systems* (Gregoriadis, G., ed.). Plenum Press, New York, In Press.

Kreuter, J. (1994) *Colloidal Drug Delivery Systems*. Marcel Dekker, Inc., New York.

Okano, T., Yui, N., Yokoyama, N. and Yoshida, R. (1994) *Advances in Polymeric Systems for Drug Delivery*, Volume 4. Gordon and Breach Science Publishers, Switzerland.

Seymour, L.W. (1992) Passive Tumor Targeting of Soluble Macromolecules and Drug Conjugates. *Critical Reviews in Therapeutic Drug Carrier Systems*, 9:135–187.

Shaw, J.M. (1991) *Lipoproteins as carriers of pharmacological agents*. Marcel Dekker, New York.

Tomlinson, E. (1987) Theory and Practice of Site-Specific Drug Delivery. *Advanced Drug Delivery Reviews*, 1:87–198.

Tyle, P. and Ram, B. (1990) *Targeted Therapeutic Systems*. Marcel Dekker, New York.

Storm, G. and Crommelin, D.J.A. (1998) Liposomes: Quo vadis? *Pharmaceutical Science & Technology Today*, 1:19–31.

5.7 SELF-ASSESSMENT QUESTIONS

1. A company selects liposomes as targeted delivery system because of their ability to exploit the EPR phenomenon for targeted delivery of its active compound. What is the preferred size range of the liposomes to be produced?

2. A particular carrier system containing a cytotastic drug is rapidly taken up by the MPS upon intravenous injection. How can one realistically extend the blood circulation time of this particulate carrier system keeping in mind that this system should be used in patients?

3. Both polymeric micelles and liposomes are being used as carrier systems for drugs. What is a common feature of these two carrier systems?

4. Human monoclonal antibodies are on the market both for therapeutic and diagnostic purposes. Why is it then necessary to develop immunotoxins?

5. In leishmaniasis, macrophages are infested by the parasite. A hypothetical anti-leishmanial drug is strongly hydrophilic and

positively charged at physiological pH. What targeting system would you recommend to develop if a fast market introduction is desirable?

6. What is a prerequisite to use the concept of "macrophage mediated release of drugs" for therapeutic purposes?

7. In an animal model of inflammation coating of an iv administered carrier system with PEG increases the therapeutic index of the carrier-associated anti-inflammatory drug. What could be the reason for this observation?

6 **Oral Drug Delivery**

Vincent H.L. Lee and Johnny J. Yang

OBJECTIVES

On completion of this chapter the reader should be able to:

- Describe those biochemical and physiological characteristics of the gastrointestinal tract pertinent to oral drug delivery,
- Understand the drug-, formulation-, and patient-related factors influencing oral drug bioavailability,
- Understand the advantages and disadvantages of oral drug delivery,
- Describe the current technologies in oral drug delivery,
- Describe the new and emerging technologies in oral drug delivery.

6.1 INTRODUCTION

The oral route is the most common and convenient of the existing administration methods for the systemic delivery of drugs. It affords high patient acceptability, compliance, and ease of administration. Moreover, the cost of oral therapy is generally much lower than that of parenteral therapy.

Nevertheless, the oral route is not without disadvantages, particularly with respect to labile drugs such as peptide- and oligonucleotide-based pharmaceuticals. During the past two decades, numerous novel oral drug delivery systems, such as mucoadhesives, matrix systems, reservoir systems, microparticulates, and colon-specific drug delivery systems have been developed to overcome some of these limitations. This chapter includes an introduction to the structure and physiology of the gastrointestinal (GI) tract, as well as a review of both conventional and novel oral drug delivery systems.

6.2 STRUCTURE AND PHYSIOLOGY OF THE GI TRACT

6.2.1 Structure of the GI tract

Figure 6.1 Anatomy of the human gastrointestinal tract. From V.C. Scanlon and T. Sanders (1995) *The digestive system. Essentials of Anatomy and Physiology*, F. A. Davis Company, Philadelphia, pp. 358–385

The GI tract consists of four main anatomical regions: the oral cavity, the stomach, the small intestine and the large intestine (Figure 6.1).

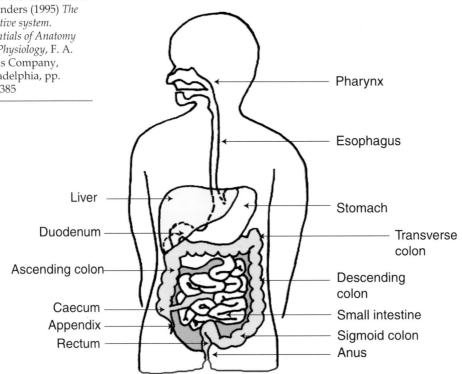

It is appropriate to consider gastrointestinal structure in relation to gastrointestinal function. The function of the digestive system is to break down complex molecules, derived from ingested food, into simple ones for absorption into the blood or the lymph. This process occurs in five main phases, within defined regions of the gastrointestinal system:

- ingestion (mouth);
- fragmentation (mouth and stomach);
- digestion (stomach and small intestine);
- absorption (small and large intestine);
- elimination of waste products (large intestine).

The various regions of the GI tract are discussed briefly below.

The mouth

Ingestion and initial fragmentation of food occurs in the oral cavity. There has recently been considerable interest in this site for the systemic delivery of drug moieties. The possibility of transmucosal delivery via the mucous membranes of the oral cavity is discussed in Chapter 7.

The stomach

The stomach is a sack that serves as a reservoir for food, where fragmentation is completed and digestion initiated. Digestion is the process by which food is progressively broken down by enzymes into molecules small enough to be absorbed; for example, ingested proteins are initially broken down into polypeptides, then further degraded into oligopeptides and finally into di- and tri-peptides and amino acids, which can be absorbed. Although the stomach does not contribute as much as the small intestine to the extent of drug absorption, the rate of gastric emptying does influence both the rate and extent of drug absorption from the small intestine.

The small intestine

The small intestine, comprising the duodenum, jejunum and ileum, is the principal site for the absorption of digestive products from the gastrointestinal tract. Extending from the stomach to the cecum of the large intestine, it is about 2.5 cm in diameter and approximately 6 meters long. The first 25 cm of the small intestine is the duodenum, the main functions of which are to neutralize gastric acid and pepsin and to initiate further digestive processes. Digestive enzymes from the pancreas (which include trypsin, chymotrypsin, amylase and lipases) together with bile from the liver, enter the duodenum via the common bile duct at the ampulla of Vater (or hepatopancreatic ampulla). Bile contains excretory products of liver metabolism, some of which act as emulsifying agents necessary for fat digestion. The next segment of the small intestine, the jejunum, is where the major part of food absorption

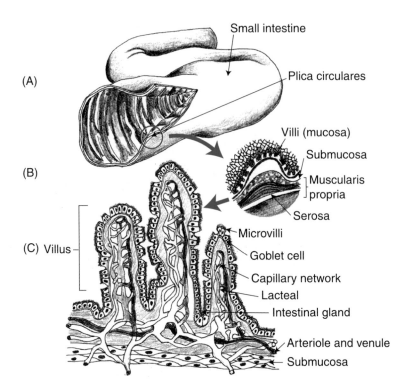

Figure 6.2 Section of the small intestine. (A) Section through the small intestine showing plica circulares. (B) Magnified view of a section of the intestinal wall showing the villi and the four layers. (C) Microscopic view of three villi showing the internal structure. From V.C. Scanlon and T. Sanders (1995) *The digestive system. Essentials of Anatomy and Physiology*, F.A. Davis Company, Philadelphia, pp. 358–385

occurs. In addition to the great length of the small intestine, the available surface area is further enhanced by the presence of (Figure 6.2):

- circularly arranged folds of the mucosa and submucosa, called *plica circulares*, or valves of Kerckring (the plica are particularly numerous in the jejunum);
- finger-like projections, or villi, in the mucosa;
- extensive microvilli (brush-border) on the surface of each intestinal lining cell;
- invaginations of the mucosa between the bases of the villi into crypts, called the crypts of Lieberkuhn.

These features boost the total surface area of the small intestine in humans 50,000 times to approximately 200 m^2, thereby massively increasing the absorption efficiency of nutrients and drug molecules. The ileum links the jejunum to the large intestine via the ileocaecal junction.

The large intestine

The large intestine (colon) is approximately 6.3 cm in diameter and 1.5 m in length and extends from the ileum of the small intestine to the anus. The large intestine has two main functions:

- to absorb water and electrolytes;
- to store and eliminate fecal matter.

6.2.2 Epithelium of the GI tract

The GI tract is essentially a muscular tube lined by a mucous membrane, possessing four distinct functional layers (Figure 6.2(B) and Figure 6.3):

The mucosa

This is divided, histologically, into three layers: an epithelial surface, a supporting connective tissue layer (the lamina propria), and a thin smooth muscle layer (the muscularis mucosae). The latter produces local movements and folding of the mucosa.

The submucosa

This is a layer of loose connective tissue that supports the epithelium and also contains blood vessels, lymphatics and nerves.

The muscularis propria

This consists of both an inner circular layer and an outer longitudinal layer of smooth muscle and is responsible for peristaltic contraction.

The serosa

This is an outer layer of connective tissue containing the major vessels and nerves.

Figure 6.3 The four distinct functional layers of the GI tract

The arrangement of the major *muscular* component of the GI tract remains relatively constant throughout the tract, whereas the *mucosa* show marked variations in the different regions of the tract, reflecting

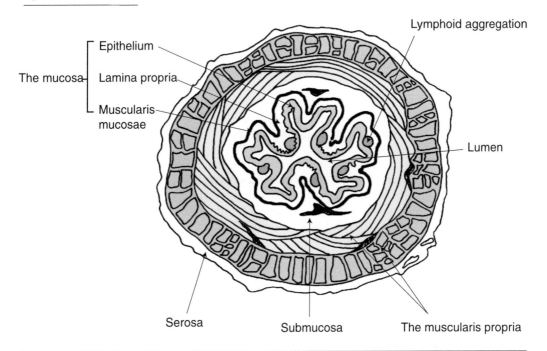

the different functions of the system at different sites. Four main types of mucosa can be identified, which can be classified according to their main function:

- *Protective*: this is found in the oral cavity, pharynx, esophagus and anal canal. The surface epithelium is stratified squamous and may be keratinized (see Section 1.3.1).
- *Secretory*: this type of epithelium is found in the stomach. The mucosa consists of long, closely packed, tubular glands which, depending on the stomach region, secrete mucus, the hormone gastrin and the gastric juices.
- *Absorptive*: this is found in the entire small intestine (Figure 6.2). The intestinal villi are lined by a simple, columnar epithelium which is continuous with that of the crypts. The cells of this epithelium are of two main types:
    (i) the intestinal absorptive cells (enterocytes), which are tall columnar cells with basally located nuclei;
    (ii) the mucus-secreting goblet cells, which are scattered among the enterocytes.

- *Absorptive/Protective*: this form lines the whole of the large intestine. The mucosa is arranged into closely packed straight glands consisting of cells specialized for water absorption and also mucus-secreting goblet cells, which lubricate the passage of feces.

A further type of epithelium is associated with the lymphoid tissue of the GI tract. This gut-associated lymphoid tissue, GALT, is distributed in four anatomical regions:

- as diffusely-scattered cells in the lamina propria;
- intra-epithelial lymphocytes;
- isolated lymphoid follicles present throughout the intestine;
- most importantly, as discrete, non-encapsulated aggregates of lymphoid follicles known as the Peyer's patches.

The Peyer's patches are found particularly in the distal ileum of the intestinal tract. The epithelium covering the Peyer's patches comprises specialized antigen-presenting epithelial cells, called M-cells (modified epithelial cells). This lymphoid tissue plays an important part in the body's immune system, as it samples antigenic material entering the GI tract and mounts an immune response as appropriate. The uptake and translocation of antigen by the M-cells of Peyer's patches can be exploited for oral drug and vaccine delivery, as described below (Section 6.7.7).

6.3 PHYSIOLOGICAL FACTORS AFFECTING ORAL BIOAVAILABILITY

Physiological factors which affect oral bioavailability include:

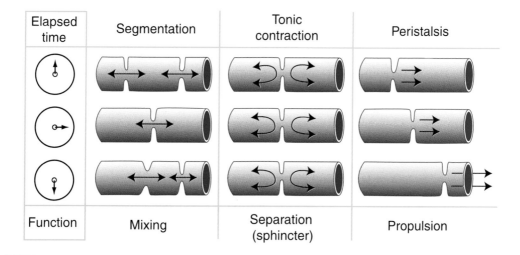

Elapsed time	Segmentation	Tonic contraction	Peristalsis
Function	Mixing	Separation (sphincter)	Propulsion

Figure 6.4 Types of intestinal motility patterns. Segmentation, tonic contraction, and peristalsis are the three major types of motility patterns observed in the gut. Each serves a specific function for digestion and processing of luminal contents. From E.B. Chang, M.D. Sitrin and D.D. Black (1996) *Gastrointestinal motility and neurophysiology. Gastrointestinal, Hepatobiliary, and Nutritional Physiology*, Lippincott-Raven, Philadelphia, pp. 27–51

6.3.1 GI motility

Gastrointestinal motility is an essential function of the digestive and absorptive processes of the gut. It propels intestinal contents, mixes them with digestive juices, and prepares unabsorbed particles for excretion. Gastric motility has been shown to be inhibited by D-glucose in the intestinal fluid.

There are three major types of motility patterns in the gut (Figure 6.4):

- Segmentation is the non-propulsive annular contraction of the circular muscle layer that is predominately found in the small and large intestine.
- Tonic contractions characterize certain regions of the gut that serve as sphincters for dividing the gut into functional segments.
- Peristalsis describes a highly integrated, complex motor pattern marked by sequential annular contraction of gut.

The length of time a drug moiety is in contact with the absorbing tissue will obviously influence the extent of drug absorption. Intestinal motility moves materials in the stomach or small intestine distally towards the large intestine and it has been estimated that in some cases residence of a drug moiety in the small intestine can be in the order of minutes, thereby severely limiting the effective contact time.

6.3.2 pH

The pH along the GI tract ranges from acidic to basic (Table 6.1). The fluid pH in the fasting stomach lies between 0.8 to 2. Following the ingestion of food, the gastric pH rises transiently to 4–5 or higher, but this provokes further acid secretion. Gastric acid is subsequently neutralized by bicarbonates in the duodenum, attaining a value of pH 5.5 at the jejunal junction. Thereafter, the pH rises slowly along the length

Table 6.1 Ranges of gastrointestinal pH in healthy subjects.	Location	pH
	Stomach	1.5–3.5
	Duodenum	5–7
	Jejunum	6–7
	Ileum	6.0–7.5
	Colon	5.5–7.0
	Rectum	7

of the small intestine to a pH of 6–7. The cecum and the ascending colon are usually more acidic than the small intestine, by one-half to one pH unit, but a higher pH of 6–7 or above is reached more distally.

The pH of the fluids throughout the GI tract plays a critical role in the dissolution, solubilization, and absorption processes of ionizable drugs. This concept is discussed further below.

6.3.3 Metabolism

Drug metabolism may occur at various sites along the GI tract, including:

- in the gut fluids;
- within the microvilli of the enterocytes;
- within the enterocytes, either within the cell cytoplasm or within cellular lysosomes;
- by colonic microflora, in the lower end of the tract

Cytochrome P450 3A4 is highly expressed in the human small intestinal mucosa, and is responsible for the metabolism of cyclosporine, midazolam, clozapine and saquinavir during passage across the intestinal mucosa. Indeed, inhibition of presystemic metabolic processes is likely to be a factor in a 34% to 103% increase in the bioavailability of nifedipine observed in individuals consuming grapefruit juice.

First-pass metabolism in the liver is another important issue for oral drug delivery. Drugs absorbed from the GI tract are initially carried in the portal circulation to the liver, where they may be metabolized. This loss of drug from the bloodstream on passage through the liver is termed the first-pass effect. In some cases, the first-pass effect may result in virtually complete elimination of the original drug. Although this is generally disadvantageous for drug delivery, first-pass metabolism can be beneficial for prodrugs, which rely on drug metabolism for activation.

Drugs that structurally resemble nutrients such as polypeptides, nucleotides, or fatty acids may be especially susceptible to enzymatic degradation. For example, the proteolytic enzymes chymotrypsin and trypsin can degrade insulin and other peptide drugs. In the case of insulin, proteolysis was shown to be reduced by the coadministration of carbopol polymers at 1% and 4% (w/v%), which presumably shifted the intestinal pH away from the optimal pH for proteolytic degradation.

In addition to enzymatic degradation, acid- or base-mediated drug breakdown is also a possibility in the GI tract. Drugs such as erythromycin, penicillin, and omeprazole are unstable in acidic media, and will therefore degrade and provide lower effective doses depending on the gastric pH, drug solubility, and residence time of the dosage form in the stomach.

6.3.4 P-glycoprotein drug efflux pump

P-glycoprotein (P-gp) is a 1,280 amino acid, 170 kDa protein that functions as an energy-dependent drug efflux pump at the apical surface of cells. It has been proposed that P-glycoprotein acts as an "hydrophobic vacuum cleaner". Thus, hydrophobic substrate molecules that enter the membrane lipid bilayer from the lumen will be extracted directly back to the extracelluar medium by the P-glycoprotein, prior to reaching the cell cytoplasm. An alternative model proposes that substrate efflux through the pump (at low substrate concentration) occurs via a four-step mechanism. The drug substrate is bound to P-glycoprotein on the cytoplasmic side of the cell membrane. The P-glycoprotein substrate complex undergoes an ATP-mediated conformational change that pumps the substrate out of the cell.

There is a high level of expression of P-gp in the epithelial cells of the small intestine. Compounds that have been found to be substrates exhibit a wide range of chemical structures. However, they tend to be lipophilic and, for some, cationic, such as anthracyclines, vinca alkaloids, cyclosporin, etoposide, and celiprolol. It has been shown that taxol, an anti-microtubule anticancer drug, was not absorbed after oral administration in pre-clinical trials. This can probably be attributed to P-gp, since the flux from the basolateral to the apical side was 4–10 times greater than in the opposite direction. Thus, P-gp may play an important role in determining the oral bioavailability of certain drugs.

6.3.5 Presence of food

Drug absorption is generally less efficient when food is present in the GI tract. Food may reduce the rate or extent of absorption by a number of mechanisms:

- By slowing down gastric emptying rate, which is a particularly important effect for compounds unstable in gastric fluids and for dosage forms designed to release drug slowly.
- Food provides a rather viscous environment, which may retard drug dissolution as well as drug diffusion to the absorptive surface.
- Drugs may bind to food constituents forming a non-absorbable complex.
- Gastrointestinal fluids are secreted in response to food. Enzymes present in these fluids may deactivate a drug moiety; similarly, increased acid secretion provoked by the presence of food may cause increased degradation of acid-labile compounds.

- Food constituents may compete with drugs for carrier-mediated absorption mechanisms.

The deleterious effects of food on drug absorption have prompted the use of dietary strategies in order to improve oral bioavailability. For example, the drug L-dopa, used in the treatment of Parkinson's disease, is absorbed via a stereospecific, saturable active transport mechanism shared by large neutral amino acids such as phenylalanine and tyrosine. The breakdown products of dietary proteins can compete with L-dopa for this active transport mechanism, thereby reducing its oral bioavailability. Taking L-dopa at least 30 min before eating and controlling dietary protein has been shown to improve L-dopa treatment in Parkinson's disease. A further example is the avoidance of milk 2 h prior to taking preparations containing tetracyclines, as these drugs chelate calcium ions in milk, forming a poorly absorbable complex.

Interestingly, the presence of food may favor drug absorption in other situations. For example, the presence of food was shown to increase the oral absorption of a novel HIV protease inhibitor (CGP57813), by increasing the intestinal bulk (dilution of the compound), slowing GI transit, and stimulating GI secretions. The positive effect of food on the absorption of this drug was also observed with Eudragit S100 nanoparticles. Whereas administration of these particles to fasted dogs resulted in no detectable plasma levels of CGP57813, the same particles administrated to fed dogs afforded high plasma concentrations.

However, for other drugs, there exists no food effect. A case in point is diclofenac. The administration of a 150 mg diclofenac hydrogel-based capsule dose within 30 min following a standardized breakfast was shown to minimally affect the bioavailability of dicolfenac relative to administration under fasted conditions.

6.3.6 Mucus

Mucus produced by submucosal glands and goblet cells located throughout the GI tract is largely made up of glycoprotein molecules called mucins, is extremely hydrophilic and can form gels that contain up to 95% water (see Section 1.3.2). Two forms of mucus are found in the stomach, a soluble and an insoluble form. Soluble mucin results from the degradation of insoluble mucus by peptic action. The insoluble fraction forms a semi-impermeant layer, which, in conjunction with bicarbonates (secreted by gastric cells at the surface and in gastric pits), protects underlying cells from damage by gastric acid.

Studies have shown that gastrointestinal mucus presents a physical barrier to the diffusion of small molecules such as urea, benzoic acid, antipyrine, l-phenylalanine and warfarin as well as to large protein molecules. Similarly, the passive absorption of testosterone was shown to be doubled upon ridding the intestinal epithelial cells of the overlying mucus layer. However, the situation regarding the effect of mucus on oral bioavailability is a complex one; for example, it has been shown that drug binding to the mucosal surface is essential to the absorption of barbituric acid derivatives from the rat small intestine.

6.3.7 Individual variations

Individual variations such as gender, race, age, and disease state affect oral bioavailability.

Gender

Gastric acid secretion is greater in men than in women, whereas gastric emptying time is slower in women. Enzyme expression is also different between men and women; for example, sex-related cytochrome P-450 isozymes and glucuronidation enzymes are more abundant in men. However, in general, gender differences are small and insufficient to warrant a modification in dosage regiments. Pregnancy results in reduced gastric acid secretion, increased intestinal motility, increased plasma volume, decreased plasma drug binding and also an additional pharmacokinetic compartment. These altered pharmacokinetic factors may require modifications in the dosage regimen for certain drugs.

Race

Racial differences in oral drug bioavailability are known to exist and may be due to environmental, dietary or genetic differences. These differences are becoming increasingly important in therapeutics, due to both the increasingly international nature of drug development and use, and also the multi-racial nature of the population of many countries. The most profound differences are found in metabolic processes. For example, the hydroxylation of debrisoquine, an adrenergic-blocker used in the treatment of hypertension, is expressed as two phenotypes, designated extensive metabolizer (EM) and poor metabolizer (PM). The hydroxylation defect for debrisoquine also applies to the oxidative metabolim of codeine, metoprolol, and perphenazine. Swedish and Spanish populations appear to be both EMs and PMs, whereas Chinese and African populations are predominantly PMs. The clinical consequnces of polymorphic oxidation have not been examined in great detail. Obviously, the small percentage of the population who are poor metabolizers may be at considerable risk of adverse effects from the usual doses of many drugs.

Age

Few pharmacokinetic studies are carried out beyond the range of 28–40 years and, consequently, there are few data on oral bioavailability for extremes of age. Gastric fluid is less acidic in newborns than in adults, which can affect the absorption of ionizable and acid-labile drugs. Neonates are also associated with a "leaky" epithelium, which permits the absorption of proteins and other macromolecules not normally absorbed from the GI tract. Decreased enzymatic activity, including hepatic first-pass metabolism, is associated with the elderly, which may result in an increased oral bioavailabiliy for drugs subject to the first-pass effect.

6.3.8 Enterohepatic shunt

A drug that is secreted into the bile is presented again to the intestine; it may thus be reabsorbed and again sequestered by hepatocytes on its passage through the portal circulation, and secreted again into the bile. This cycle of events is termed an enterohepatic shunt. The effect of the shunt is to increase the presistence of the drug in the body and, provided the concentrations of the drug at its sites of action are sufficiently high, to prolong its duration of action.

6.3.9 Transport routes and mechanisms

As discussed extensively in Chapter 1 (Section 1.3.3), the organization and architecture of epithelial mucosa restricts drug permeation across the epithelial barrier to two main routes (Figure 6.5):

- the paracellular route: *between* adjacent epithelial cells;
- the transcellular route: *across* the epithelial cells, which can occur by any of the following mechanisms: passive diffusion, carrier-mediated transport and via endocytic processes.

Figure 6.5
Mechanisms of drug transport across gastrointestinal epithelium

It is important to remember that although a drug molecule may be *predominantly* absorbed via one particular route/mechanism, it is also likely that *suboptimal* transport will occur via alternative routes and mechanisms.

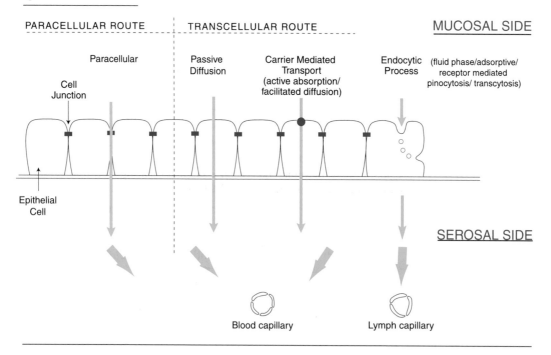

Chapter Six

6.3.9.1   *The paracellular route*

Low molecular weight, water-soluble drugs may be absorbed by passive diffusion between the epithelial cells. Diffusion is driven by a concentration gradient and is inversely related to molecular weight. The paracellular route of drug absorption in the GI tract is limited by the presence of junctional complexes, which encircle the cells, preventing access of luminal contents to the intercellular spaces. The junctional complexes begin immediately below the luminal surface and are made up of three components (Section 1.3.2 and Figure 1.2):

- a tight junction;
- an adherent junction;
- a desmosome.

Thus only small hydrophilic molecules, such as, for example, mannitol, are capable of squeezing through the junctional complexes to be absorbed via the paracellular route.

6.3.9.2   *The transcellular route*

Transcellular passive diffusion

Conventional drug molecules, which tend to be low molecular weight and lipophilic, are usually absorbed transcellularly, by passive diffusion across the epithelial cells. The rate of absorption is governed by Fick's Law and is determined by the physicochemical properties of the drug as well as the concentration gradient across the cells (Section 1.3.3.2).

Carrier-mediated transport

Amino acid transporters, oligopeptide transporters, glucose transporters, lactic acid transporters, monocarboxylic acid transporters, phosphate transporters, bile acid transporters and other transporters present on the apical membrane of the epithelial cells serve as carriers to facilitate nutrient absorption by the intestine. On the basolateral membrane, amino acid and oligopeptide transporters also exist. Drug moieties possessing similar structures to nutrients that are absorbed by such carriers may also be absorbed in this manner.

Endocytic processes

Considerable evidence has accumulated indicating that macromolecules and microparticulates can be taken up by the intestinal enterocytes, generally via pinocytosis. In some cases, transcytosis, i.e. passage through the cells, has been observed, with microparticles subsequently gaining access to the lymphatics of the mucosa. For example, studies have shown that receptor-mediated endocytosis via enterocytes is a major pathway for the internalization of certain antisense oligonucleotides.

However, in general, endocytic uptake is a minor process for the enterocytes. In contrast, endocytic uptake of macromolecules and microparticles is carried out extensively by the M cells of the Peyer's patches. Transcellular shuttling through the M cells to the underlying Peyer's patch may involve an adsorptive and/or receptor-mediated process, with membrane-bound vacuoles or vacuoles already present in the apical cytoplasm of the cells (see below, Section 6.7.7).

6.4 FORMULATION FACTORS AFFECTING ORAL BIOAVAILABILITY

6.4.1 Physicochemical factors associated with the drug moiety

The effect of physicochemical properties of the drug on bioavailability has been discussed in general terms in Section 1.3.4; the following constitutes a brief summary of some of the factors of specific relevance to the intestinal route.

6.4.1.1 Drug pKa

The majority of drugs are either weak acids or weak bases. Therefore, they are ionized to a certain extent, determined by their pKa and the pH of the biological fluid in which they are dissolved; the extent of ionization can be quantified by the Henderson-Hasselbalch Equation (see Section 1.3.4.2). According to the pH-partition hypothesis, the nonionized form of a drug, with a more favorable oil/water partition coefficient ($K_{o/w}$) than the ionized form, is preferentially absorbed. Therefore, acidic drugs are best absorbed at pH < pKa (i.e. acidic drugs are absorbed to a greater extent from the acidic gastric fluids of the stomach, where they are predominantly unionized), while basic compounds are best absorbed at pH > pKa (i.e. basic drugs are preferentially absorbed from the relatively more alkaline intestinal fluids, where they are predominantly unionized). For example, the absorption of salicylic acid, a weakly acidic drug, is approximately twice as high at pH 4 than at pH 7. By contrast, quinine, a weakly basic drug, is absorbed approximately four times higher at pH 7 than at pH 4 (Table 6.2).

Table 6.2 Influence of pH on drug absorption from the small intestine of the rat

Drug	PKa	Percentage absorbed			
		pH 4	pH 5	pH 7	pH 8
Acids					
5-Nitrosalicylic acid	2.3	40	27	<2	<2
Salicylic acid	3.0	64	35	30	10
Acetylsalicylic acid	3.5	41	27	–	–
Benzoic acid	4.2	62	36	35	5
Bases					
Aniline	4.6	40	48	58	61
Aminopyrine	5.0	21	35	48	52
p-Toluidine	5.3	30	42	65	64
Quinine	8.3	9	11	41	54

Figure 6.6 Linear correlations between log cellular permeability (P_c), determined from apparent permeabilities at two different stirring rates in the Caco-2 model and the partition coefficients. The numbers refer to 1, atenolol; 2, practolol; 3, pindolol; 4, metoprolol; 5, oxprenolol; and 6, alprenolol. Each point represents mean ± SD (n = 4). Modified from K. Palm, K. Luthman, A. Ungell, G. Strandund and P. Artursson. *J. Pharm. Sci.*, 85:32–39 (1996).

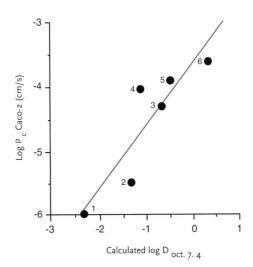

Calculated log D oct. 7. 4

6.4.1.2 Lipid solubility and partition coefficient

The oil/water partition coefficient is an index of the probability of partitioning of a drug into the phospholipid bilayers that comprise biological membranes (see Section 1.3.4.1). Generally, the larger the partition coefficient, the more lipophilic is a compound, and the more readily would it partition into biological membranes. As shown in Figure 6.6, alprenolol, with the highest partition coefficient of the β-adrenergic antagonists studied, shows the highest cellular permeability across the Caco-2 intestinal cell model. By contrast, hydrophilic atenolol, with the smallest partition coefficient, shows the lowest permeability. Figure 6.7 shows that, generally, the higher the drug's partition coefficient the higher the drug absorption. Some drugs exhibit a lower absorption than expected on the basis of their partition coefficient. This reduced absorption is thought, in some cases, to be due to the P-glycoprotein efflux effect (see above, Section 6.3.4).

6.4.1.3 Drug solubility

As drugs must generally be in aqueous solution for them to be absorbed, drugs with limited solubility often exhibit poor absorption and large inter- and intra-subject variation in blood levels following oral administration.

The ionized form of a drug displays a higher dissolution rate and greater solubility than the nonionized form (see Section 1.3.4.4). Therefore, drug solubility is critically dependent on the pKa of the drug moiety and the prevailing pH of the GI tract.

Drug solubility is also a function of the crystalline, hydrate and salt form (see Section 1.3.4.4). For example, the amorphous form of a drug moiety is usually more soluble than the corresponding crystalline form (e.g. novobiocin). The anhydrous form is usually more soluble than the

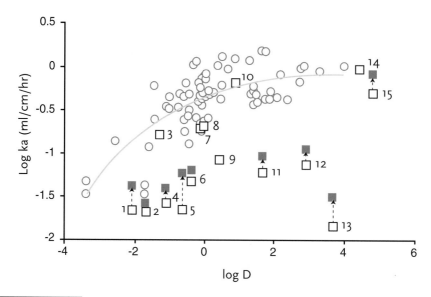

Figure 6.7
Relationship between rat intestinal absorption clearance and lipid solubility. The results shown with the squares represent the relationship between intestinal absorption clearance (ka) observed from the *in situ* jejunum loop in the presence (■) and absence (□) of cyclosporin A in rats and octanol-buffer (pH 7.0) partition coefficients (log D) determined in this study. The numbers refer to 1, atenolol; 2, nadolol; 3, acetamide; 4, celiprolol; 5, acebutolol; 6, doxorubicin; 7, timolol; 8, sulfathiazole; 9, quinidine; 10, sulfamethoxazole; 11, digoxin; 12, cyclosporin A; 13, vinblastine; 14, b-estradiol; 15, verapamil. Modified from A. Tsuji and I. Tamai. *Pharm. Res.*, 13:963–977 (1996).

hydrate (e.g. ampicillin). The solubility of a salt form of a lipophilic drug is higher than the free form and conversion of the free base to the corresponding salt represents a common method of increasing drug solubility.

6.4.2 Formulation factors affecting oral bioavailability

Formulation factors affecting the oral bioavailability from *conventional* dosage forms such as solutions, suspensions, emulsions, capsules and tablets are described here.

6.4.2.1 Particle size

Particle size is a key factor that influences drug dissolution rate. The smaller the particle size, the greater is the surface area for dissolution. The Noyes-Whitney equation describes the influence of surface area (S) and other factors on the dissolution rate:

$$dC/dt = kS(C_s - C_t) \qquad \text{(Equation 6.1)}$$

where dC/dt is the dissolution rate;
             k is the dissolution rate constant;
             S is the surface area of the particles;
             C_s is the solubility of the drug;
             C_t is the drug concentration in the bulk fluid.

A reduction in particle size results in an increase in the surface area, which facilitates an increase in the dissolution rate and therefore, also, an increase in the rate of absorption. Drugs administered as suspension are generally rapidly absorbed because of the large available surface area of the dispersed solid. For solid dosage forms such as tablets and capsules, decreasing the particle size facilitates dissolution and thus absorption. Figure 6.8 shows the effect of particle size on

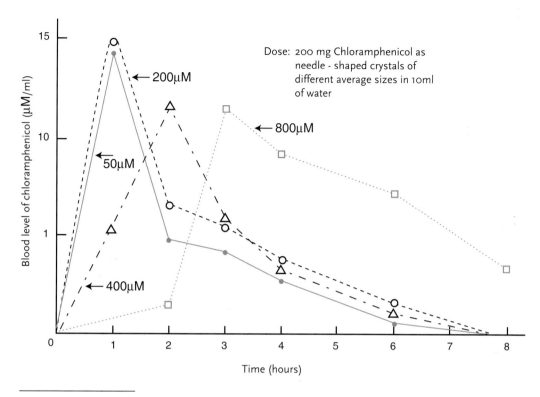

Dose: 200 mg Chloramphenicol as needle - shaped crystals of different average sizes in 10ml of water

Figure 6.8 Effect of particle size on absorption and resultant blood levels of chloramphenicol in rabbits. Modified from K. Kakemi. Symposium on Drug Absorption, Metabolism and Excretion, Scientific section of the American Pharmaceutical Asso., Las Vegas. (1962)

absorption and resultant blood levels after oral administration of chloramphenicol in rabbits. Peak blood levels occurred much faster with the smaller particles (50 μm) than with large ones (800 μm), confirming that particle size must be considered in order to optimize absorption. For this reason, many poorly soluble, slowly dissolving drugs for oral drug delivery are marketed in a micronized or microcyrstalline form.

6.4.2.2 *Formulation additives*

Various formulation additives are employed to enhance the release and dissolution of drugs from formulation matrices. These include:

Wetting agents

Wetting agents are surfactants that lower the interfacial tension and contact angle between solid particles and liquid vehicles. These agents are therefore commonly used to improve the wettability of hydrophobic compounds. Typical wetting agent concentrations that are used range from 0.05% to 0.5%. Polysorbate 80 is the most widely used wetting agent because of its low toxicity and high compatibility with most formulation ingredients.

Wetting agents can also affect the absorption of drugs. For example, the common pharmaceutical wetting agent, sodium dodecyl sulfate, has been shown to increase the absorption of drugs and peptides across the human intestinal epithelium. Studies have confirmed that such agents enhance absorption via the paracellular pathway.

Diluents

Diluents are inert substances added to the active ingredient to bulk up the formulation, in order to make a reasonably sized tablet, or to fill a capsule. Carbohydrates are commonly used, such as lactose, dextrose, sucrose, and microcrystalline cellulose. Hydrophilic diluents promote rapid tablet disintegration and therefore liberate the drug quickly from the dosage form, which promotes absorption. Some diluents dissolve very slowly and therefore release of the drug occurs by tablet erosion, rather than tablet disintegration. Similarly for capsules, on dissolution of the capsule shell, particles of hydrophilic diluent dissolve rapidly in the gastrointestinal fluids, leaving a porous mass of drug which can be readily penetrated by the GI fluids. The effective surface area of drug and hence dissolution rate is increased. However, a hydrophobic diluent impedes penetration of gastrointestinal fluids, so that dissolution of drug occurs only from the surface of the plug-shaped mass.

Binders (adhesives)

In tableting, binders are used to bind powders together in the wet granulation process. They also help to bind granules together during compression. Common binding agents include starch mucilage, gelatin solution and polyvinylpyrrolidone (PVP). These agents coat the drug particles and therefore the rate of binder dissolution can determine the drug release rate. It has been shown that chlorpropamide tablets containing soluble binders (such as hydrolysed gelatin and PVP) have rapid dissolution rates, whereas the use of hydrophobic starch paste as a binder resulted in slow and incomplete tablet disintegration and delayed drug release.

Disintegrants

The purpose of a disintegrant is to cause the tablet to disintegrate rapidly, so as to generate an increased surface area which facilitates rapid drug dissolution. Disintegrants act by swelling in the presence of water, to burst open the tablet. An alternative mechanism involves capillary action, in which liquid is drawn up through capillary pathways within the tablet and ruptures the interparticulate bonds, which serves to break the tablet apart. Common disintegrants include starch and cation exchange resins. Obviously, disintegrants with high swelling and hydrating capacities promote rapid dissolution and thus a high bioavailability.

Lubricants

Lubricants act by interposing an intermediate layer between the tablet constituents and the die wall, to prevent adherence of the granules to the punch faces and dies. Thus, they ensure smooth ejection of the tablet from the die. In addition, many lubricants also enhance the flow properties of the granules. Stearic acid and its magnesium and calcium salts are widely used. The most effective lubricants, such as magnesium stearate, are very hydrophobic and can also prevent wetting of powders and hence retard dissolution (Figure 6.9).

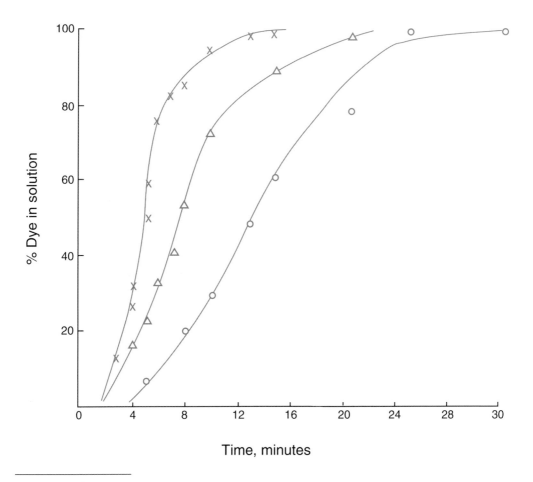

Figure 6.9 The dissolution of dye from capsules containing lactose (x), and capsules containing lactose with 2% (△) or 5% (○) of magnesium stearate. Modified from R.R. MacGregor and A.L. Graziani. Clin. Infect. Diseases 24:457–467 (1997)

Oral dosage forms may contain various other additives to increase the solubility and hence oral bioavailability of the drug, such as co-solvents, buffers and surfactants. Newer technologies may also incorporate additives such as enzyme inhibitors, to prevent premature degradation of enzymatically labile drugs. For example, the inclusion of trypsin inhibitors, such as soyabean trypsin inhibitor and aprotinin, have been shown to be effective in enhancing the effect of insulin in rats. Penetration enhancers may also be included to facilitate the uptake of poorly absorbed moieies. These are discussed below in Section 6.7.4.

6.5 ADVANTAGES AND DISADVANTAGES OF ORAL DRUG DELIVERY

Oral drug delivery offers several advantages, but also disadvantages, depending on the nature of the drug being delivered. A brief overview of both the advantages and disadvantages of oral drug delivery is given below.

6.5.1 Advantages

The advantages of the oral route for drug delivery include:

Patient acceptability and compliance

Compared to all other possible routes of drug delivery, oral drug administration is the most common and convenient administration method and demonstrates high patient acceptability and compliance.

Large surface area

The total surface area of the small intestine in humans is approximately 200 m^2, which represents a large effective surface area for drug absorption.

Rich blood supply

The highly vascular surface of the gastrointestinal mucosa ensures rapid absorption and onset of action, as well as the maintenance of sink conditions.

Prolonged retention

Prolonged retention of the drug moiety is possible within the GI tract, if the appropriate delivery system is used. This allows a lowering of the dosing frequency.

Zero-order controlled release

Oral drug delivery offers the potential to achieve zero-order controlled release. As described in Section 1.5.1, controlled release offers the further advantages of:

- avoiding the peaks (risk of toxicity) and troughs (risk of ineffectiveness) of conventional therapy;
- reducing the dosing frequency;
- increasing patient compliance.

Commercial advantages

The cost of oral therapy is generally much lower in comparison to parenteral and other routes of delivery.

6.5.2 Disadvantages

However, oral drug delivery systems also have some disadvantages:

Variability

The rate and extent of drug absorption from conventional dosage forms are affected by many factors, including fluctuating pH in the stomach and small intestine, the presence or absence of food, esophageal transit and gastric emptying rates, posture, diurnal rhythms, drug interactions and gastrointestinal or other pathology. In addition, a number of patient variables (gender, race, age, and disease state) can also drastically alter the absorption of orally administered drugs. As so many variables influence the availability of the drug at the target site, there is great potential amongst orally administered drugs for bioinequivalence.

Adverse reactions

Locally irritating or sensitizing drugs must be used with caution in this route. For example, some drugs are gastro-toxic, causing damage to the mucosal lining of the stomach.

Adverse environmental effects

The nature of the gastrointestinal environment also limits the types of drugs that may be administered via this route.
Adverse environmental effects include:

High metabolic activity
The high metabolic activity creates a formidable biochemical barrier to the delivery of enzymatically labile drugs. In particular, the oral bioavailability of therapeutic peptides and proteins is very low (typically < 1%). Metabolic activity within the GI tract is further compounded by first-pass metabolism in the liver.

Extreme of pH
Some drugs are acid-labile and are degraded by the highly acidic conditions of the stomach. Delays in gastric emptying rates can prolong the residence time of drugs in the stomach, increasing the potential for acid-mediated degradation. Base-labile drugs are susceptible in the lower GI tract.

Intestinal motility
Intestinal motility can severely constrain the contact time of a drug moiety with the absorbing surface.

Mucus barrier
Drug diffusion may be limited by the physical barrier of the mucus layer and the binding of drugs to mucus.

P-glycoprotein efflux pump
By restricting the transcellular flux of some molecules, this pump serves as further barrier to drug absorption.

Impermeable epithelium
The organization and architecture of the gastrointestinal epithelium provides a substantial physical barrier to the absorption of large, hydrophilic molecules such as therapeutic peptides, proteins and oligonucleotides.
The adverse environmental effects encountered in the GI tract compound to make the oral route highly unsuitable for the delivery of many macromolecules. For example, although insulin was com-

mercially introduced in 1923, despite intensive research efforts directed towards attaining its oral delivery, all approaches have proven unsuccessful, and an oral form of insulin is as yet not commercially available.

6.6 CURRENT TECHNOLOGIES IN ORAL DRUG DELIVERY

6.6.1 Conventional dosage forms: tablets, capsules, suspensions, emulsions and solutions

Conventional dosage forms for oral drug delivery comprise:

- liquid-dosage forms, such as solutions, suspensions and emulsions;
- solid-dosage forms, such as soft and hard gelatin capsules, and tablets.

When rapid, efficient absorption of drugs is desired, aqueous solutions represent the oral dosage form of choice. Drugs in suspension are also readily absorbed because, as described above, the large available surface area of the dispersed solid facilitates rapid dissolution and absorption. Suspensions are also suitable for young children and patients who have difficulty in swallowing tablets and capsules. Emulsions are potentially useful for improving the bioavailability of lipid-soluble drugs.

Soft gelatin capsules have been shown to be efficient and reliable dosage forms, and their use has grown in recent years. However, with regard to solid dosage forms, tablets dominate the market. The most common tablet type is designed to be swallowed whole, disintegrating and releasing its components in the GI tract. Effervescent tablets are less common, but provide a convenient method for supplying sufficient amounts of a drug for relatively rapid dissolution. They are based on an acidic material in combination with a dry carbonate salt, which react in water to liberate carbon dioxide. Buccal and sublingual tablets are also available for both local and systemic drug delivery and are described in Chapter 7.

The various formulation factors which affect oral absorption from conventional oral dosage forms, such as:

- particle size, and
- the presence of additives (wetting agents, diluents, binders, etc.), which facilitate or impede the processes of disintegration, dissolution and the penetration of GI fluids

have been described above (see Section 6.4.2). These conventional dosage forms are not considered as advanced drug delivery systems and are therefore not discussed here in further detail.

6.6.2 Enteric-coated tablets

Coatings can be applied to tablets, which are resistant to gastric juices, but which readily dissolve in the small intestine. These "enteric" coatings have traditionally been reserved for drug substances that:

- cause gastric irritation;
- produce nausea if released in the stomach;
- are destroyed by acid or gastric enzymes.

More recently, enteric coating has also found application in delaying drug release to the distal region of the GI tract. Common polymers used for enteric coating include methacrylic acid and ethyl acrylate copolymers (Eudragit L 30D), cellulose acetate phthalate (Aquateric), and polyvinyl acetate phthalate (Coateric). Such polymers possess free carboxylic acid groups on the polymer backbone and therefore demonstrate a highly pH-dependent solubility, being insoluble in gastric acid but soluble at intestinal pH. Depending on the number of carboxylic acid groups present, different polymers exhibit different solubilities at different pHs; for example, a sharp increase in the solubility of cellulose acetate phthalate occurs at pH 5.2.

Enteric-coated dosage forms have been shown to provide a more desirable therapeutic effect. For example, a new enteric-coated formulation of sodium ursodeoxycholate, in which the barrier film disintegrates and releases the drug only at pH $\geq$ 5.5, was shown to give a much higher bioavailability than that of either ursodeoxycholic acid or sodium ursodeoxycholate administered in a conventional gelatin capsule. Enteric-coated sulodexide tablets administered once daily demonstrated greater efficacy and similar tolerability to a standard capsule formulation administered twice daily. Compared to slow release formulations of diclofenac sodium (Voltaren-XR and the internationally marketed formulation Voltaren Retard), the enteric coated form (Voltaren) has a higher C_{max} and a shorter T_{max}.

However, it should be remembered that enteric-coated formulations are not suitable in some situations. Enteric-coated tablets contain indigestible solids and are often of considerable size. Thus, seriously ill patients, who may have gastric hypomotility or pyloric channel narrowing, are probably not good candidates for therapy with large enteric-coated dosage forms. A further disadvantage of this approach is the uncertainty of the location in which the enteric coating starts to dissolve. Large inter- and intra-patient variations exist in such parameters as GI motility and pH profile. Thus, there is a lack of control associated with the system, so that depending on the prevailing GI motility pattern, pH profile within the GI tract and fed-state, drug release may occur within the small intestine or deep within the colon.

6.6.3 Matrix and reservoir systems

Matrix and reservoir systems are used to effect controlled release of the drug within the gastrointestinal tract. In some cases, near zero-order release can be achieved using these systems. In general, synthetic water-soluble polymers tend to be widely used for reservoir and

Hydrophilic	Hydrophobic
Acrylic acid	
Acrylic acid derivatives/esters	Glyceryl monostearate
Carboxymethyl cellulose (CMC)	Glyceryl behanate
Ethylcellulose (EC)	Hydrogenated vegetable oil
Hydroxypropylmethyl cellulose (HPMC)	Paraffin
Hydroxypropyl cellulose (HPC)	White wax
Hydroxyethylcellulose (HEC)	
Methylcellulose (MC)	
Polvinyl alcohol (PVA)	
Polyacrylic acid (PAA)	
Poly (meth) acrylic acid ester (PMAA)	
Polyvinyl pyrrolidone (PVP)	
Polyethylene glycols (PEG)	

Table 6.3 Some commonly used controlled-release polymers

matrix oral controlled release dosage forms, although hydrophobic polymers are also used (Table 6.3).

These systems have been described in Section 3.2 and also in Chapter 4, Sections 4.4 and 4.5; in summary, the drug is either:

- distributed throughout a polymer matrix (matrix system), or
- surrounded by a rate-controlling polymer membrane (reservoir system).

In a matrix system, drug release is facilitated by the gradual dissolution of the matrix and is controlled by solubility and porosity of the matrix. In a reservoir system, drug release is facilitated by the gradual dissolution of the coat and is controlled by thickness and solubility of the coating.

The Indas (insoluble drug absorption system) is a matrix tablet designed to improve the solubility and absorption characteristics of poorly water-soluble drugs. The gel-forming erodible tablet system facilitates controlled release of the active moiety. A further system from Elan is the Modas (multiporous oral drug absorption system), which is specifically designed to control absorption of highly water-soluble drugs. Modas tablet formulations are reservoir systems which employ a permeable membrane which controls drug dissolution and allows diffusion from the tablet into the gastrointestinal tract.

Matrix and reservoir systems are also available as multi-dose formulations. For example, in a reservoir multi-dose system, individual drug particles/pellets are coated with a poorly soluble polymer. The coated pellets are either compressed into a tablet, or filled into a capsule. Controlled release can be achieved by using a spectrum of pellets, containing different coating thicknesses. In a matrix system, individual drug particles/pellets are dispersed in a slowly dissolving polymeric matrix. Again, the matrices can be compressed into a tablet or put in a capsule. Controlled release can be achieved by using a mixture of free and matrix-entrapped drug.

The advantage of such multi-dose formulations is that they are not subject to the vagaries of gastric emptying. Gastric emptying is an "all-

or-nothing" process, so that a single-dose solid dosage form (typically a tablet) is either all in the stomach or all in the duodenum. There is a large inter- and intra-subject variation in the rate of gastric emptying, which can range from approximately 30 min to several hours; this can result in extreme variability in bioavailability with this type of dosage form. The tablet is also subject to unpredictable variations in the rate of passage through the intestine, so that the tablet may, for example, have passed beyond the absorption site before its release mechanism has been completed.

In contrast, when the gelatin capsule of a multi-dose formulation dissolves, hundreds of coated pellets are released, these pellets are small enough to pass through the pyloric sphincter even if the sphincter is actually closed. Thus, this type of formulation is not subject to the vagaries of gastric emptying. Furthermore, the pellets are widely dispersed throughout the gastrointestinal tract, which tends to reduce the effect of variations in gastrointestinal motility. However, multi-dose formulations suffer from the disadvantage that they are often less sophisticated, because of the small size of the individual dosage units.

6.6.4 Prodrugs

A prodrug (see also Section 1.3.4.1) is a compound resulting from the chemical modification of a biologically active compound, that will liberate the active compound *in vivo* by enzymatic or hydrolytic cleavage. The prodrug approach can offer various advantages for oral drug delivery.

Prodrugs that are more lipophilic than the parent drug can increase membrane pentration and thus oral drug absorption. Thus it was shown that phenytoin 2-monoglyceride, a lipophilic phenytoin prodrug, afforded a 4-fold increase in oral bioavailability in the rat.

The prodrug form can protect the parent compound from hydrolysis or enzymatic attack. A series of ester prodrugs of propranolol were synthesized by incorporating substituents (straight alkyl, branched alkyl, acyloxyalkyl and cycloalkyl) into the β-hydroxyl function of propranolol (Figure 6.10), in order to protect the drug from first-pass metabolism. The prodrugs were rapidly absorbed and regenerated propranolol to attain peak plasma level at 0–0.5 hour, with absolute bioavailabilities about 2–4-fold that of an equivalent dose of propranolol. Prodrug strategies are also being developed to protect enzymatically labile peptide and protein drugs, as well as nucleosides and nucleotides, from premature degradation.

Prodrugs may reduce the GI irritation and other side effects of the parent drug. Orally administered dexamethasone and a prodrug, dex-

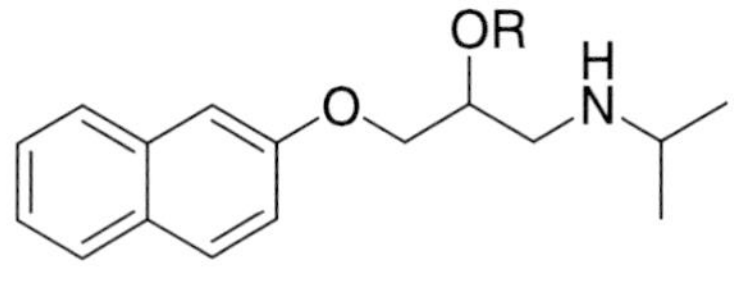

Figure 6.10 Ester prodrugs of propranolol

Propranolol (R=H)

amethasone-D-glucoside, demonstrated no significant differences in the anti-inflammatory effect, but few side-effects were observed for the prodrug. Similarly, oral budesonide-D-glucuronide was shown to have enhanced anti-inflammatory activity than free budesonide, but did not result in adrenal suppression, whereas free budesonide treatment did. Morpholinoalkyl ester (HCl salts) prodrugs of diclofenac were shown to be significantly less irritating to gastric mucosa than the free drug.

Prodrugs can be used to exploit natural transport mechanisms (see below, Section 6.7.3) and to achieve targeted drug delivery to the colon (see below, Section 6.7.6).

6.7 NEW AND EMERGING TECHNOLOGIES IN ORAL DRUG DELIVERY

New and emerging technologies in oral drug delivery are concentrated in three main areas, which focus on improving:

- the retention of drug delivery devices in the GI tract, via the use of mucoadhesives;
- the absorption of poorly absorbed drug moieties, via the use of lipidization strategies, targeting endogenous drug transporters, and penetration enhancers;
- targeted drug release, via the use of osmotic pumps, colonic specific delivery systems, and systems targeted to the Peyer's patches of the GALT and the lymphatics.

6.7.1 Improvements in retention: mucoadhesives

Mucoadhesive polymers possess properties that facilitate their interaction with the mucus layer overlying the gastrointestinal epithelium. Their most important physicochemical features include:

- They are generally hydrophilic molecules with numerous hydrogen bond forming groups.
- They possess surface tension characteristics suitable for wetting mucus/mucosal tissue surface.
- They are predominantly anionic in nature containing many carboxyl groups.
- They are usually of high molecular weight, i.e. >100,000 Da.
- They possess sufficient flexibility to penetrate the mucus network or tissue crevices.

Several mechanisms of the polymer/mucus interaction have been suggested, including the electronic, adsorption, wetting, diffusion, and fracture theories.

A mucoadhesive drug delivery system can enhance oral drug absorption in a variety of ways, by:

- localizing drug delivery in specified regions of the GI tract;

- promoting intimate contact of the formulation with the absorptive surface;
- prolonging the residence time of the dosage form in the GI tract;
- increasing the local drug concentration at the site of adhesion/ absorption;
- protecting the drug from dilution and possible degradation by gastrointestinal secretions.

Considerable work has been carried out on the mucoadhesive polymer, polycarbophil, a poly(acrylic acid) lightly cross-linked with divinyl glycol, in order to promote absorption in the gastrointestinal tract and also at other mucosal sites. Carbopol (carboxypolymethylene) is a further mucoadhesive poly(acrylate), comprising a totally synthetic co-polymer of acrylic acid and allyl sucrose. Both these mucoadhesive polymers have been shown to increase the oral absorption of poorly absorbed drugs, including insulin, the peptide drug buserelin and the model peptide drug 9-desglycinamide, 8-arginine vasopressin. In the latter case, the absorption across rat intestinal tissue was increased by 330% by polycarbophil. A new mucoadhesive delivery system has been developed for the oral delivery of the peptide desmopressin acetate. The system is based on an oil-in-water mucoadhesive (Carbopol) submicron emulsion, and preliminary reports are encouraging.

Recent studies have shown that in addition to their mucoadhesive effects, these polymers can also enhance oral bioavailability by inhibiting enzymes which deactivate the drug moiety in the GI tract. Both polymers have been shown to be potent inhibitors of the intestinal proteolytic enzyme trypsin. Trypsin inhibition was found to be time-dependent upon addition of Ca^{2+} and both polycarbophil and carbomer showed a strong Ca^{2+} binding ability. The amount of Ca^{2+} depleted out of the trypsin structure and the reduction of enzyme activity were comparable.

6.7.2 Improving the absorption of poorly absorbed drug moieties

6.7.2.1 Lipidization strategies

Increasing the lipid character of a hydrophilic drug molecule may enhance its membrane-penetrative properties and thus improve oral bioavailability. In particular, lipidization strategies have been investigated for the oral absorption of therapeutic peptides and proteins, which are generally hydrophilic compounds.

One such strategy involves the conjugation of a fatty acid to a peptide or protein drug. For example, the conjugation of palmitic acid with Bowman-Birk protease inhibitor (BBI) resulted in a 140-fold higher uptake of the drug into Caco-2 cell monolayers, in comparison to unconjugated BBI. This strategy has also been applied to thyrotropin-releasing hormone, tetragastrin, calcitonin, and insulin.

6.7.3 Exploiting natural transport mechanisms

As described above (Section 6.3.9.2), a family of endogenous ligand transporters exist in the intestinal epithelial cells, including the amino acid transporter, oligopeptide transporter, glucose transporter, mono-carboxylic acid transporter, phosphate transporter, and bile acid trans-porter. These transporters may be of use in facilitating oral drug absorption, as such transporters may take up drugs possessing a similar structure to endogenous nutrients. Several successful examples of this approach exist in the literature:

- *Pravastatin*: a hydroxymethylglutaryl coenzyme A (HMG-CoA) reductase inhibitor is a substrate for the intestinal H^+-coupled monocarboxylic acid-specific transporter.
- *Stavudine*: a nucleoside analog of thymidine, used in the treatment of AIDS, is a substrate of the intestinal nucleoside transporter.
- L-α-methyldopa: a substrate for the amino acid transporter. In Caco-2 cells, the active transport of this drug by the amino acid trans-porter was seven times higher than transport by passive diffusion. Its absorption may be further increased by upregulating the amino acid transporter, as has been observed in the 20–70% stimulation of carrier-mediated amino acid transport by treatment of 0.2 mg/kg growth hormone.

Prodrugs (see above, Section 6.6.4) may also be prepared, in order to exploit the ligand transporters: the dipeptide prodrug of α-methyl-dopa, α-methyldopa-L-phenyl-alanine (Figure 6.11), is transported by the intestinal H^+/oligopeptide transporter resulting in enhanced bioavailability of the parent drug. Utilizing the same transporter, the

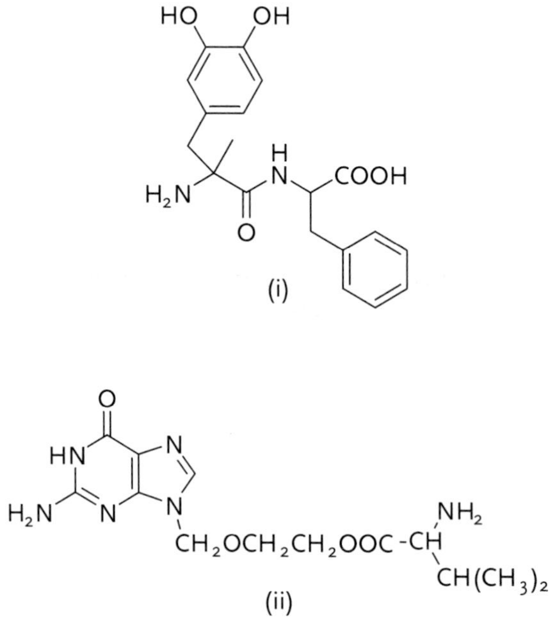

Figure 6.11 (i)α-Methyldopa-L-phenyl-alanine (ii)Valaciclovir

(i)

(ii)

bioavailability of acyclovir, an antiviral drug, can be increased 3-fold by administering its L-valyl ester prodrug, valaciclovir (Figure 6.11). The H^+/oligopeptide transporter is also responsible for the oral absorption of several beta lactam antibiotics (e.g. cephalexin and loracarbef) and ACE inhibitors (e.g. lisinopril, quinapril, and benzazepril). Utilizing monosaccharide transporters, p-nitrophenyl-D-gluco-pyranoside and p-nitrophenyl-D-mannopyranoside-insulin have been shown to afford a hypoglycemic effect after intra-intestinal administration in rats.

6.7.4 Penetration enhancers

Penetration enhancers are substances that can increase the absorption of a co-administered drug, and include surfactants, bile salts, chelating agents, and fatty acids. Penetration enhancers are widely used in drug delivery to potentiate absorption across various types of epithelia, including the epithelium of the gastrointestinal tract. However, a major limiting factor in the general acceptance of absorption enhancers for improving oral drug absorption is the non-specific nature of their effects.

Absorption can be enhanced via several mechanisms. These include increased membrane fluidity, chelation of the calcium ions that serve to maintain the dimension of the intercellular space, solubilization of the mucosal membrane, enhancement in water flux, and reduction of the viscosity of the mucus layer adhering to the epithelial cells. A discussion of various types of pentration enhancers and their mechanism(s) of action is given in Chapter 8 (Section 8.7.1). Table 6.4 summarises the oral absorption enhancers that have been tested for oral drug delivery.

6.7.5 Improvement in targeted drug release

6.7.5.1 Osmotic pump

Osmotic-controlled drug release is described in detail in Chapter 4 (Section 4.6.1). Figure 6.12 illustrates the configuration of the Osmet pump for oral delivery, which resembles a rigid capsule in outer appearance and consists of:

- an outer, rigid, semi-permeable membrane, which is permeable to water but not to drug solutes;
- the osmotic chamber, which contains sufficient contents of an osmotic agent;
- the drug reservoir wall, which is flexible and impermeable to water molecules;
- the drug reservoir, which contains the drug in solution/suspension;
- a fine laser-produced orifice, which traverses both membranes.

In the GI tract, water is absorbed across the semi-permeable membrane, causing the osmotic chamber to expand. This force compresses the flexible drug reservoir, discharging the drug through the orifice.

Table 6.4 Examples of oral mucosal permeation enhancement.	Drug	Enhancer	Results
	Insulin	Sodium glycocholate	Absorption only in presence of enhancer (F 0.5%)
		5% sodium glycocholate	F sublingual from 0.3% to 12% F buccal from 0.7% to 26%
		5% laureth-9, 5% sodium salicylate, 5% sodium EDTA, aprotinin 40 mM sodium taurocholate, 40 mM dextean sulfate, 40 mM linoleic acid, 5% Labrafil, 5% Transcutol, 1% urea	F sublingual from 0.7% to 27% with laureth-9. Others had no effect. F 22% at pH 7.5, not with enhancers
		Various bile salts and derivatives, nonionic surfactants, sulfoxides, lauric acid/PG	F from < 1-4% to 30% maximum. Most effective were deoxycholate, sodium glycholate CHAPS and laureth-9
		Sodium lauryl sulfate, sodium taurocholate, deoxycholate, EDTA, POE 23 lauryl ether, ethoxysalicylate, dextran sulfate	Maximum F 12%
		2% sodium cholate, 3% sodium taurocholate, 2% lysophosphatidyl choline	blood glucose, glucose back diffusion
		Various alkylglycosides (0.1 – 0.2 M)	F from 0.8% to 30% maximum
	Calcitonin	Various saponins, bile salts, fatty acids, sucrose esters, sodium lauryl sulfate	pharmacological effect
		Various bile salts	pharmacological effect, stability in mucosal homogenate
	Octreotide	3% Azone, 4% sodium glycocholate, sodium taurocholate, sodium taurocholate + EDTA	Azone F from 1.5% to 6%, sodium glycocholate F from 0.4% to 4.2%

F = Bioavailable Dose (see section 1.2)
Modified from B. J. Aungst (1996) Oral mucosal permeation enhancement: possibilities and limitations. M.J. Rathbone, (ed.). *Oral Mucosal Drug Delivery*. Marcel Dekker, New York, pp. 65–83.

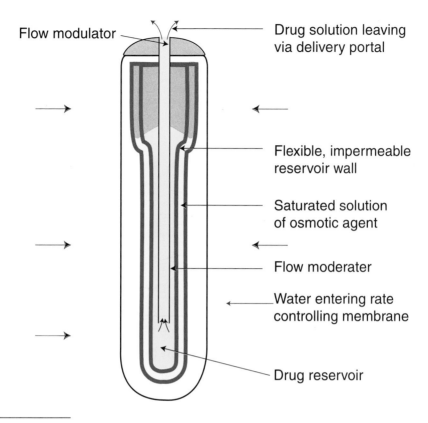

Flow modulator

Drug solution leaving
via delivery portal

Flexible, impermeable
reservoir wall

Saturated solution
of osmotic agent

Flow moderater

Water entering rate
controlling membrane

Drug reservoir

Figure 6.12 The
Osmet osmotic pump

The delivery profile of the pump is controlled by the characteristics of
the semi-permeable membrane (such as permeability, pore size, and
thickness), the osmotic pressure difference across the membrane and
the dimensions of the orifice.

An important consideration here is that osmotic-controlled devices
require only an osmotic pressure to be effective, thus such devices
operate essentially independently of the drug formulation and also the
surrounding environment. Hence, for oral delivery, changes in pH or
ionic strength in the gastrointestinal tract will not affect the drug
release rate. Thus, far less variability in drug release is achieved with
this system, in comparison to traditional coating strategies.

The most notable example of the application of the osmotic pump in
improving oral drug delivery is that of nifedipine (Procardia XL),
which allows once daily dosing while minimizing certain side-effects.
Relatively constant plamsa drug concentrations were achieved within
6 h and maintained for at least 24 hours (Figure 6.13). Simvastatin, a
potent HMG-CoA reductase inhibitor for the lowering of cholesterol,
is another drug whose oral delivery also benefits from the osmotic
pump system. A two-fold improvement in cholesterol lowering
efficacy was realized by using osmotic pump technology for the oral
delivery of simvastatin.

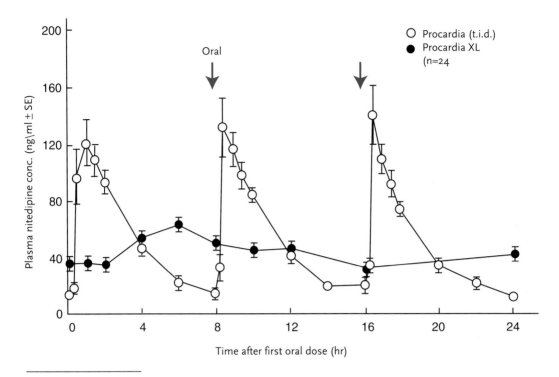

Figure 6.13
Comparative
pharmacokinetic
profiles of nifedipine
delivered from
Procardia XL, an
osmotic pressure-
controlled drug
delivery system, once-
a-day versus that from
Procardia, an
immediate-release
dosage form, taken on
time 0, 8 and 16 in
human volunteers.
Modified from Y.W.
Chien. Oral drug
delivery and delivery
systems. Y.W. Chien
(ed.) (1992) *Novel Drug
Delivery Systems.*
Marcel Dekker, Inc.
New York, pp. 139–196

6.7.6   Targeted drug delivery to the colon

A major indication for colon-specific drug delivery is in the treatment
of local disorders of the colon, such as inflammatory bowel disease
(IBD; which includes ulcerative colitis and Crohn's disease) and carcinoma of the colon. The colon can also be used as an absorption site for
the delivery of drugs to the systemic circulation. Although absorption
from the colon is generally considerably lower than from the small
intestine, systemic drug delivery via the colon is associated with a
number of advantages, including:

- prolonged residence time, thus the drug is allowed prolonged
  contact with the absorbing surface;
- relatively low enzyme secretion and low brush border enzyme
  activity, which makes it a particularly attractive site for the absorption of enzymatically labile drugs such as therapeutic peptides and
  proteins;
- drugs absorbed from the proximal colon are delivered directly into
  the systemic circulation, avoiding hepatic first-pass effect.

Numerous strategies have been developed to achieve colon-specific
drug delivery. Some approaches, such as the use of sustained release
formulations, enteric-coated dosage forms and osmotic pumps, were
not originally designed for colon-specific drug delivery. However, it is
possible to increase the proportion of the drug delivered to the colon
by modifying the original formulations.

A further colonic drug delivery strategy involves the use of a prodrug which is metabolized by enzymes found only in the colon. An example is menthol-β-D-glucuronide, which is stable at various pHs and in the luminal contents of the rat stomach, proximal small intestine, and distal small intestine, but which undergoes accelerated hydrolysis in the rat cecum and colon. The glucoside and glucuronide prodrugs of dexamethasone are another example. These prodrugs are relatively poorly absorbed in the upper gastrointestinal tract but are rapidly hydrolyzed into dexamethasone and glucuronic acid once in the colon. Specificity of colonic delivery in humans should be even greater due to lower levels of β-D-glucuronidase activity in the small intestine.

Azoreduction is another important approach that has been used for targeted drug delivery to the colon. Classical examples include prontosil and sulphasalazine; on reaching the colon anaerobic bacteria reductively cleave the azo bond and release the active agent (sulphanilamide and 5-aminosalicylic acid, respectively) and a carrier moiety. Newer approaches include the development of an azo polymeric system, consisting of poly(2-hydroxyethylmethacrylate), poly(styrene) and the azoaromatic compound 4,4-divinylazobenzene, which is claimed to act as a cross-linker between the polymer chains. The polymer was used to coat gelatin capsules and pellets and it was hypothesized that on arrival in the colon, the azo bonds in the coating would be reduced by the colonic bacteria, disrupting the polymer network and making it permeable to the GI fluids and the drug. Azo polymer coated pellets and capsules have been shown to promote the oral administration of insulin and desmopressin in rats. Other azo polymer systems have demonstrated potential for the systemic delivery of vitamin B_{12} and ibuprofen.

Hydrogels are aqueous gels, usually made of hydrophilic polymers, which are cross-linked either by chemical bonds or other cohesive forces such as hydrogen bonding, or ionic or hydrophobic interactions (see Chapter 16). Although insoluble in water, they are able to swell rapidly in water and retain large volumes of water in their swollen structures. Different hydrogels can afford different drug release patterns and the use of hydrogels to facilitate colonic delivery have been investigated. For example, hydrogels and xerogels have been prepared using a high-viscosity acrylic resin gel, Eudispert hv, which have excellent staying properties in the lower part of the rectum, over a fairly long period. These gels have demonstrated potential in potentiating the absorption of salicylamide and propentofylline, a new cerebral microcirculation-improving agent.

The Pulsincap system was designed to release its drug at a predetermined time or place within the GI tract. The device comprises an impermeable capsule body fitted with a hydrogel plug (Figure 6.14). In aqueous media, the plug hydrates, swells and after a time period defined by the plug's dimensions, is ejected from the device, thereby allowing a bolus drug release from the capsule. The device may be configured to target drug release to the colon by application of an enteric coat, which prevents hydration of the plug while it is in the stomach. Once in the small intestine, the enteric coating dissolves,

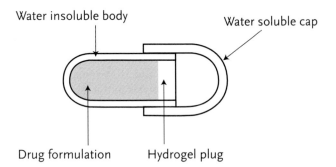

Figure 6.14 The
Pulsincap colonic drug
delivery device

Water insoluble body

Water soluble cap

Drug formulation

Hydrogel plug

thereby allowing plug hydration to take place. Plug ejection and therefore release from the capsule can be controlled to take place after transit through the small intestine and entry into the colon.

There are two possible limitations of colonic drug delivery. First, the colonic epithelia are practically impermeable to all but low molecular weight lipophilic drugs; second, the transit time to the colon is long.

A pharmaceutical preparation taken on an empty stomach is likely to arrive in the ascending colon about 5 hours after dosing, with the actual arrival dependent largely on the rate of gastric emptying. Drug delivery *within* the colon is greatly influenced by the rate of transit through this region. In healthy men, capsules and tablets pass through the colon in 20–30 hours on average. Solutions and particles usually spread extensively within the proximal colon and often disperse throughout the entire large intestine. Colonic transit of such preparations is slower than for large single units (approximately 30–40 hours). In order to avoid the build-up of drugs from successive doses in patients with relatively slow colonic transit, the duration of drug release should be limited to about 15 hours. This will allow 5 hours for the formulation to reach the colon and 10 hours for the delivery in this region.

6.7.7 Drug targeting to the Peyer's patches

As described above (Section 6.2.2), the Peyer's patches belong to the gut-associated lymphoid tissue (GALT) and participate in the process of antigen sampling and presentation to the immune system. Specialized antigen-presenting epithelial cells cover the patches, called M-cells (modified epithelial cells). Unlike the intestinal enterocytes, the M cells of the Peyer's patches are capable of extensive endocytic uptake of macromolecules and microparticles (Figure 6.15).

The efficiency of uptake is dependent on many factors, including:

- *Particle size*: it would appear that particles of certain compositions in the size range 50–3,000 nm are capable of uptake by the Peyer's patches and subsequent translocation through the lymphatics. Particles of 3–10 μm are often retained within the Peyer's patches and do not subsequently move through the lymph. Particles larger than 10 μm are generally not taken up by the GI tract.

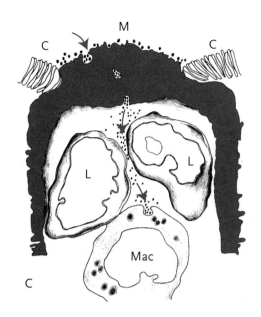

Figure 6.15 Schematic diagram of a portion of the epithelium covering above a lymphatic nodule in a Peyer's patch (mouse). Attenuated M cells (M) extend as membranelike cytoplasmic bridges between the absorptive columnar epithelial cells present on either side (C). Beneath the M cell lies a small nest of intraepithelial lymphocytes (L) together with a central macrophage (Mac). The M cell provides a thin membrane-like barrier between the lumen above and the lymphocytes in the intercellular space below. This M cell has taken up the macromolecules and particulate matter that reach it and macrophages (Mac) may ingest them. Modified from D.H. Cormack. Lymphatic tissue and the immune system. D.H. Cormack (ed.) (1987) *Ham's Histology*, J. B. Lippincott Company, Philadelphia, pp. 234–263

- *Surface hydrophobicity*: greater uptake is generally observed for more hydrophobic microparticles.
- *The presence of specific targeting ligands*: monoclonal antibodies with specificity for M cells, or lectins which bind to specific carbohydrate residues found on M-cells, can increase the uptake of microparticulate delivery systems.

Microparticles taken up by the Peyer's patches may migrate through the underlying lymphatics and ultimately reach the blood via the thoracic lymph duct. Therefore, various microparticulate delivery systems (including PLGA microparticles, polymerized liposomes and microparticles composed of polyanhydride copolymers of fumaric and sabacic acid) are being investigated as drug carriers for the oral delivery of poorly absorbed moieties.

Microparticulate uptake by the GALT is also being investigated for the oral delivery of vaccines. The mucosal surfaces of the intestinal, respiratory and urogenital tracts are the most common sites of pathogen entry, and over 90% of all infections are acquired by mucosal routes. However, effective vaccination at mucosal surfaces requires the *localized* production of secretory immunoglubulin A (sIgA). Parenteral vaccines, which induce predominantly immunoglobulin G and M responses in the blood (rather than sIgA responses at the mucosal surface), are thus of limited efficacy in the treatment of the majority of infectious diseases.

In contrast, oral vaccines offer the ability to induce a local sIgA response and therefore offer greater efficiency than parenteral vaccines in the treatment of infectious diseases. Oral vaccines also offer the advantages of increased compliance in comparison to parenteral delivery, and the access of antigen to the common mucosal immune system (CMIS). Via this system, antigen-activated lymphocytes from the

GALT can disseminate to various other mucosal and glandular tissues, producing a disseminated mucosal immune response (Figure 6.16). Thus through the CMIS, oral vaccines offer the potential to protect, not only against enteric pathogens, but also a wide range of pathogens infecting other mucosal membranes, such as the respiratory and genital tracts.

Considerable success in the oral delivery of vaccines has been achieved using PLG nanoparticulate carriers; other carriers demonstrating potential include alginate microspheres and cochleate vesicles (i.e. stable protein-phospholipid-calcium precipitates). Although the potential of microparticulates as drug/vaccine delivery systems has thus far focused on the oral route of delivery, there is now increasing attention being paid to their potential for alternative mucosal routes, in particular, the nasal route and the vaginal route (see Section 11.7.4).

6.7.8 Drug targeting to the lymphatics

A variety of diseases affect the lymphatic system early in their time course. For example, many cancers spread by lymphatic dissemination, and HIV, fungal, and bacterial infections are located primarily in the lymph nodes. The high prevalence of lymph node involvement in disease is due to the role of lymphatic tissue in the provision of the body's immune response. Intralymphatic and interstitial administration are two efficient access routes. However, the oral route may also prove to be important for the lymphatic uptake of lipophilic drugs and macromolecules.

In addition to the treatment of diseases of the lymphatics, drug targeting to the lymphatics may be used to facilitate sustained release effects, as the drug must distribute from the lymphatics into the general circulation. Delivery into the systemic circulation following oral lymphatic delivery is also a means of avoiding first-pass liver metabolism.

Strategies are being developed to selectively redirect drug absorption into the lymphatics. Formulation of drugs in lipid-based particles or oil increases lymphatic uptake, while macromolecules and colloidal particles may enter the lymphatic system through clefts in the terminal vessels or by pinocytosis. Oral delivery of lipophilic drugs to lymph nodes is associated with the transport of chylomicrons, which are formed following the absorption of lipid digestion products in enterocytes. The colloids accumulate in the mesentric lymph nodes after oral administration and the development of carriers with enhanced intestinal drug delivery may result in efficient drug transport to the abdominal lymph nodes.

Milk fat globule membrane (MFGM) emulsion was shown to enhance the absorption of epidermal growth factor (EGF) from the intestine, especially to intestinal lymph. The oral bioavailability of propanolol was shown to increase when administered in oleic acid and other lipid media. It is thought that the oleic acid forms an ion-pair with the drug and the entire complex is incorporated into chylomicrons. A further factor in the absorption enhancing effects may be that oleic acid *per se* stimulates chylomicron production.

Figure 6.16 The common mucosal immune system (CMIS). Uptake of antigen by the M cells of the Peyer's patches stimulates the production of Ig-A committed B cells and T helper cells. These cells migrate through the lymphatics and enter the blood via the thoracic lymph duct. The cells then "home" to various mucosal sites where they undergo maturation and antibody secretion

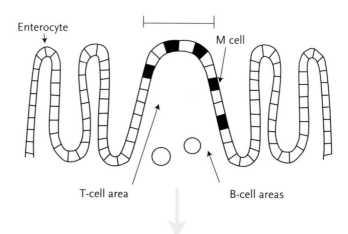

Dome region of Peyer's patch sharing overlying M cells and under-lying T and B - cell regions

Enterocyte

M cell

T-cell area

B-cell areas

Precursor IgA committed B cells
and CD4+ T helper cells

Mesenteric lymph node

Blood

Common mucosal immune system

Lamina propria
GI tract
Respiratory tract
Genitourinary tract

Glandular tissue
Mammary gland
Lacrimal gland
Salivary gland

Maturation and antibody secretion

6.8 CONCLUSION

The efficiency of oral drug absorption is dependent on many factors related to the physicochemical properties of the drug, formulation factors associated with the dosage form and the physiological conditions prevailing in the GI tract. In this chapter, both conventional and novel approaches to achieving oral drug delivery have been reviewed. Targeted drug delivery to specific regions within the gastrointestinal tract, prolonging drug release to longer than one day, and manipulating the interplay of polymer-epithelial cell interactions for the optimization of drug absorption, are examples of promising oral drug delivery opportunities awaiting future development.

6.9 FURTHER READING

Aungst, B.J. (1996) Oral mucosal permeation enhancement: possibilities and limitations. In: *Oral mucosal drug delivery* (M.J. Rathbone, ed.). Marcel Dekker, New York, pp. 65–83.

Chien, Y.W. (1992) Oral drug delivery and delivery systems. *Novel drug delivery systems* (Y.W. Chien, ed.). Marcel Dekker, New York, pp. 139–196.

Fletcher, C.V., Acosta, E.P. and Strykowski., J.M. (1994) Gender differences in human pharmacokinetics and pharmacodynamics. *J. Adolescent Health*, 15:619–629.

Gu, J.M., Robinson, J.R. and Leung S.H.S. (1988) Binding of acrylic polymers to mucin/epithelil surfaces: Structure-property relationships. *Crit. Rev. Ther. Drug Carrier Sys.*, 5:21.

Kalow, W. (1991) Interethnic variation of drug metabolism. *TIPS*, 12:102–107.

Lee, V.H.L. (1987) Enzymatic barriers to peptide and protein absorption and the use of penetration enhancers to modify absorption. In: *Delivery systems for peptide drugs* (S.S. Davis, L. Illum and E. Tomlinson, eds). Plenum Press, New York.

MacGregor, R.R. and Graziani, A.L. (1997) Oral adminstration of antibiotics: A rational alternative to the parenteral route. *Clin. Infect. Diseases*, 24:457–467.

Michelson, E.L. (1991) Calcium antagonists in cardiology: update on sustained-release drug delivery systems. *Clin. Cardiol.*, 14:947–950.

Moes, A.J. (1993) Gastroretentive dosage forms. *Crit. Rev. Ther. Drug Carrier Sys.*, 10:143–195.

Muranishi, S. and Yamamoto, A. (1994) Mechanisms of absorption enhancement through gastrointestinal epithelium. In: *Drug Absorption Enhancement: Concepts, Possibility, Limitation and Trends* (A.G. de Boer, ed.). Harwood Academic Publishers, Poststrasse, pp. 67–100.

Shalaby, W.S. and Park, K. (1990) Biochemical and mechanical characterization of enzyme-digestible hydrogels. *Pharm. Res.*, 7:816–823.

Ritschel, W.A. (1996) Microemulsion technology in the reformulation of cyclosporine: The reason behind the pharmacokinetic properties of Neoral. *Clin. Transplantation*, 10:364–373.

Rudnic, E.M. and Kottke, M.K. (1995) Tablet dosage forms. In: *Modern Pharmaceutics* (G.S. Banker and C.T. Rhodes, eds). Marcel Dekker, New York, pp. 333–394.

Tsuji, A. and Tamai, I. (1996) Carrier-mediated intestinal transport of drugs. *Pharm. Res.*, 13:963–977.

Watkins, P.B. (1997) The barrier function of CYP3A4 and P-glycoprotein in the small bowel. *Adv. Drug Delivery Rev.*, 27:161–170.

6.10 SELF-ASSESSMENT QUESTIONS

1. Where are Peyer's patches found in the gastrointestinal tract, and what is their major function? How can they be exploited in drug delivery and targeting?

2. How does the pH of the fluid vary along the length of the gastrointestinal tract?

3. What is the principal mechanism of drug metabolism in the small intestine?

4. What is the P-glycoprotein pump and how would it affect oral drug absorption?

5. How does food affect oral drug bioavailability?

6. Name the physicochemical factors affecting oral bioavailability.

7. Name the formulation factors affecting oral bioavailability.

8. When would enteric-coated tablets be preferred to uncoated tablets?

9. How can a matrix system be differentiated from a reservoir system?

10. Describe three ways by which the oral absorption of poorly absorbed drug moieties may be improved?

7 Oral Trans-mucosal Drug Delivery

Janet Hoogstraate, Luce Benes, Sophie Burgaud, Françoise Horriere
and Isabelle Seyler

OBJECTIVES

On completion of this chapter the reader should be able to:

- Compare the buccal mucosa with other absorptive sites for drugs in the body
- Give a general overview of the structure of the oral mucosa
- List the advantages and disadvantages of buccal administration
- Give some examples of buccal and sublingual dosage forms

7.1 INTRODUCTION

Localized drug delivery to the mouth is used for the treatment of conditions of the oral cavity, principally aphthous ulcers, fungal conditions and periodontal disease. However, in addition to topical delivery, there has been considerable interest in the possibility of oral transmucosal delivery in order to achieve the *systemic* delivery of drug moieties via the mucous membranes of the oral cavity. It is this latter possibility that is the subject of this chapter.

Oral transmucosal drug delivery can be subdivided into:

- sublingual drug delivery: via the mucosa of the ventral surface of the tongue and the floor of the mouth under the tongue;
- buccal drug delivery: via the buccal mucosa – the epithelial lining of the cheeks, the gums and also the upper and lower lips.

Various physiological differences between the buccal and sublingual regions (described below) mean that the types of dosage forms appropriate for these two routes are very different.

7.2 STRUCTURE AND PHYSIOLOGY OF THE ORAL MUCOSA

Microscopically, the oral mucosa consists of three main layers (Figure 7.1):

- the oral epithelium;
- the lamina propria;
- the submucosa.

7.2.1 The oral epithelium

The epithelium of the mouth consists of stratified, squamous epithelium, which can be keratinized, or non-keratinized.

Keratinized epithelium is dehydrated, mechanically tough and chemically resistant. It is found in areas of the oral cavity subject to mechanical stress such as the mucosa of the gingiva (gums) and hard palate (roof of mouth). Non-keratinized epithelium is relatively flexible and is found in areas such as the soft palate, the floor of the mouth, the lips and the cheeks. Thus the regions of the oral cavity pertinent to drug delivery (i.e. the sublingual and buccal regions) have a non-keratinized epithelium.

In common with all epithelial interfaces (see Section 1.3.2), the epithelium of the oral cavity is supported by a basement membrane, which separates the epithelium from the underlying connective tissue layer (the lamina propria) (Figure 7.1). Oral epithelium is broadly similar to stratified squamous epithelia found elsewhere in the body, for example the skin (see Section 8.2.1), in that cells are produced by mitosis in the basal layer of the epithelium and these proliferating cells push existing cells towards the surface. The phases of this dynamic process are represented in four morphological layers:

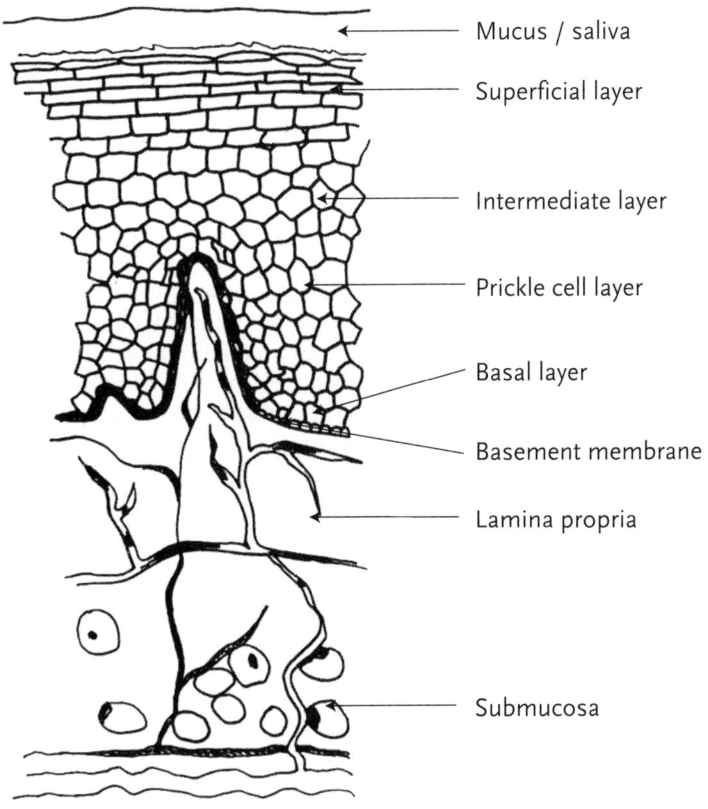

Figure 7.1 Structure of non-keratinized oral epithelium, as found in the sublingual and buccal regions of the oral cavity. (Note: keratinized epithelium has a broadly similar structure; however, the epithelial cell layers comprise: basal layer, prickle cell layer, granular layer and keratinized layer)

- basal layer;
- prickle cell layer;
- intermediate layer;
- superficial layer.

Structural changes that occur during this upward transit, from basal to superficial layer, include the cells becoming:

- larger in size;
- more flattened: the cuboidal cells of the basal layer assume a more polygonal shape in the prickle cell layer, become slightly flattened in the intermediate layer and more flattened in the superficial layer (this flattening effect is more extreme in keratinised epithelium);
- more proteinaceous: increasing amounts of protein are found in the cells (for both keratinized and non-keratinized epithelium) towards the epithelial surface, in the form of protein monofilaments;
- less viable: there is an absence of organelles in superficial cells, indicating that these cells are no longer viable.

This maturation and differentiation process is broadly similar to the process for keratinized epithelium, although obviously cells of keratinized epithelium also show increasing amounts of the fibrous protein, keratin, in the upper layers.

The process of maturation from basal cell through to desquamation (shedding) has been estimated at 13 days for the buccal epithelium and this process is probably representative of the oral mucosa as a whole. Thus the rate of cell turnover in the oral cavity is considerably faster than that of skin, which takes approximately 30 days (see Section 8.2.1).

The cells of the oral epithelia are surrounded by an intercellular ground substance, the principal components of which are carbohydrate–protein complexes. This matrix is thought to play a role in cell–cell adhesion, as well as acting as a lubricant to allow cells to move relative to one another. Membrane coating granules present in both keratinized and non-keratinized oral epithelium are first evident in the prickle cell layer. These same organelles are also evident in the epidermis of the skin (see Section 8.2.1). The granules fuse with the plasma membrane in approximately the upper third quarter of the epithelium and extrude their lipidic contents into the intercellular space. Keratinized epithelium shows a lipid pattern of mainly neutral lipids such as ceramides, whereas the non-keratinized epithelium contains predominantly polar lipids, particularly cholesterol sulfate and glucosylceramides.

7.2.2 The lamina propria

The lamina propria constitutes a continuous sheet of connective tissue containing collagen, elastic fibres and cellular components in a hydrated ground substance. It also carries blood capillaries and nerve fibres that serve the mucosa. It is through the blood vessels in the lamina propria that drug moieties can gain entry to the systemic circulation.

7.2.3 The salivary glands

Saliva is produced by three pairs of major salivary glands:

- the parotid
- the sublingual
- the submandibular

and numerous minor accessory glands scattered throughout the oral mucosa. Saliva is a hypotonic, watery secretion containing variable amounts of mucus, enzymes (principally amylase and the antibacterial enzyme lysozyme), antibodies and inorganic ions. Two types of secretory cells are found in the salivary glands: serous cells and mucous cells. The parotid glands consist almost exclusively of serous cells and produce a thin, watery secretion rich in enzymes and antibodies. The sublingual glands have predominantly mucous secretory cells and produce a viscid mucous secretion. The submandibular glands contain both serous and mucous secretory cells and produce a secretion of intermediate consistency. The overall composition of saliva varies according to the degree of activity of each of the major gland types.

The watery component of saliva moistens and lubricates the masticatory process. Salivary mucus helps to bind the food bolus ready for swallowing. The surface coating of mucus also serves to protect the epithelium from potentially harmful substances. Enzymes present in the saliva initiate the digestive process.

7.3 PHYSIOLOGICAL FACTORS AFFECTING ORAL TRANSMUCOSAL BIOAVAILABILITY

A primary function of the oral epithelium is to provide a safety barrier, to protect the oral cavity against injury. However, this protective role means that the oral epithelium also presents a considerable barrier to systemic drug delivery.

Physiological factors which affect oral transmucosal bioavailability are discussed below.

7.3.1 Inherent permeability of the epithelium

Permeation studies using a number of tracers, including horseradish peroxidase and lanthanum nitrate, have confirmed that the outer third of the epithelium is the rate-limiting barrier for mucosal penetration. When applied to the outer surface of the epithelium, these tracers are seen to penetrate only through the outermost layers of cells. Thus the compacted, flattened cells of the lower superficial layer and intermediate layer present a major physical barrier to transport. The intercellular lipids also play an important role, since extraction of these lipids results in more permeable tissue. Generally, keratinized epithelium appears to be more impermeable than non-keratinized epithelium.

The permeability of the oral mucosal epithelium is intermediate between that of the skin epithelium, which is highly specialized for a barrier function (see Section 8.1) and the gut, which is highly specialized for an absorptive function. Within the oral cavity, the buccal mucosa is less permeable than the sublingual mucosa.

7.3.2 Thickness of the epithelium

The thickness of the oral epithelium varies considerably between sites in the oral cavity:

- The buccal mucosa measures approximately 500–800 μm in thickness.
- The sublingual mucosa is much thinner, approximately 100–200 μm. The thin epithelium of the sublingual mucosa means that extremely rapid absorption is possible via this route.

7.3.3 Blood supply

A rich blood supply and lymphatic network in the lamina propria serve the oral cavity, thus drug moieties which traverse the oral epithelium are readily absorbed into the systemic circulation. The blood flow in the buccal mucosa is 2.4 mL min^{-1} cm^{-2} whereas that to the sublingual mucosa is 0.97 mL min^{-1} cm^{-2}.

7.3.4 Metabolic activity

Drug moieties absorbed via the oral epithelium are delivered directly into the blood, avoiding first-pass metabolism effects of the liver and gut wall. Thus oral mucosal delivery may be particularly attractive for the delivery of enzymatically labile drugs such as therapeutic peptides and proteins.

The oral mucosa, in common with other mucosa, shows enzymatic activity, in particular esterase and peptidase activity. Depending on the animal species and substrates used, buccal homogenates have shown enzyme activites between a few and several hundred percent of the activities of intestinal homogenates.

In general, it can be said that enzyme levels are generally lower in the mouth than, for example, levels present in the gastrointestinal tract. Again, this lower metabolic activity makes the oral mucosa an attractive route for the delivery of enzymatically labile biopharmaceuticals.

7.3.5 Saliva and mucus

The activity of the salivary glands means that the oral mucosal surfaces are constantly washed by a stream of saliva, approximately 0.5–2 L per day. The sublingual area, in particular, is exposed to a lot of saliva which can enhance drug dissolution and therefore increase bioavailability. However, there are also negative aspects for drug delivery associated with salivary flow, including:

- a drug moiety may be diluted by the saliva;
- excessive salivary flow may cause too rapid dissolution and absorption;
- a drug delivery system (e.g. adhesive patch) may be washed away in the saliva and inadvertently swallowed;
- variations in the amount of saliva produced between individuals gives rise to inter-patient variability;
- enzymes present in the saliva may degrade a labile drug.

The mucous secretions may also limit drug delivery via the oral cavity, via a number of mechanisms:

- clearance of the drug prior to drug absorption;
- forming a physical barrier through which the drug must diffuse, prior to reaching the absorbing surface;
- binding drugs specifically, or non-specifically (via electrostatic, hydrophobic- and hydrogen-bonding interactions).

7.3.6 Ability to retain delivery systems

The buccal mucosa comprises an expanse of smooth and relatively immobile surface and thus is ideally suited to the use of retentive delivery systems. In contrast, the sublingual mucosa is unsuitable for adhesive dosage forms for a number of reasons, including:

- the mucosa is exposed to a lot of saliva;
- the mucosa is highly flexible and moving constantly;
- an adhesive dosage form in this region would be uncomfortable and rather disturbing for the patient.

7.3.7 Species differences

Rodents contain a highly keratinized epithelium and thus are not very suitable as animal models when studying buccal drug delivery. Suitable animal models for studying oral mucosal drug delivery include pigs and dogs, as their oral mucosa is quite similar to the human counterpart, both in morphology and permeability characteristics.

7.3.8 Transport routes and mechanisms

As discussed in Chapter 1 (Section 1.3.3), drug permeation across the epithelial barrier is via two main routes (Figure 1.3):

- the paracellular route: between adjacent epithelial cells;
- the transcellular route: across the epithelial cells, which can occur by any of the following mechanisms: passive diffusion, carrier-mediated transport and via endocytic processes.

7.3.8.1 *The paracellular route*

Low molecular weight, water-soluble compounds may traverse the mucosa via the paracellular route, moving between the junctions of the epithelial cells. The major junctional attachment between the epithelial cells is the desmosome, which displays minimal impedence to intercellular diffusion. Tight junctions are rare in oral epithelia. Thus in the majority of cases, drug absorption for small hydrophilic moieties is thought to occur via paracellular penetration, moving between the cells, as claimed for drug transport through the epidermis of the skin.

However, it should also be remembered that the intercellular space of the epithelial cells of the oral cavity contains lipidic material, deposited from the membrane coating granules. Lipidic moieties (depending, as always, on their physicochemical properties) may be able to permeate through this lipidic environment between the cells, thereby being absorbed via the paracellular route.

7.3.8.2 *The transcellular route*

Transcellular passive diffusion

Low molecular weight, lipophilic drugs may be absorbed transcellularly, by passive diffusion across the cells of the epithelium. Again, movement occurs down a concentration gradient, according to Fick's Law (see Section 1.3.3.2). The stratified nature of the epithelium means that lipophilic moieties must permeate across several layers of cells to reach the underlying blood capillaries (Figure 7.1).

Carrier-mediated processes

It has also been suggested that the oral mucosa contains active or carrier-mediated systems for small molecules such as mono-saccharides and amino acids. However, these processes have not been fully characterized in terms of location, transport capacity or specificity.

Endocytic processes

These are presently poorly characterized in the oral mucosa. However, as the oral cavity becomes increasingly important as a potential site of systemic absorption, particularly for high molecular weight drugs which are generally thought to cross epithelial cells endocytically, future studies will tend to focus on attempting to better understand these processes.

7.4 Formulation factors affecting oral transmucosal bioavailability

7.4.1 Physicochemical factors associated with the drug moiety

The physiochemical factors which influence the mechanism and rate of drug absorption (see above) through the oral cavity epithelium are the same as those described in Section 1.3.4.

Studies using FITC labelled dextrans have shown that permeability across the buccal mucosa is dependent on molecular weight of the permeant, leading to a lower permeability for higher molecular weight permeants, followed by a permeability restriction for compounds with a molecular weight above 20 kDa. The degree of ionization of a drug species in the oral cavity will depend on the pK_a of the drug and the pH at the mucosal surface; salivary pH is in the region 6.2–7.0. The degree of ionization can be quantified using the Henderson-Hasselbalch Equation (see Section 1.3.4.2).

7.4.2 Factors associated with the dosage form

The type of dosage form that is appropriate for oral transmucosal drug delivery is dependent on whether the sublingual or buccal region is to be used as the absorption site. Physiological differences between these two regions means that they are suitable for different applications and thus different types of dosage forms.

As discussed above the sublingual route is:

- relatively permeable;
- capable of giving rapid and appreciable absorption of low-molecular weight lipophilic drugs;
- unsuitable for retentive systems, due to high salivary flow, excessive movement and patient discomfort.

As a result of salivary flow, drug concentrations in this region are sustained only for a relatively short period of time, probably in the order of minutes. For these reasons, the sublingual route is ideally suited to the delivery of low molecular weight lipophilic drugs where rapid onset of action is required (e.g. nitroglycerin). Dosage forms that have been developed that are suitable for these types of applications include:

- sublingual sprays;
- sublingual fast-dissolving tablets.

In contrast, as discussed above, the buccal route is:

- relatively less permeable than the sublingual route;
- does not generally give the rapid onset of absorption seen with sublingual delivery;
- highly suited to retentive systems.

These attributes make the buccal mucosa ideally suited for sustained-delivery applications, delivery of poorly permeating molecules, and perhaps peptide and protein drugs. Such formulations include:

- adhesive tablets;
- adhesive patches.

Specific physicochemical properties of the various dosage forms are discussed below.

7.5 ADVANTAGES AND DISADVANTAGES OF ORAL TRANSMUCOSAL DRUG DELIVERY

Transmucosal drug delivery offers several advantages, but also disadvantages, as drug delivery systems, depending on the nature of the drug being delivered. A brief overview of both the advantages and disadvantages of oral transmucosal drug delivery is given below.

7.5.1 Advantages

The advantages of oral transmucosal drug delivery can be summarized as follows:

Relatively large surface area

The oral cavity offers a relatively large surface area (the total area of the buccal cavity is approximately 100 cm^2) for drug absorption.

Accessibility

The oral cavity offers a very accessible surface for drug delivery, both for the application and removal of drug delivery systems. This accessibility obviates the need for complex delivery devices to enable the drug to reach its absorption site. Thus devices for oral delivery are simpler in design than those intended to deliver drugs to, for instance, the alveolar region of the lung.

Ease of use

Oral transmucosal devices, such as sprays, tablets or patches, are also simple for the patient to use and might be expected to be more acceptable to the patient than the use of pessaries or suppositories for the intravaginal and rectal delivery routes respectively.

Rich blood supply

The highly vascular surface of the oral mucosa ensures rapid absorption and onset of action, as well as the maintenance of sink conditions. In particular, the sublingual route is characterized by a rapid onset of action. The buccal cavity offers the combined advantages of a relatively rapid onset of action, with the potential for sustained delivery over several hours.

Low metabolic activity

The metabolic activity of the oral cavity is thought to be less than that of the GI tract, making this route an attractive alternative to the oral delivery of enzymatically labile drugs such as therapeutic peptides and proteins. Furthermore, this route avoids first-pass effects of degradation in the intestinal wall or the liver, prior to the drug reaching the systemic circulation.

Low variability

This route has less variability than, for example, the oral route, where factors such as intestinal motility, presence of food and extremes of pH combine to make oral drug delivery highly variable. However, factors such as salivary flow and certain disease states can contribute to a degree of variabiliy associated with this route.

Robust

The oral mucosa is routinely exposed to a multitude of different foreign compounds and is relatively robust and less prone to irritation than, for example, the nasal mucosa.

Prolonged retention

Prolonged retention of the drug is possible in the buccal cavity, if the appropriate delivery system is used. This allows a lowering of the dosing frequency.

Intestinal alternative

The buccal cavity is a useful alternative to the intestinal route for drug absorption in situations where the gastrointestinal route is unfeasible. Examples include:

- patients with nausea and vomiting;

- patients with swallowing difficulties;
- drugs that cause gastric irritation;
- drugs that are unstable in the gastrointestinal fluids;
- drugs that undergo extensive first-pass effects in the gut wall or liver.

Zero-order controlled release

Buccal drug delivery offers the potential to achieve zero-order controlled release. As described in Section 1.5.1, zero-order controlled release offers the further advantages of:

- avoiding the peaks (risk of toxicity) and troughs (risk of ineffectiveness) of conventional therapy;
- reducing the dosing frequency;
- increasing patient compliance.

7.5.2 Disadvantages

The disadvantages of oral mucosal drug delivery include:

Limited to potent molecules

For drugs of a high molecular weight (which thus are poorly absorbed), the route is limited only to potent drug molecules; typically those with effective plasma concentrations within or below the ng mL^{-1} range.

Adverse reactions

Locally irritating or sensitizing drugs must be used with caution in this route. However, as described above, the oral epithelium is relatively robust and this factor is not as limiting as in other highly sensitive mucosal sites, such as the nasal cavity.

Metabolic activity

While the metabolic activity of the oral cavity towards peptides and proteins is less than that of the GI tract, it should be recognized that the oral mucosa and secretions do have the ability to degrade drugs and that measures might be necessary to overcome this.

Mucus and salivary clearance

Mucus and salivary clearance reduces the retention time of drugs within the oral cavity and thus the opportunity for absorption. This may be overcome by the use of mucoadhesive systems.

Mucus barrier

Drug diffusion may be limited by the physical barrier of the mucus layer and also the specific or non-specific binding of drugs to the mucus layer.

Patient acceptance

A buccal patch comprises a relatively novel dosage form, which is placed in an unconventional drug delivery site. As such, there may be difficulties encountered in trying to get patients to accept this route. It can be imagined that patients may be more reluctant to use a buccal patch in comparison to, for example, a transdermal patch, which has become a well-known and well-established dosage form.

Commercial

Novel approaches, such as the use of buccal adhesive patches for the systemic delivery of large molecular weight drugs, require a huge input of time, effort and money, and are also associated with a large amount of risk. These issues can contribute to significant delay in the development and marketing of a new delivery system and can also make these systems relatively expensive.

7.6 CURRENT TECHNOLOGIES FOR ORAL TRANSMUCOSAL DRUG DELIVERY

7.6.1 Sublingual route

7.6.1.1 *Sublingual nitroglycerin*

Extensive first-pass hepatic metabolism results in nitroglycerin being largely inactive by the oral route. In sublingual tablet form nitroglycerin is highly effective, usually relieving the pain within 2 min of dissolution. Sublingual tablets are composed of soluble excipients (lactose, mannitol, sucrose) to achieve fast dissolution and thus aid rapid onset of drug action. However, the time taken to dissolve can be variable and prolonged, particularly in the presence of mouth dryness. Furthermore, the tablets have stability problems and extreme care must be taken to avoid their exposure to heat, light, moisture and inappropriate packing material, which leads to a requirement for the tablets to be discarded 8 weeks after opening.

Lipid aerosol formulations of nitroglycerin are also available, which are far more stable than the tablets, with a prolonged (3-year) shelf life. Sprayed directly onto the tongue, they produce relief of anginal pain within 2 min with a duration of effect of up to 30 min. However, it has been shown that the use of different aerosol vehicles markedly influences the bioavailability of the drug, which obviously has important therapeutic implications.

7.6.1.2 *Delivery of other drugs via the sublingual route*

Fast-dissolving tablets containing soluble excipients have also been used to achieve sublingual delivery of the opioid analgesic, fentanyl. The tablets were shown to produce satisfactory pre-surgical sedation in children. Fast-dissolving molded tablets consisting of drug and poly(ethyleneglycol) blends with a melting point around the body temperature have also been investigated for the delivery of nitroglycerin and progesterone. Recently, fast-dissolving tablets based on freeze-drying techniques have been developed and are described further below.

7.6.2 Buccal route

7.6.2.1 Buccal prochlorperazine

Prochlorperazine is widely used for its anti-emetic activity and its effectiveness in suppressing dizziness due to labrintine disorder. Oral bioavailability is very low, due to extensive intestinal and hepatic first-pass metabolism. Furthermore, the oral route is impractical in patients with nausea and vestibular disturbance, who have been demonstrated to have impaired gastric emptying.

Buccastem tablets are a form of prochlorperazine for buccal administration, containing 3 mg of prochlorperazine in a polysaccharide base. When placed in position the tablet softens over a period of a few minutes to form a gel which adheres to the gum and gradually releases the drug.

Prochlorperazine fulfils the criteria for efficient transmucosal delivery; it is a highly lipid soluble base with a pKa of 8.1 and is therefore largely non-ionized at salivary pH. Because first-pass metabolism is avoided, the bioavailability via the buccal route is much higher than via the oral route (Figure 7.2).

7.6.2.2 Buccal nitroglycerin

The acute onset of anti-anginal effect with sublingual nitroglycerin occurs within 2 min, but the effect is short-lived, decreasing to negligible levels after 1 h. By contrast, oral long-acting nitrates have a prolonged but slow onset of action, restricting their use to angina prophylaxis. Sustained release buccal nitroglycerin (Suscard Buccal)

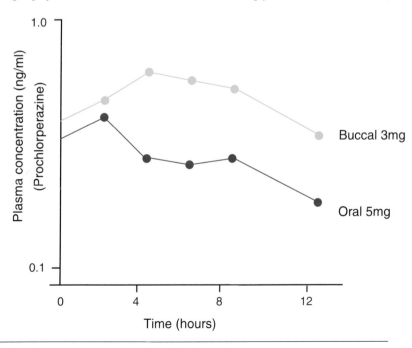

Figure 7.2 Mean plasma levels of prochlorperazine versus time in 12 volunteers for the buccal (Buccastem) or oral (Stemetil) delivery of prochlorperazine

was developed to provide both a rapid onset and a prolonged effect, in a single formulation.

Suscard Buccal tablets are formulated so that the drug particles are entrapped within a meshwork of cellulose fibres. On contact with the moist mucosa the outer layer of the tablet hydrates and swells, becoming gel-like in consistency. This has the dual effect of:

• promoting firm adherence of the tablet to the mucosa;
• causing the outer layer of the cellulose meshwork to rupture, immediately releasing some of the drug for absorption.

Gradual erosion of the tablet matrix allows slow release of the entrapped active moiety. Release from this system has been shown to be linear throughout the period of tablet dissolution.

7.6.2.3 *Other dosage forms for buccal delivery*

Recently, adhesive patches have been developed for transmucosal delivery. Such systems are discussed further in Section 7.7.

7.7 NEW AND EMERGING TECHNOLOGIES FOR ORAL TRANSMUCOSAL DRUG DELIVERY

7.7.1 Sublingual delivery

7.7.1.1 *Freeze-dried fast-dissolving forms*

The Zydis fast-dissolving dosage form is a novel oral dosage form consisting of a freeze-dried porous wafer containing the drug substance and other fast-dissolving excipients. The high porosity of the system means that it dissolves instantaneously on the tongue and does not require water to aid swallowing. A number of products are currently available which use the Zydis technology including Dimetapp Quick Dissolving Tablets, Feldene Melt and Pepdine.

However, it is important to note that the system does not actually facilitate oral transmucosal delivery *per se*, rather it allows rapid release of the drug in the mouth. The drug is then washed down with the saliva for subsequent absorption in the gastrointestinal tract.

The convenience and acceptability of a Zydis formulation make it particularly suitable for patients who find it difficult or inconvenient to swallow solid dosage forms. In trials, up to 90% of patients expressed a preference for taking the Zydis formulation compared with a conventional tablet.

7.7.2 Buccal delivery

Special formulations are now in development to provide prolonged mucosal adhesion and sustained delivery of drug through the buccal membrane. Such formulations comprise flexible adhesive patches and films. Important features for drug delivery associated with these novel buccal patches include:

7.7.2.1 *Patch type*

Patches can be divided into two main types, with respect to the directions available for drug release (Figure 7.3).

Multi-directional release

The type of patch allows release of the drug moiety to the underlying mucosa (and thus the systemic circulation) and also to the saliva bathing the oral cavity (Figure 7.3). Drug released into the saliva may also be absorbed systemically through the mucus membranes of the oral cavity and/or remain locally. However, disadvantages associated with this approach include:

- the drug becomes substantially diluted in the saliva;
- substantial loss of the drug may occur when the saliva is swallowed;
- release of drug into the mouth means that the drug is not protected from the physiological environment.

Unidirectional release

In this type of system, drug loss to the saliva can be decreased by using an impermeable backing layer (Figure 7.3). An additional advantage of these systems is that the effect of additives can be restricted to the site of application. However, this approach also means that the drug moiety is confined to the site of application, thus the available absorption area is quite small. Furthermore, presence of a backing layer can also decrease the flexibility of the dosage form leading to increased patient discomfort and reduced patient compliance.

Drug release rate can be controlled by the use of:

Matrix or drug-in-adhesive systems

The drug is distributed throughout a polymer matrix. Such a system can be relatively easy to manufacture, the simplest case being

Figure 7.3 Types of release possible from a buccal patch

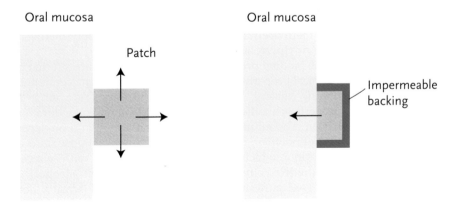

Oral mucosa

Patch

Oral mucosa

Impermeable backing

Multi - directional release

Unidirectional release

when the drug is dispersed directly in a blend composed of, for example, a mixture of poly(acrylic acid) and elastomeric compounds such as poly(isobutylene) and poly(isoprene).

Reservoir systems

The reservoir patch has a similar bioadhesive component but pharmaceutical formulations containing certain excipients, such as penetration enhancers and enzyme inhibitors, can be placed in the center of the design. A rate-controlling polymer membrane can be designed to control the drug release.

Matrix and reservoir systems, and their drug release profiles (first-order, and square-root time order, respectively), have been discussed in detail in Chapters 3 and 4.

7.7.2.2 Patch area

For drugs absorbed via passive diffusion mechanisms (paracellular or transcellular), increasing the area of the patch should increase the amount of drug absorbed. However, patch size must always be considered with respect to patient comfort and acceptability and must not be too large so that these factors are compromised. Thus the size of adhesive patches is generally in the range 2–5 cm^2, with 10–15 cm^2 being the upper limit.

7.7.2.3 Patch adhesion

Bioadhesion is necessary:

- to maximize the intimacy of contact of the patch with the mucosa;
- to retain the delivery system in the oral cavity.

The principal mechanism for bioadhesion of oral patches appears to be physical entanglement of the adhesive polymer of the patch in the mucus glycoprotein chains, with secondary (electrostatic, hydrogen, hydrophobic) chemical bonding playing a minor role.

Adhesive polymers used in oral patches include poly(hydroxyethylcellulose), poly(hydroxypropylcellulose), poly(sodium carboxymethylcellulose), poly(acrylic acid), poly(methacrylic acid), poly(vinylpyrrolidone) and poly(vinyl alcohol).

The binding properties of a given polymer are affected by physicochemical properties such as its molecular weight, configuration, cross-linking density, charge and concentration. As well as initial tack properties, another important consideration is the duration of bioadhesion. The influence of viscosity on adhesion time depends on the type of polymer, for example poly(vinylpyrrolidone) affords an adhesion time which increases exponentially with viscosity grade. Poly(hydroxyethylcellulose) and poly(vinyl alcohol) also show increased adhesion times with increasing viscosity; however, the reverse is true for hydroxypropylcellulose. The basis for this behavior has yet to be determined.

Regardless of the viscosity, increasing the amounts of polymer in the patch increases the adhesion time. Patches with backing layers that are permeable to water generally show shorter adhesion times than those with impermeable backing layers. This is due to the slower erosion of the hydrocolloid when one side of the patch is protected against water uptake.

7.7.2.4 *Patch hydration*

Patch hydration affects buccal drug delivery in a number of ways:

- Water uptake by patches is a primary parameter determining solubilization of the drug.
- Water uptake by patches affects the duration of bioadhesion.
- The degree of swelling of the patches influences their comfort and acceptability.

7.7.2.5 *Penetration enhancers*

As discussed above, patient acceptability and comfort requirements dictate that the surface area of a buccal patch is not greater than 15 cm^2. The limited surface area available for absorption often means that a penetration enhancer is necessary to ensure:

- an effective dose can be delivered from a patch of reasonable size;
- the range of transmucosal drug delivery candidates can be extended, for example, to include poorly absorbed moieties such as therapeutic peptides and proteins.

Penetration enhancers are discussed extensively for the transdermal nasal route in Sections 8.6.1 and 9.7.1. Comparatively few penetration enhancers have been tested for buccal absorption enhancement; those which have been investigated include bile salts. Various investigators have demonstrated the absorption-promoting effect of bile salts on the oral mucosal absorption of drugs such as calcitonin, insulin, α-interferon, GnRH and low molecular weight heparin in laboratory animals. For example, 2% sodium cholate and 3% sodium taurocholate are effective in facilitating the buccal absorption of insulin in beagle dogs to some degree and sodium glycodeoxycholate (10 mM) has been shown to be effective in enhancing the buccal absorption of FITC-dextran 4,000 and the peptide buserelin in pigs.

In addition, the buccal delivery of insulin in rabbits has been shown to be increased from approximately 3–5% by co-administration of edetate (least effective), sodium dextransulfate, sodium methoxysalicylate, sodium deoxycholate, sodium lauryl sulfate, sodium taurocholate and Brij 35 (most effective); with Brij 35 increasing the bioavailability of insulin to 12% by this route.

7.7.2.6 *Patient acceptability and compliance*

Two critical aspects of developing a patch for transmucosal drug delivery in the mouth are:

- The device must be reasonably comfortable, interfering as little as possible with usual daily activities (eating, drinking, talking, sleeping etc.).

- It must be tolerated by the tissues with which it is in contact. A smooth surface and good flexibility are prerequisites to prevent mechanical irritation or local discomfort.

Adequate evaluation of patient acceptability and compliance of buccal patches should include a clinical examination to observe local tolerance, and the incidence and degree of irritation. Trials should also involve the use of questionnaires, in order to determine a subject assessment of such factors as:

- overall comfort;
- sensation (taste, movement, swelling);
- pain (during wear, on removal);
- whether the patch interferes with normal activities (talking, eating, drinking, sleeping).

Various systems are presently under development, including:

7.7.3 The Cydot delivery system

3M, whose experience in adhesive technology has been put to use in the transdermal field, has similarly built on its adhesive expertise in the development of a proprietary mucosal patch formulation (Cydot), which has demonstrated considerable potential for oral transmucosal delivery. The pill-sized patch uses a new bioadhesive which sticks to the gum, the cheek or the lip without causing irritation and is designed to deliver drugs for short and extended periods (up to 24 h). The small size, 0.5 to 3 cm^2, helps patient compliance significantly.

Cydot technology accommodates both uni-directional and multi-directional release, and both reservoir- and matrix-type systems are possible. Two specific applications of the Cydot technology have been described recently:

- delivery of melatonin;
- delivery of low molecular weight (LMW) heparins.

7.7.3.1 *Melatonin delivery*

Melatonin (N-acetyl-5-methoxytryptamine) is an indolamine neuro-hormone synthesized in the pineal gland and secreted rhythmically, with greatest secretion occurring during times of darkness. Among various actions ascribed to the hormone, it has also been implicated in the etiology of the symptoms of jet-lag, seasonal affective disorders (SAD) and sleep disorders; although it should be noted that, as yet, there have been no therapeutic ramifications of these suggestions.

Melatonin is available in the US (although not in Europe) as an oral dosage form for the treatment of the symptoms of jet-lag. However, when administered orally, melatonin shows low and variable bioavailability, presumably due to the extensive first-pass metabolism and/or variable absorption. Its low molecular weight (Mw = 232 Da) and the fact that it is largely non-ionized at salivary pH make this drug a suitable candidate for transmucosal delivery. Gingival delivery of mela-

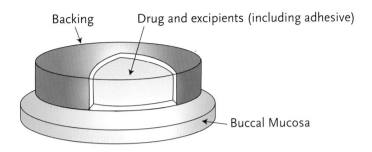

Figure 7.4 Cydot matrix system for the transmucosal delivery of melatonin (Courtesy of 3M Pharmaceuticals)

Figure 7.5 Melatonin kinetics after 10 h diurnal Cydot patch application in 12 healthy subjects. TMD = transmucosal delivery, TDD = transdermal delivery, ORAL-CR = oral controlled release delivery. (Courtesy of 3M Pharmaceuticals)

tonin has been investigated using Cydot technology, using a uni-directional, matrix-type patch (Figure 7.4).

Various pharmacokinetic evaluations in humans, including those illustrated in Figure 7.5, have demonstrated that Cydot melatonin provides:

- rapid therapeutic onset;
- sustained delivery;
- rapid decline on patch removal;
- good dose response and reproducibility;
- low inter-subject variability;
- delivery/metabolism mimics endogenous secretion.

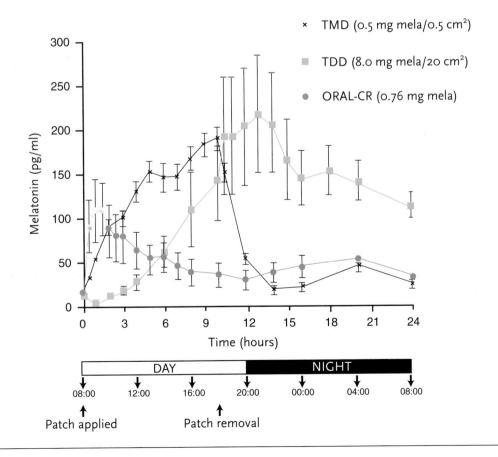

In contrast, trans*dermal* delivery of melatonin results in a significant delay in systemic melatonin levels and a gradual decline in drug delivery after patch removal, possibly due to deposition of melatonin in the skin (Figure 7.5). Moreover, plasma levels tend to be lower after transdermal delivery and inter-subject variability to be higher. Pharmacokinetic evaluations comparing transmucosal, oral-controlled release and transdermal delivery of melatonin clearly demonstrated that the transmucosal route is the best dosage form to mimic endogenous secretion of this drug (Figure 7.5).

Further studies have investigated the tolerance and acceptability of the patch. The Cydot melatonin patches have been shown to demonstrate good adhesion (e.g. overnight) with negligible irritation in humans. Acceptability and compliance studies have shown that the patch is accepted favorably by patients.

7.7.3.2 *LMW heparin delivery*

LMW heparins are mixtures of sulfated glycosaminoglycan chains, produced by the fractionation of native heparin. They are recommended for use in the post-operative prevention of thromboembolic disorders and are conventionally administered via the subcutaneous route. The LMW heparins do not possess ideal properties for transmucosal delivery, as they have a relatively large molecular weight with a broad molecular weight distribution around 4,000 Da, they are also hydrophilic molecules. To maximize transmucosal absorption, the active was incorporated in a Cydot uni-directional *reservoir* system. LMW heparin patch was applied on the cheek. Use of a reservoir system allows a high degree of drug loading and also permits absorption enhancers to be included with the drug in the central reservoir compartment.

Studies have demonstrated that the patches:

* possess prolonged adhesion properties;
* are of low irritancy;
* have bioavailabilites ranging from 50% to 75%.

7.7.4 TheraTech buccal delivery system

The drug delivery company TheraTech, which has developed a number of transdermal formulations, has also been working on a special buccal tablet to deliver glucagon-like insulinotropic peptide (GLP-1) through the oral mucosa, as an alternative to injection, in the treatment of type II diabetes. GLP-1 is a 30 amino acid endogenous peptide which lowers fasting and postprandial blood glucose, stimulates insulin secretion, inhibits glucagon secretion, slows gastric emptying, reduces insulin requirements and increases insulin sensitivity. The TheraTech buccal delivery system comprises a bilayer tablet, with an adhesive layer on one side, and an active layer on the other side, which lies in contact with the cheek mucosa. Preliminary studies with this system have proven highly encouraging.

7.8 Conclusions

The market for oral transmucosal delivery systems is still very small, and its growth over the next five years will depend on the drugs which are approved for delivery by this route and the prevalence of the conditions for which they are intended.

However, the route is associated with many advantages for drug delivery and there is clearly considerable ongoing research in this area. In the past decade, new and highly sophisticated formulations have been developed; drug delivery using the new types of retentive systems for buccal absorption is a particularly promising area. Some success has also been attained in the transbuccal delivery of peptides and proteins. Thus it can be expected that a more exponential growth phase will develop in the coming years.

7.9 Further reading

Lee, V.H.L. (1988) Enzymatic barriers to peptide and protein absorption. *Crit. Rev. Ther. Drug Del. Syst.*, 5:69–97.

Merkle, H.P. and Wolany, G. (1992) Buccal delivery for peptide drugs. *J. Control. Rel.*, 21:155–164.

De Vries, M.E., Boddé, H.E., Verhoef, J.C. and Junginger, H.E. (1991) Developments in buccal drug delivery. *Crit. Rev. Ther. Drug Carrier Syst.*, 8:271–303.

Rathbone, J. and Hadgraft, J. (1991) Absorption of drugs from the human oral cavity. *Int. J. Pharm.*, 74:9–24.

Aungst, B.J. and Rogers, N.J. (1989) Comparison of the effects of various transmucosal absorption promoters on buccal insulin delivery. *Int. J. Pharm.*, 53:227–235.

Meyer, J. Squier, C.A. and Gerson, S.J. (eds) (1984) *The structure and function of oral mucosal*, Pergamon Press.

Ebert, C.D., Heiber, S.J., Dave, S.C., Kim, S.W. and Mix, D. (1994) Mucosal delivery of macromolecules. *J. Control. Rel.*, 28:37–44.

Nagai, T. and Konishi, R. (1987) Buccal/gingival drug delivery systems. *J. Control. Rel.*, 6:353–360.

Degrande, G., Bénès, L., Horrière, F., Karsenty, H., Lacoste, C., McQuinn, R., Guo, J-H. and Scherrer, R. (1996) *Oral mucosal drug delivery*. Ed. Rathbone, Marcel Dekker, New York.

Motwani, J.G. and Lipworth, B.J. (1991) Clinical pharmacokinetics of drugs administered buccally and sublingually. *Clin. Pharmacokin.*, 21:83–94.

Ponchel, G. (1994) Formulation of oral mucosal drug delivery systems for the systemic delivery of bioactive materials. *Adv. Drug Del. Rev.*, 13:75–87.

Harris, D. and Robinson, J.R. (1992) Drug delivery via the mucous membranes for the oral cavity. *J. Pharm. Sci*, 81:1–10.

Hoogstraate, A.J. and Boddé, H.E. (1993) Methods for assessing the buccal mucosa as a route of drug delivery. *Adv. Drug Del. Rev.*, 12:99–125.

7.10 SELF-ASSESSMENT QUESTIONS

1. Name 3 differences between the buccal mucosa and the mucosa of the gastrointestinal tract.
2. What advantages does the buccal route offer for the systemic delivery of peptides?
3. When is buccal administration not an appropriate route of administration?
4. Name 3 possible buccal or sublingual dosage forms.
5. What is the main structural difference between the gingival and the cheek epithelium?
6. Rank the permeability of the gastrointestinal mucosa, the skin and the buccal mucosa in the order lowest to highest.
7. Name 4 properties of a drug which affect its transmucosal permeability.

Transdermal Drug Delivery

M. Begoña Delgado-Charro and Richard H. Guy

OBJECTIVES

On completion of this chapter the reader should be able to:

- Compare the skin with other absorptive sites for drugs in the body
- Give a general overview of the structure of the skin
- List the advantages and disadvantages of transdermal drug delivery
- Give examples of commercial transdermal delivery systems
- Describe approaches for enhancing transdermal drug delivery

8.1 INTRODUCTION

On initial inspection, the skin is an unlikely route for systemic drug administration. Evolution has provided the mammalian organism with an external covering, the principal function of which is to act as a barrier, specifically to the loss of tissue water. Think about it: the concentration of water inside the human body is on the order of 50 M, while that in the atmosphere is clearly very much less. Thus, there is a strong driving force for water to be lost from the body and, to prevent desiccation, an efficient barrier at the interface is therefore required. The skin, and more specifically skin's outermost layer, the *stratum corneum*, provides this shield. Of course, in so doing, the skin also presents a formidable resistance to the absorption, either deliberate or accidental, of chemicals which contact the external surface.

Nevertheless, the challenge of transdermal drug delivery has been accepted by pharmaceutical scientists and, over the past 25 years, considerable progress and achievement have been recorded. So, what led to the investigation of the skin as a potential route for systemic drug input in light of the formidable challenges posed by the stratum corneum? First, the skin offers a large (1–2 m^2) and very accessible surface for drug delivery. Second, transdermal applications, relative to other routes, are quite noninvasive, requiring the simple adhesion of a "patch" much like the application of a Band-Aid. As a result, thirdly, patient compliance is generally very good – that is, in general, people are quite comfortable with the use of a simple-looking patch (no matter how complex the interior machinery). And, fourth, with again a positive aspect for the patient, a transdermal system is easily removed either at the end of an application period, or in the case that continued delivery is contra-indicated – with the exception of intravenous infusions, no other delivery modality offers this advantage.

Although transdermal administration is limited at present to relatively few drugs, it has proven to be a considerable commercial success when compared to other "controlled release" technologies. The current worldwide market for transdermal systems is about $2 billion annually. In the US alone, there are more than 30 different products for sale, but only seven active agents (scopolamine, nitroglycerin, clonidine, estradiol, fentanyl, nicotine and testosterone) and a combination estrogen–progestin product have actually been approved by the Food & Drug Administration; that is, there are many manufacturers with competing products that contain the same drug.

8.2 STRUCTURE AND PHYSIOLOGY OF THE SKIN

In discussing skin structure, we limit ourselves to those features of the membrane which are pertinent to drug delivery; in particular, to the stratum corneum (SC), the outermost layer wherein skin's barrier function principally resides. Macroscopically, skin comprises two main layers: the epidermis and the dermis (~0.1 and 1 mm in thickness, respectively) (see Figure 8.1). The dermal-epidermal junction is highly

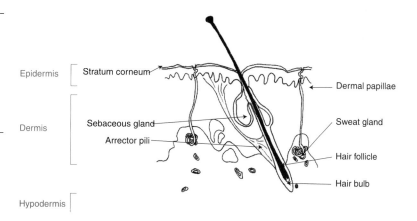

Figure 8.1 Schematic structure of the skin, highlighting the dermis, the epidermis and the stratum corneum (outermost layer of the epidermis)

convoluted ensuring a maximal contact area. Other anatomical features of the skin of interest are the appendageal structures: the hair follicles, nails and sweat glands.

8.2.1 Epidermis: structure and differentiation

The epidermis is a stratified, squamous, keratinizing epithelium. The keratinocytes comprise the major cellular component (> 90%) and are responsible for the evolution of barrier function. The epidermis *per se* can be divided into five distinct strata which correspond to the consecutive steps of keratinocyte differentiation. The ultimate result of this differentiation process is formation of the functional barrier layer, the stratum corneum (~0.01 mm).

The stratum basale or basal layer is responsible for the continual renewal of the epidermis (a process occurring every 20–30 days). Proliferation of the stem cells in the stratum basale creates new keratinocytes which then push existing cells towards the surface. During this upward transit, given that the epidermis is avascular, the keratinocytes begin to differentiate, finally achieving terminal differentiation in the stratum corneum.

The next layer of the epidermis is the stratum spinosum, named for the numerous spiny projections (desmosomes) on the cell surface. The keratinocytes maintain a complete set of organelles and also include membrane-coating granules (or lamellar bodies) which originate in the Golgi. Subsequently, we encounter the stratum granulosum or granular layer, characterized by numerous keratohyalin granules present in the cytoplasm of the more flattened, yet still viable, keratinocytes. More lamellar bodies are also apparent and concentrate in the upper part of the granular cells. The lamellar bodies contain stacks of flattened lipid vesicles.

The transition layer, the stratum lucidum, comprises flattened cells which are not easy to visualize microscopically. The cellular organelles are broken down leaving only keratin filaments in the stratum granulosum an interfilament matrix material in the intracellular compartment. The membrane coating granules fuse with the cell membrane and release their contents into the intercellular space. These intercellular lipids organize into multilamellar domains. Finally, in the stratum corneum, the outermost layer, protein is added to the inner surface of the cell membrane to form a cornified envelope that further strengthens the resistance of the cell.

8.2.2 Stratum corneum: structure and barrier function

The stratum corneum is usefully thought of as a "brick wall", with the fully differentiated corneocytes comprising the "bricks", embedded in the "mortar" created by the intercellular lipids. A layer of lipid covalently bound to the cornified envelope of the corneocyte contributes to this exquisite organization. The intercellular lipids of the stratum corneum include no phospholipids, comprising an approximately equimolar mixture of ceramides, cholesterol and free fatty acids. These non-polar and somewhat rigid components of the stratum corneum's "cement" play a critical role in barrier function. On average, there are about 20 cell layers in the stratum corneum, each of which is about $0.5~\mu m$ in thickness. Yet, the architecture of the membrane is such that this very thin structure limits, under normal conditions, the passive loss of water across the entire skin surface to only about 250 mL per day, a volume easily replaced in order to maintain homeostasis.

The link between skin barrier function and stratum corneum lipid composition and structure has been clearly established. For example, changes in intercellular lipid composition and/or organization typically result in a defective and more permeable barrier. Lipid extraction with organic solvents provokes such an effect. Skin permeability at different body sites has been correlated with local variations in lipid content. And, most convincingly, the conformational order of the intercellular lipids of the stratum corneum is correlated directly with the membrane's permeability to water. Taken together, it has been deduced that the stratum corneum achieves its excellent barrier capability by constraining the passive diffusion of molecules to the intercellular path. This mechanism is tortuous and apparently demands a diffusion path length at least an order of magnitude greater than that of the thickness of the stratum corneum. Thus, the stratum corneum is most convincingly viewed as a predominantly lipophilic barrier (this makes perfectly good sense as it was designed to inhibit passive loss of tissue water in an arid environment), which manifests a high degree of organization, and which constrains permeating molecules to a long and convoluted pathway of absorption. These characteristics dictate the permeability of the membrane and determine the extent to which drugs of various physicochemical properties may be expected to transport.

8.2.3 Dermis and appendageal structures

The dermis, the inner and larger (90%) skin layer, comprises primarily connective tissue and provides support to the epidermis. The dermis incorporates blood and lymphatic vessels and nerve endings. The extensive microvasculature network found in the dermis represents the site of resorption for drugs absorbed across the epidermis; that is, it is at this point that transdermally absorbed molecules gain entry to the systemic circulation and access to their central targets. The dermis also supports skin's appendageal structures, specifically the hair follicles and sweat glands. With respect to drug delivery, interest in these structures has centered upon the possibility that they may provide "shunt" pathways across the skin, circumventing the need to cross the full stratum corneum. However, surface area considerations mean that the appendages cannot contribute significantly to the overall drug flux.

8.3   FACTORS AFFECTING TRANSDERMAL BIOAVAILABILITY

8.3.1   Physiological factors

8.3.1.1   *Stratum corneum*

This is the primary barrier to drug absorption across the skin. Transdermal bioavailability therefore and strategies to improve delivery often involve changing the composition or the organization of the intercellular lipids. Such enhancing technologies are of course feasible, but not without problems (see below).

There are situations for which the stratum corneum is not rate-determining. For very lipophilic compounds (say, those with octanol-water partition coefficients greater than 10^4), it is generally believed that transport is limited not by diffusion across the stratum corneum, but rather by the kinetics with which the molecule leaves this membrane and enters the underlying (and much more aqueous in nature) viable epidermis. Compounds exhibiting this behavior also manifest two other problems with respect to transdermal bioavailability. First, the "lag-time" observed prior to their appearance at useful levels in the blood may be significantly prolonged by the slow partitioning kinetics (see Figure 8.2). Second, these substances, because of their strong attraction for the lipophilic environment of the stratum corneum, often form significant reservoirs in the membrane from which release may continue even after removal of the delivery system.

8.3.1.2   *Anatomic site*

Dogma states that skin absorption "varies widely from site to site on the body". In fact, there is variability but, over most of the surface, this is not greater than the normal inter-individual variability observed at a specific site. Certain regions are significantly more permeable – the genitalia, especially the scrotum, the axilla, the face, the scalp, and post-auricularly. Indeed, these high-permeability sites have been used to optimize transdermal delivery of particular drugs: e.g. the first testosterone patch was designed to be worn on the scrotum; and the scopolamine system is placed behind the ear. However, room for manoeuvre is limited; most transdermal systems usually function equivalently at many different sites, and the recommended location usually depends primarily upon convenience (e.g. choosing a discreet site for an estradiol system) and/or psychology (e.g. placing a nitroglycerin patch over the heart).

8.3.1.3 Skin condition and disease

Changes in barrier function due to skin disease generally result either from alteration of the lipid/protein composition of the stratum corneum or from abnormal epidermal differentiation (e.g. in psoriasis). As far as transdermal bioavailability is concerned, however, patches intended for systemic therapy are labelled for application only at "normal" skin sites, free from dermatologic pathology.

8.3.1.4 Age

It is known that from soon after birth (assuming at-term) until early "old age", there is little change in the rate of transepidermal water loss across normal, intact skin. In older subjects, there are data pointing to changes in barrier function, but these are not dramatic when viewed in the context of typical variability across the entire population. What is perhaps more important is that as the skin ages, it becomes progressively more fragile (and therefore more sensitive to the removal of a well-adhered transdermal patch, for example) and requires a progressively longer period of time for recovery after injury. Thus, the chronic application of transdermal systems to elderly patients should be carefully monitored. It should also be noted that premature neonates, on the other hand, particularly those born at less than 30 weeks gestational age, have poorly developed barriers and are at risk for many problems including percutaneous intoxication due to inadvertent chemical absorption.

8.3.1.5 Skin metabolism

Presystemic metabolism in the skin can obviously modify transdermal drug bioavailability. The "cutaneous first-pass effect" for nitroglycerin, for example, has been estimated to be 15–20%. The viable epidermis is a biochemically active tissue with metabolic capability. Indeed, a multitude of enzymes have been identified in the skin, including a Cytochrome P450 system. However, the capacity of the viable epidermis below a transdermal patch to metabolize a delivered drug is limited (it must be remembered that nitroglycerin is an exceptionally sensitive compound, with a systemic half-life of only a few minutes), and the role of biodegradation is likely to be minor. Indeed, one of the advantages of transdermal delivery is avoidance of presystemic metabolism and an excellent illustration of this attribute is found with estradiol.

8.3.1.6 Desquamation

As stated above, the epidermis undergoes complete renewal every three weeks or so. This corresponds, therefore, to the shedding (or desquamation) of one layer of the stratum corneum per day. How does this affect drug bioavailability from a transdermal patch? Probably not too much for those systems designed for 24 hours of wear, but potentially more significant as the duration of patch wear is extended, because of problems of adhesion. That is, after one day, a transdermal system is attached primarily to a layer of skin which under normal circumstances would have fallen off and, as time progresses, the situation is likely to deteriorate.

8.3.1.7 Skin irritation and sensitization

A biological facet of skin's barrier function is that insult to the membrane is often, if not always, followed by an inflammatory response that is non-immunologic or immunologic (i.e. characterized broadly as a classic irritation or sensitization reactions). When a drug is a frank irritant, there is little to save its candidacy for transdermal delivery. Sensitization is an equally great problem, often made worse by the fact that it can be more difficult to uncover during transdermal patch development, becoming clear only when the system is used on a much larger patient population (e.g. clonidine). In the case of sensitization, however, progress with respect to the structure–activity relationships involved has been made allowing some measure of pre-screening to identify potential sensitizers.

8.3.2 Formulation factors

8.3.2.1 Physical chemistry of transport

Drug bioavailability depends upon both the rate and extent of absorption. Permeation through the stratum corneum occurs by passive diffusion, a process well described by Fick's 1st and 2nd laws. Consider the steady-state situation shown in Figure 8.2. Assume that the drug concentration in the formulation (C_v) is constant and that, on the other side of the membrane, "sink conditions" prevail (i.e. due to the efficient uptake of drug by the dermal microcirculation, the local concentration there (C_d) is much less than C_v, and hence (C_v -C_d) ~ C_v). At steady-state, the concentration gradient across the membrane is linear, Fick's 1st law of diffusion applies, and the flux ($J(t) = J = $ constant) is given by:

$$J = \{DK/h\}C_v = K_p C_v \qquad \text{(Equation 8.1)}$$

where D is the drug's apparent diffusivity in the stratum corneum, which we assume for the moment to be the rate-determining step for absorption, K is the stratum corneum–formulation partition coefficient of the drug, and h is the thickness of the barrier. K_p (= $D \cdot K/h$)[1] is defined as the drug's permeability coefficient across the skin from the formulation in question (note that K_p is formulation-dependent because it includes the applicable stratum corneum–formulation partition coefficient).

The role of the formulation, and that of the physicochemical properties of the drug, on transdermal bioavailability can now be readily appreciated because, at steady-state, there is a direct relationship between J and the plasma concentration (C_{ss}) achievable:

$$\text{Rate in} = A \, J = \text{Rate Out} = Cl \, C_{ss} \qquad \text{(Equation 8.2)}$$

---

1 Note, K_p here is described elsewhere as P, the permeability constant, in the discussion of Ficks law of diffusion (see for example section 1.3.3.1).

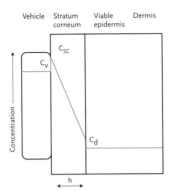

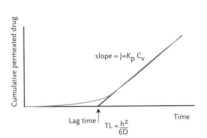

Figure 8.2 The steady-state concentration profile of a drug across the skin following application of a vehicle in which the concentration of the active agent is C_v (left panel). The discontinuity at the vehicle–SC interface indicates that the drug favors the SC over the vehicle; the ratio C_{sc}/C_v equals the drug's SC-vehicle partition coefficient (K). The linear profile across the SC, of thickness h, is described by Fick's 1st law of diffusion, and the steady-state flux per unit area, $J = K_p C_v$, where $K_p = K D/h$ and D is the drug's diffusivity across the barrier. The diagram on the right shows the cumulative amount per unit area of drug arriving in the viable epidermis as a function of time. At times shortly after application of the vehicle, very little drug has reached this layer because the molecules are diffusing across the SC and establishing the concentration profile. Eventually, once the linear gradient is established, the amount permeating per unit time becomes constant, and Fick's 1st law applies. The slope of the line equals J. Extrapolation of the linear part of the curve to the x-axis intercept yields the so-called lag-time (see text)

where Cl is the drug's clearance. It follows that J, which depends upon two parameters linked to the properties of the formulation and of the drug (i.e. K_p and C_v), directly determines whether the target plasma concentration is attainable or not when the area of contact between the delivery system and the skin (A) is reasonable.

The flux can be maximized by manipulating C_v and/or K. The most straightforward approach is to maximize C_v, i.e. to use a formulation saturated with the drug. One must be careful, however, to ensure that the formulation, under these conditions, has appropriate stability. The partition coefficient is a little trickier, since here one really wants to formulate the drug so that its affinity for the stratum corneum is much greater than that for the vehicle. The risk is that one might find oneself in a situation where the drug loading in the formulation is insufficient to provide delivery for the length of time desired (i.e. if one makes the drug dislike the formulation so much, its solubility therein may be quite low). So, one has to strike a balance between K and C_v so that the leaving tendency of the drug from the formulation favors its efficient movement into the skin, but that the saturation solubility of the drug in the vehicle is high enough that sustained delivery can be achieved for the intended time of application.

It should be pointed out that, under ideal conditions (specifically, when there is no interaction between the formulation and the stratum corneum), all formulations which are saturated with a particular drug will produce the identical steady-state, and maximal flux (J_{max}) across the skin. This is because, under these conditions, the gradient of the chemical potential of the drug across the skin is the same, and it is this gradient that determines the flux. Simplistically, we can understand this phenomenon in the following way: the partition coefficient of the drug between the stratum corneum and the vehicle is the ratio of its concentrations in the two phases at equilibrium. At this point, the thermodynamic activity of the drug in the stratum corneum exactly equals that in the vehicle. If the formulation is saturated with the drug then, at equilibrium, the drug concentration in the stratum corneum will also arrive at its saturation value ($C_{sc,sat}$) in that phase and the partition coefficient is given by:

$$K = C_{sc,sat}/C_{v, sat} \qquad \text{(Equation 8.3)}$$

Substitution of Equation 8.3 into Equation 8.2, when $C_v = C_{v, sat}$ yields:

$$J = J_{max} = (D/h) (C_{sc,sat}/C_{v, sat}) C_{v, sat} = (D/h) C_{sc,sat} \quad \text{(Equation 8.4)}$$

from which it is clear that J_{max} is independent of the vehicle.

With respect to the physicochemical properties of the drug, lipophilicity and molecular size are the dominant determinants of the stratum corneum permeability coefficient (via, respectively, their impact upon K and D). Lipophilicity is a key feature for drug "acceptance" by the stratum corneum, and the current transdermally delivered drugs have log octanol-water partition coefficients (Table 8.1) in the range of 0.8–3.3. The stratum corneum is not a welcoming environment for either very polar or charged substances, and the percutaneous penetration of such species is usually so low as to preclude their useful passive delivery. However, excessive lipophilicity is problematic too, since successful transport into the systemic circulation (or even into viable cellular targets in the skin for dermatological therapy) requires that the drug partition from the stratum corneum into the aqueous, underlying epidermal layers. Thus, in order that this "phase transfer" not become rate-limiting, it is important that the drug have at least some degree of aqueous solubility (otherwise it has to be extremely potent such that it can elicit a pharmacological effect at a very low concentration at the site of action).

Drug diffusivity, in general, is size-dependent, i.e. large molecules diffuse more slowly than small ones. It is to be noted that the existing transdermal drugs all have MW < 350 Da (Table 8.1). It must also be realized that there is a relationship, at least for conventional drug molecules, between K (oil-water) and MW – specifically, as MW increases, it is quite usual that K also increases (since, typically, molecules are made larger by adding -CH_2-groups or aliphatic or aromatic rings, etc.). It follows that, in terms of the permeability coefficient, K and MW act in opposite ways – that is, increased lipophilicity means an increasing effect on K_p, whereas increasing MW has the opposite effect. A practical result of this observation is that small polar compounds often have better permeabilities than might be expected, based only on

Table 8.1
Physicochemical and pharmacokinetic properties of transdermally administered drugs

Drug	MW	log $K_{o/w}$[a]	Cl[b] (L/h)	$t_{1/2}$[c] (h)	Oral bioavailability (%)	Efficacious blood level (ng/mL)
Scopolamine[d]	303	1.24	67.2	2.9	27	0.04
Clonidine[d]	230	0.83	13	6–20	95	0.2–2.0
Nitroglycerine	227	2.05	966	0.04	< 1	1.2–11.0
Estradiol	272	2.49	615–790	0.05	–	0.04–0.06
Fentanyl[d]	337	2.93	27–75	3–12	32	1
Nicotine	162	–	77.7	2	30	10–30
Testosterone	288	3.31	–	–	< 1	10–100

[a] Octanol–water partition coefficients
[b] Total clearance
[c] Biological half–life
[d] Base form of the drug

their lipophilicity, because of the compensation from a rather high diffusivity.

An additional ramification of the size-dependence of the diffusion coefficient is the question of the time necessary post-application of a transdermal system for the target plasma concentration to be attained. While this may be determined, at least in part, by the elimination kinetics of the drug from the body, for compounds of relatively short biological half-life (a characteristic of most of the drugs presently given by the transdermal route), this "lag-time" is usually the result of slow diffusion across the stratum corneum. That is, a certain time is required to establish the necessary concentration gradient across the barrier membrane (Figure 8.2). The classical diffusional lag-time (T_L) is defined as: $T_L = h^2/6D$. T_L is about one-third of the time required to set up a linear concentration profile across the stratum corneum. Given that D is inversely dependent upon the drug's molecular size, it follows that T_L is longer for compounds of higher molecular weight.

8.4 ADVANTAGES AND DISADVANTAGES OF TRANSDERMAL DRUG DELIVERY

8.4.1 Advantages

The positive features of delivering drugs across the skin to achieve systemic effect are:

- Avoidance of significant presystemic metabolism (for example, that due to degradation in the gastrointestinal tract or by the liver), and the need, therefore, for a lower daily dose.
- Reduced inter- and intra-patient variability – this is particularly true for those situations in which drug release from the transdermal patch is slower than drug diffusion across the stratum corneum.
- Drug levels can be maintained in the systemic circulation, within the therapeutic window (i.e. above the minimum effective concentration, but below the level at which side-effects become apparent), for prolonged periods of time.
- Thus, the duration of drug action following a single administration of the drug can be extended, and the frequency of dosing reduced.
- Improved patient compliance and acceptability of the drug therapy.
- Drug input can be terminated simply by removal of the patch.

8.4.2 Disadvantages

The limitations of transdermal drug delivery are principally associated with the skin's barrier function, which severely constrains the absolute amount of a drug that can be absorbed across a reasonable area of skin during a dosing period. Thus, the major disadvantage of the method is that it is limited only to potent drug molecules, typically those requiring a daily dose on the order of 10 mg or less. Usually, this translates into drugs with effective plasma concentrations in the ng mL^{-1} (or lower) range.

Even if the drug is sufficiently potent, it must yet satisfy other criteria to be considered a viable candidate for transdermal delivery. First, its physicochemical properties must allow it to be absorbed percutaneously. This means that its molecular weight should be reasonable (see above), and that it should have adequate solubility in both lipophilic and aqueous environments since, to reach the dermal micro-circulation and gain access to the systemic circulation, the molecule must cross the stratum corneum (a lipoidal barrier) and then transfer through the much-more-aqueous-in-nature viable epidermis and upper dermis. Absence of either oil or water solubility will preclude permeation at a useful rate.

Second, the pharmacokinetic and pharmacodynamic characteristics of the drug must be such that the relatively sustained and slow input provided by transdermal delivery makes sense. Tolerance-inducing compounds, for example, are not an intelligent choice for this mode of administration unless an appropriate "wash-out" period is programmed into the dosing regimen (see the discussion of nitroglycerin below). Drugs with short biological half-lives, that are subject to large first-pass metabolism, necessitating inconvenient and frequent oral or parenteral dosing (with the concomitant problems of side-effects and poor compliance), are good candidates. On the other hand, drugs that can be given orally once a day, with reproducible bioavailability, and which are well tolerated by the patient, do not really need a patch formulation.

Third, the drug must not be locally irritating or sensitizing, since provocation of significant skin reactions beneath a transdermal delivery system will most likely prevent its regulatory approval.

8.5   CURRENT TECHNOLOGIES FOR TRANSDERMAL DRUG DELIVERY

8.5.1   Conventional dosage forms

The use of conventional topical formulations for transdermal drug delivery is presently limited to classic ointments for nitroglycerin, and some gel formulations of estradiol and progesterone. Although of demonstrated efficacy, these vehicles are often inelegant and result in poor reproducibility of the delivered dose (and hence of the provoked pharmacological effect). This variability, of course, originates in the application procedure: the amount of formulation applied, the area to which it is applied, the amount of inunction used, and the potential for subsequent depletion to clothing, etc., all contributing to the observed inconsistency in dosage control. There is a concern, furthermore, about the inadvertent transfer of material from the treated individual to another person via bodily contact. On the other hand, these conventional delivery systems are relatively simple and inexpensive to manufacture.

8.5.2 Transdermal delivery systems

The seven drugs and the combination estrogen–progestin product presently approved in the US for delivery by the transdermal route were all well known and available in more conventional dosage forms before their formulation into "skin patches". All of these drugs are extremely potent, none requiring more than about 20 mg per day (and some, much less) for effective therapy.

8.5.2.1 *Transdermal patch design, composition and manufacture*

There is a wide variety of transdermal systems on the market at present. These patches are diversely referred to as "reservoir", "monolithic", "membrane-controlled", "adhesive", "matrix", and so on. Unfortunately, these terms are not always used consistently and, worse, they are sometimes used inaccurately. In all cases, however, the idea is that the system offers a means to hold a "payload" of the drug and a configuration (or "platform") to ensure presentation of the active agent to the skin surface at a rate sufficient to ensure a systemic pharmacological effect after the drug has crossed the skin's barrier. Most simplistically, one can divide the transdermal formulations presently available into three categories (Figure 8.3):

- adhesive systems,
- layered systems, and
- reservoir systems.

Upon removal from their package, all these devices present common exterior surfaces. On one side, they have an impermeable backing layer across which neither the drug nor any other component can diffuse. On the other face which will contact the skin, there is a peel strip which is removed prior to application. In between these two layers, however, the composition and design of the device varies considerably.

Adhesive patches

The adhesive patches are simplest in concept, consisting only of a layer of drug-containing adhesive polymer which serves, therefore, as a

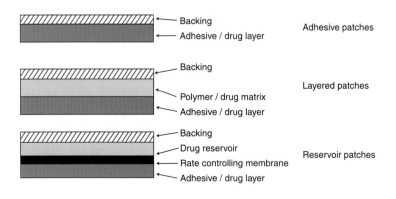

Figure 8.3 Schematic diagrams of the three main categories of transdermal delivery system. It should be noted that these representations of the patches greatly exaggerate their real thicknesses, which are in fact similar to that of a normal Band-Aid

reservoir of the compound and the means by which the device is held to the skin. These systems can hold substantial amounts of the active agent, often in considerable excess of that delivered during the designated application of the patch (e.g., the Nitrodur device for nitroglycerin). Not infrequently, the degree of control offered by these systems is relatively small (see below), and it is the stratum corneum that ultimately regulates the absorption rate of the drug into the body.

Layered patches

The layered devices are a little more complex than the simple adhesive systems in that they use different polymer compositions or different polymers to provide the functions of drug-containing matrix and adhesive. (For a detailed discussion of drug release for matrix systems, see chapter 4.) The matrix "layer" may consist of more than a single sub-layer, with drug loading in the different layers adjusted to optimize the ultimate delivery characteristics. It should also be noted that some layered systems have been developed in which the drug-containing matrix contacts the skin directly and the patch is held to the skin by a peripheral adhesive. While effective, these devices suffer from the drawback that the area of contact between patch and skin is significantly greater than the "active" area, i.e. the area through which drug is actually delivered.

Reservoir patches

The reservoir systems were pioneered by Alza Corporation, who have been involved in the development of transdermal patches for each drug presently marketed in the US. These devices are characterized by two particular features: first, an enclosed reservoir of the drug, which may be liquid in nature; and, second, a polymeric membrane separating the reservoir from the adhesive layer, itself made from a different polymer. The idea, naturally, behind this design is that the membrane acts as a rate-controlling element for drug delivery to and across the skin (i.e. that transfer of drug through the membrane is slower than drug diffusion across the stratum corneum) – indeed, the membrane in such reservoir devices is frequently called the "rate-controlling membrane". There are, in fact, situations for which this claim is true; however, it must also be noted that there are others where the control lies, at least in part, elsewhere (see below).

The essential components of a transdermal system are the drug, one or more polymers, the "vehicle", and other excipient(s). Polymers are used in transdermals as pressure-sensitive adhesives, release liners, backings and laminates, and for speciality films and supports. A pressure-sensitive adhesive may be defined as a solvent-free, permanently tacky, viscoelastic substance, capable of adhering instantaneously to most solid surfaces with application of slight pressure, and removable without leaving perceptible residue. Typically, pressure-sensitive adhesives are acrylate, silicone or rubber-based. Release liners are usually silicone and fluorocarbon coatings on paper, polyester or poly-carbonate films. Backing and other membranes are fabricated with diverse polymers including ethylene vinyl acetate, polypropylene, polyester, polyethylene, polyisobutylene and polyvinyl chloride. Special films in current use include foams, non-wovens, micro-porous membranes, etc. In cases where the drug is not dissolved in one or more polymer layer (i.e. in the reservoir devices, or certain matrix systems with a peripheral adhesive), the "vehicles" used are mineral oil, isopropyl myristate, isopropyl palmitate, poly (ethylene glycol), glycerin, water, ethanol and silicone oil. Additional excipients, present for stability and other purposes, may be lactose, silicon dioxide, cross-linking agents, and hydroxyethylcellulose.

The manufacture of a transdermal drug delivery system is a complex and sophisticated process requiring specialized equipment and facilities. In the most basic and generic sense, two procedures can be identified, one for "solid-state" patches (adhesive and layered systems), the other for reservoir devices. In the former case, the import-ant steps are: (a) Mixing of drug, excipients, polymers and solvent to make a coating solution (or solutions). (b) Casting the coating solu-tion(s) onto the protective liner, evaporating the solvent, and laminat-ing the backing film. (c) Die-cutting the drug laminate to the desired patch size. (d) Packaging. For reservoir systems, the components of the reservoir (drug, excipients, viscous liquid) are first mixed. Separately, the adhesive polymers and solvent are mixed to make a solution, which is then cast onto a protective liner. The solvent is evaporated and the membrane is laminated onto the adhesive. The system is then assembled by forming the backing film, pumping in the drug reser-voir, and then heat-sealing the laminate to the backing. The patch is then die-cut and packaged.

8.5.2.2 *Rate-control in transdermal delivery*

One of the obvious goals of using the skin as a route of drug adminis-tration is to eliminate or reduce, as far as possible, pharmacokinetic (and hence pharmacodynamic) variability due to inter- and intra-subject differences in absorption. That is, if the delivery system truly controls the rate of absorption of drug into the body, then only the variability in clearance remains as a factor to influence the resulting plasma concentration achieved (Equation 8.2). Given, however, that there now exist on the market many different patches for one specific drug, all of which are approved for the same therapeutic indication (and the same delivered dose), it is appropriate to ask to what extent does the control of delivery rest with the patch as opposed to the skin. To illustrate this point, consider three of the presently marketed nitro-glycerin systems that are labeled to deliver drug at 0.4 mg/hr, Nitrodur (an adhesive device), Deponit (a layered patch) and Transderm-Nitro (a reservoir system)(Table 8.2).

First of all, it should be noted that, despite the differences in design, drug loading and surface area, these patches are considered to be bio-equivalent. Thus, one cannot use drug content nor mechanism of release as useful parameters with which to assess the comparability of different transdermal systems (by contrast, for oral delivery, a generic

Table 8.2	System	Drug content (mg)	Area (cm²)	Delivery rate (mg/hr)
Characteristics of three approved transdermal nitroglycerin delivery systems	Nitrodur	80	20	0.4
	Deponit	32	32	0.4
	Transderm-Nitro	50	20	0.4

tablet must by definition contain the same drug quantity as the market standard in order to be considered for bioequivalency).

So, do these three patches all control delivery into the body, or not? To address this issue, two very simple experiments can be performed. In the first (Experiment A), drug release from the patch directly into an aqueous receptor solution is measured as a function of time; one can think of this experiment as a model for the release of drug into the body across an area of skin that has no stratum corneum (i.e. no barrier function). In the second (Experiment B), drug release into the same aqueous receptor is again measured, but now the skin is interposed between the patch and the receiver medium. If the patch is perfectly rate-controlling, the rates of appearance of drug into the receptor phase in the two experiments will be identical. On the other hand, if the drug arrives more slowly in Experiment B than in Experiment A, it can be concluded that the skin is playing at least some role in controlling the drug's flux into the body. The results of these experiments for the three nitroglycerin patches are shown in Figure 8.4. It is immediately apparent that the release of drug from Nitrodur is much greater in the absence of skin than when skin is present (compare nearly 76 mg released in Experiment A in 24 hours with 10 mg released in Experiment B). By contrast, for Deponit, the amounts reaching the receptor phase in 24 hours in Experiments A and B are quite similar, about 11 and 10 mg, respectively. Transderm-Nitro falls in between, with ~22 mg released in Experiment A, compared to 10 mg in Experiment B. Notice that all three systems deliver on the order of 0.4 mg/hr (~10 mg/day), as labeled, when applied to intact skin. However, the differences between the amounts released in Experiment A clearly reveal that the degree to which each patch controls transport

Figure 8.4 The results of two experiments designed to determine the relative degree to which transdermal nitroglycerin systems control delivery into the body. In left panel, drug release from the patch into an aqueous receptor is measured ("Experiment A"). In the right panel ("Experiment B") the transport kinetics are re-assessed when excised skin is interposed between the patch and the receiving medium (Modified from Hadgraft J. *et al.*; *Int. J. Pharm.*, 73 (1991) 125–130)

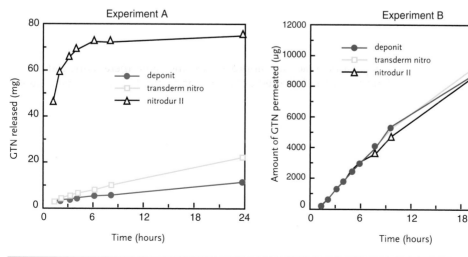

across the skin is different. In fact, the Deponit device exerts considerable control over the input rate of nitroglycerin (nearly 90% patch control), whereas Nitrodur lets the natural barrier function of the skin determine drug absorption into the systemic circulation (approximately 90% skin control). For Transderm-Nitro, despite the presence of the so-called "rate-controlling" membrane, the responsibility for metering the delivery is, on average, shared between patch and skin.

How does Deponit achieve the major share of the control of drug delivery? The answer lies simply in the surface area of the different systems. The maximum rate that nitroglycerin can diffuse across intact human skin is on the order of 20 $\mu g/cm^2/hr$. Hence, if the target delivery rate is 0.4 mg/hr (i.e. 400 $\mu g/hr$), then a minimum surface area of about 20 cm^2 is required. However, this does not leave much chance to build a rate-controlling element into the patch, since one needs the maximum flux possible across the skin (i.e. the drug must be presented at its maximum thermodynamic activity) to reach the target plasma concentration. This is the Nitrodur solution to the challenge. On the other hand, if a larger surface area is used (say 40 cm^2), then rate-control can be an integral part of the patch such that nitroglycerin is presented to the skin at only 10 $\mu g/cm^2/hr$. The target rate of 0.4 mg/hr is still met, but now it is the patch exerting control over delivery, not the skin. This is the Deponit strategy.

In conclusion, it is evident that transdermal delivery is very much determined by the area of contact between patch and skin. Indeed, dose titration with transdermal delivery is achieved not by altering the formulation but rather by adjusting the size of the system (Figure 8.5). It is also apparent that delivery is not particularly sensitive to the loading of the patch, especially when the input rate is controlled by the skin. The loading does need to be sufficient, however, to ensure that delivery is maintained for the desired period, and to sustain a diffu-

Figure 8.5 Linear relationships between the steady-state plasma concentrations achieved and the active surface areas of the transdermal drug delivery systems applied (Modified from MacGregor *et al., Clin. Pharmacol. Ther.* 38 (1978) 278; Good W.R. *et al., Drug Dev. Ind. Pharm.* 9 (1983) 647–670; McLeskey, C., *et al.;* American Society of Anesthesiology Annual Meeting, 1989)

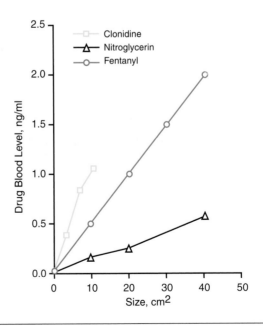

sional driving force. Next, it must be emphasized that the design of the patch does not necessarily guarantee that it will control the overall delivery (for example, the presence of a membrane in a reservoir system does not ensure 100% control by the patch). Thus, drug loading and the mechanism of drug release from a transdermal delivery system are *inappropriate* measures for bioequivalence assessment. Finally, it is worth noting that the discussion of rate-control as presented is most applicable during the period of what might be termed "steady-state" delivery. Clearly, at the early stages of drug delivery (i.e. just after patch application), control rests more or less entirely with skin and the only resistance encountered by the first molecules to cross the stratum corneum is the membrane's diffusional barrier. In other words, as the patch is applied there are drug molecules waiting at the external surface of the adhesive that become instantaneously available for transport. At the opposite extreme, if a patch remains in contact with the skin for sufficient time that the drug loading is almost completely depleted then, at this point, delivery control is fully in the hands of the patch (i.e. the concentration gradient is so small that the release of drug from the patch must now be much less than its transport rate across the stratum corneum). Of course, with almost all the systems presently used, this situation does not arise as the designated application is such that significant amounts of the "payload" remain in the device when it is replaced with a fresh system. However, it is not inconceivable that such depleting systems may become more common in the future, especially for drug substances which are exquisitely potent or expensive or potentially subject to abuse.

Scopolamine

Scopolamine was the first drug to be marketed as a transdermal delivery system (Transderm-Scop) to alleviate the discomfort of motion sickness. After oral administration, scopolamine has a short duration of action because of a high first-pass effect. In addition, several side-effects are associated with the peak plasma levels obtained. Transderm-Scop is a reservoir system that incorporates two types of release mechanims: a rapid, short-term release of drug from the adhesive layer, superimposed on an essentially zero-order input profile metered by the microporous membrane separating the reservoir from the skin surface. The scopolamine patch is able to maintain plasma levels in the therapeutic window for extended periods of time, delivering 0.5 mg over 3 days with few of the side-effects associated with (for example) oral administration.

Nitroglycerin

This drug has been used to treat angina pectoris for over 100 years. It is a potent compound with a high clearance (266 L/hr), short half-life (1–4 minutes) and extremely low oral bioavailability (<1%). Percutaneous transport of nitroglycerin is relatively efficient, and conventional ointment formulations were the first modern-day transdermal formulations available. In the early 1980s, however, three patches appeared more or less simultaneously (Transderm-Nitro NitroDisc,

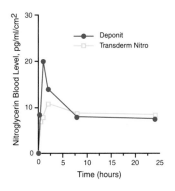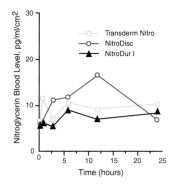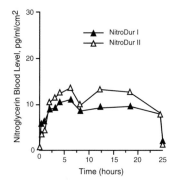

and NitroDur), and transdermal delivery became widely recognized as an alternative route of administration for appropriate drugs. Since that time, numerous new and modified patches have been approved which differ considerably in design, composition, drug loading and release mechanism. Nevertheless, it is possible to demonstrate a bio-equivalence between these patches, in terms of the resulting plasma concentration versus time profiles (Figure 8.6). When nitroglycerin is delivered via the skin, a sustained concentration can be achieved over an extended period of time. This profile contrasts sharply with those obtained following administration of sublingual and ointment dosage forms. Despite this apparently clear pharmacokinetic advantage, however, it turns out that zero-order delivery of nitroglycerin for 24 hours, on a chronic basis, poses a pharmacodynamic problem: namely, tolerance. That is, even though the delivered amount of drug per unit time remains constant, the pharmacological effect of the drug decreases progressively, to the point that there is essentially no benefit to the patient. The problem is resolved by imposing a drug-free period during each dosing interval of 24 hours. Thus, presently, the patches are applied in the morning, after showering, and worn for 12–16 hours, with a "resting" or wash-out period overnight when patients are less susceptible (although not immune) to angina attacks.

Clonidine

Clonidine is a potent antihypertensive agent which is well absorbed from the GI tract (95%). The drug has a relatively long half-life (6–20 h) and a modest clearance (13 L h^{-1}). The rationale for the development of transdermal clonidine was to reduce side-effects and to improve patient compliance. Catapres-TTS, a reservoir-type patch, reached the market in 1985 in a form designed to remain in place and to deliver drug for 7 days. Dose titration was possible via the use of systems of different active areas (3.5, 7.0, and 10.5 cm^2). The control of drug delivery over 7 days is impressive, and avoids the "peaks and valleys" of conventional (twice-a-day) oral administration (Figure 8.7). However, this system has not achieved as wide a success as first seemed likely because of skin sensitization. Clonidine itself, when administered transdermally on a chronic, repetitive basis, induces in a significant fraction of patients a classic immunologic skin reaction, and this has severely attenuated its use.

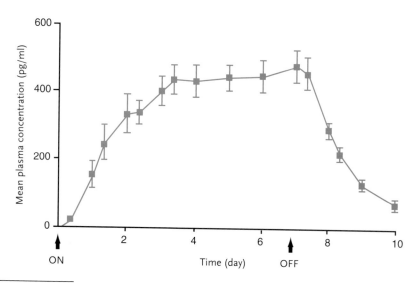

Figure 8.7 Plasma concentration of clonidine versus time profile during and subsequent to the 7-day application of a 5 cm^2 Catapres-TTS patch (Modified from Knepp, V.M.; Hadgraft, J. and Guy, R.H. (1987) *CRC Critical Reviews in Therapeutic Drug Carrier Systems.* **4**, 13–37)

Estradiol

Transdermal estradiol is indicated for postmenopausal hormone replacement therapy. Estradiol is a potent, high clearance (600–800 L/hr) and short half-life (1 hr) drug. Due to the very high hepatic first-pass effect, conventional oral hormone replacement therapy results in an artificially elevated and, in the long term, therapeutically unfavorable ratio of estrone (the major metabolite of estradiol) to the drug itself – the normal (i.e. premenopausal) ratio of estrone to estradiol is about 1. Transdermal delivery of estradiol, however, results in sustained plasma concentrations over several days (Figure 8.8) and allows normalization of the estrone to estradiol ratio. Pharmacologically, beneficial effects on the frequency of hot flushes, sleep disturbance, irritability and mental accuity have been documented. The first patch approved was a reservoir system worn over 3–4 days. More recently, other simpler, and more elegant, monolithic systems have reached the market, and perform as well as, if not better than, the original system.

Because the postmenopausal woman is usually treated concomitantly with an oral progestin (i.e. in addition to the need for estrogen replacement), there have been, and continue to be, attempts to formulate a combination estrogen–progestin patch. One of the first of these systems containing estradiol and levonorgestrel has recently been approved for marketing.

Fentanyl

This very powerful analgesic had been limited to parenteral use during and after surgery. Accurate dose titration is necessary because of the drug's very narrow therapeutic window (1–2 ng mL^{-1}). The potential of fentanyl, however, to significantly improve the treatment of acute post-operative pain and chronic cancer pain provoked the development of the now-approved Duragesic transdermal system. This reservoir system can be used for up to 3 days and is available in

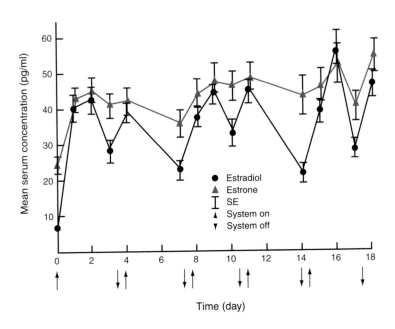

Figure 8.8 Serum levels of estradiol and its major metabolite, estrone, during the continuous wearing of consecutively-applied transdermal systems (Ciba-Geigy, 0.05 mg/day) (Modified from *Topical Drug Bioavailability, Bioequivalence, and Penetration* (Shah, V.P. and Maibach, H.I. eds). Plenum Press, New York, 1993, pp. 17–68)

four "doses" (10, 20, 30 and 40 cm^2 delivering, respectively, 25, 50, 75 and 100 μg hr^{-1}).

Nicotine

Nicotine is generally believed to be the principal addictive component in tobacco. Patches containing nicotine are targeted at smoking cessation and compete with other nicotine-based systems, including chewing gum, lozenges and a nasal spray. Nicotine has a relatively short half-life (2 hr) and high clearance (78 L hr^{-1}), which means that nicotine replacement via the gum, for example, requires almost constant chewing of about 10 pieces per day to match the bioavailability of the "drug" achieved by smoking one cigarette per hour. Transdermal delivery, therefore, was designed to provide sustained input over the course of 24 hours (or, in the case of one system, for ~16 hours – the argument being that not even the heaviest smoker lights up when asleep!). Several patches reached the market (such as Nicotrol, Nicoderm, Prostep and Habitrol) representing examples of each of the basic system designs, and all of which are pharmacokinetically bioequivalent. There are differences, though, in the degree of irritation induced by the different patches and this seems to be related to the relative thermodynamic activity of nicotine in the different systems. Drug loading also varies appreciably between the different patches, as does the efficiency of drug usage. Short-term efficacy has been established by showing that the use of the patches reduces tobacco withdrawal symptoms and increases abstinence. Longer-term studies reveal that the patches can be effective but require supplemental pyschological and motivational aid and counseling to minimize the chances that a subject returns to smoking. Recently, in many countries, nicotine patches have become available "over the counter" without a prescription.

Testosterone

These patches (Testoderm, Testoderm with Adhesive, and Androderm) are approved for the treatment of hormonal insufficiency in diseases such as primary hypogonadism and hypogonadotropic hypogonadism. The systems are applied daily to mimic the endogenous profile of serum testosterone in the normal male. Testoderm (4 mg and 6 mg) and Testoderm with Adhesive (6 mg) release controlled amounts of testosterone upon daily application to scrotal skin. These systems have contact areas of 40 or 60 cm^2, and contain 10 and 15 mg of testosterone, respectively. The matrix system, Androderm, also provides continuous delivery of testosterone for 24 hours, but is applied to non-scrotal skin. Permeation enhancers are essential for this patch to ensure the efficient delivery of drug through skin sites which are less permeable than scrotal skin. However, these adjuvants significantly increase the incidence of irritation. The Androderm systems have a central drug delivery reservoir surrounded by a peripheral adhesive and are available in doses of 2.5 mg and 5 mg. The smaller system has an active area of 7.5 cm^2 (total area 44.5 cm^2) and a drug loading of 12.2 mg. The larger patch (15 cm^2 active area, 59 cm^2 in total) contains 24.3 mg of testosterone upon application.

These testosterone systems illustrate two different approaches to solve the problem of inadequate percutaneous absorption rate. In the former case, the patch must be applied to the body's most permeable skin site, the scrotum (which has been shown to be at least five times more permeable than any other site). In the latter, the difficulty is resolved by creating a transdermal formulation which includes excipients to reduce barrier function. Neither solution is ideal: scrotal application is clearly not preferred from a patient compliance standpoint; on the other hand, permeation enhancers, by their very nature, tend to be irritating (and the more effective they are, the greater the irritation they provoke). This general problem, which presently limits the application of transdermal delivery, is now discussed in more detail.

8.5.3   The need for penetration enhancement

Consider a drug candidate for transdermal delivery. The effective steady-state concentration of the drug is C_{ss} (mg cm^{-3}) and its systemic clearance is Cl (cm^3 hr^{-1}). It follows that the required transdermal input rate (R mg hr^{-1}) is:

$$R = Cl\, C_{ss} \qquad \text{(Equation 8.5)}$$

Assuming that zero-order input is acceptable for this drug, then:

$$R = A\, k_o \qquad \text{(Equation 8.6)}$$

Drug	Cl (L/hr)	C_{ss} (µg/mL)	A_{min} (cm^2)
Acetaminophen	23	15	13,850
Cimetidine	49	1.0	1,940
Clonidine	12	0.001	0.48
Digoxin	6.8	0.002	0.54
Estradiol	67	0.0001	0.27
Indomethacin	9	0.5	181
Isosorbide dinitrate	175	0.001	7.0
Nitroglycerin	4,210	0.0001	17
Propranolol	49	0.02	39
Scopolamine	43	0.0002	0.35

Table 8.3 "Transdermal feasibility" screen for representative drugs

where A (cm^2) is the area of the delivery system and k_o (μg cm^{-2} hr^{-1}) is the steady-state delivery rate into the body. Ideally, A is relatively small (say 50 cm^2 or less) and k_o is determined by the device and is less than the maximum drug flux (J_{max}) possible across intact stratum corneum. However, the latter (i.e. $k_o < J_{max}$) is not generally the case and C_{ss} cannot be attained without an unacceptably large skin surface being covered. This point is illustrated in Table 8.3, where a "feasibility screen" has been conducted for a number of well-known drugs. Their clearance values and target steady-state plasma concentrations have been taken from the literature, and it has been assumed that, for each compound, a steady-state delivery rate (k_o) into the body of 25 μg cm^{-2} hr^{-1} can be achieved. Of course, for many compounds, such a high flux (which is typical only for such rapidly permeating drugs as nitroglycerin and nicotine) is completely unrealistic. As can be seen by the resulting estimations of the minimum patch area (A_{min}) necessary to arrive at the target blood concentration (determined using Equations 8.5 and 8.6), even with the artificially elevated value of k_o proposed, only a handful of drugs are reasonable candidates (for example, an acetaminophen patch would have to cover nearly the entire surface of the adult body in order to alleviate a mild headache!). Consequently, considerable effort is being directed at approaches to increase J_{max}, i.e. to reduce the stratum corneum (skin) barrier function to the extent that: (a) an effective dose can be delivered from a patch of reasonable size, and (b) the delivery system maintains input rate control.

By what means can a chemical cause enhanced percutaneous absorption? Possibilities include:

- increasing the amount of drug in the vehicle and hence increasing the total delivered dose from a single application (but this does not necessarily mean that the *rate* of absorption is enhanced);
- increasing drug solubility in the stratum corneum, i.e. facilitating partitioning of drug from the vehicle into the skin;
- reducing the diffusional barrier of the stratum corneum by either perturbing the intercellular lipid domains, or perturbing the intracellular keratin networks, or amplifying transport via the

appendages (sweat glands, follicles), or by combinations of two or more of the above; and

- promoting drug partitioning at the stratum corneum/viable tissue interface.

8.6 NEW AND EVOLVING TECHNOLOGIES FOR TRANSDERMAL DRUG DELIVERY

8.6.1 Chemical penetration enhancers

The following criteria have been proposed for a successful penetration enhancer. It should:

- elicit no pharmacological effect;
- be specific in its action;
- act quickly, with a predictable duration, and its action should be reversible;
- be chemically and physically stable, and be compatible with all components of the drug delivery system;
- be odorless and colorless;

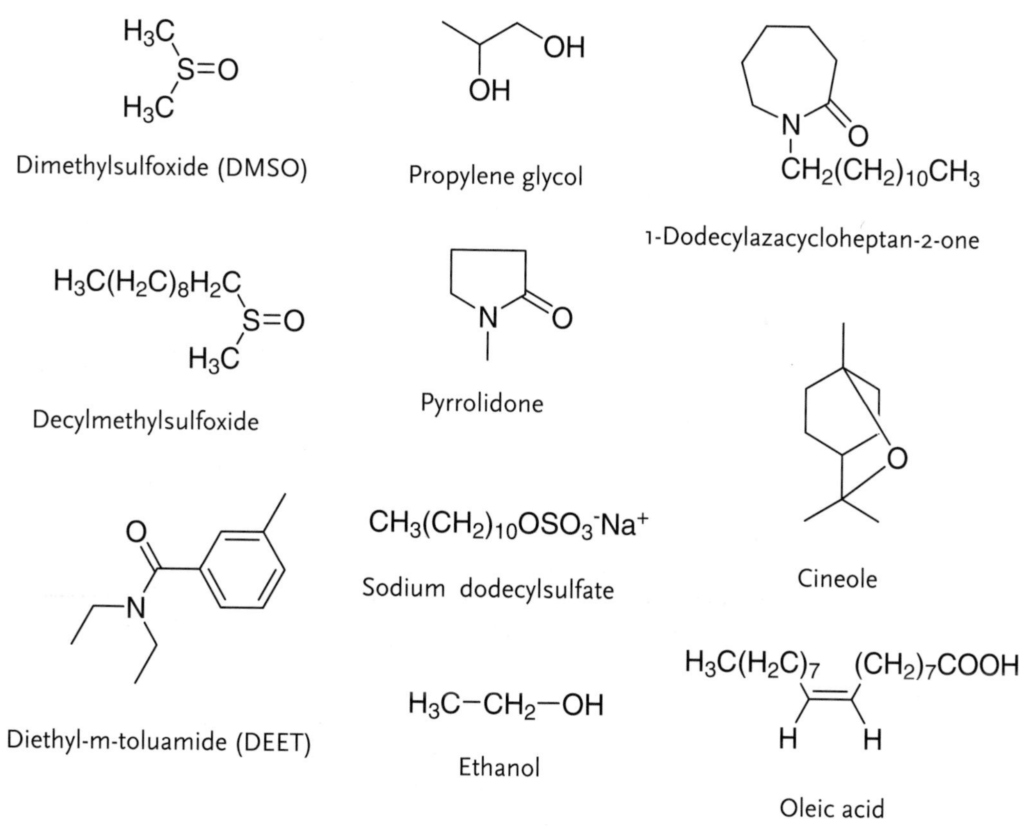

Figure 8.9 Structures of selected chemical penetration enhancers

Dimethylsulfoxide (DMSO)

Propylene glycol

1-Dodecylazacycloheptan-2-one

Decylmethylsulfoxide

Pyrrolidone

$CH_3(CH_2)_{10}OSO_3^-Na^+$

Sodium dodecylsulfate

Cineole

Diethyl-m-toluamide (DEET)

H_3C-CH_2-OH

Ethanol

Oleic acid

- be non-toxic, non-allergenic and non-irritating.

These stringent requirements are demonstrated by few chemicals other than water. It remains to be seen to what extent the limitations can be relaxed for a chemical promoter to be acceptable (to patients and to the regulatory authorities). Enhancers include a wide range of chemical entities that increase skin permeability (Figure 8.9), such as sulphoxides, alcohols, polyols, pyrrolidones, alkanes, fatty acids, esters, amines and amides, terpenes, surfactants, cyclodextrins, water, etc.

Outstanding issues which need to be resolved include questions about the mechanism of action of the different enhancers in use at present, and the reversibility of their effects *in vivo*. The question: "Is it possible to impair the SC without irritating the skin?" needs to be seriously addressed, as does skin toxicity of theses substances, in general. The synergism of enhancer (e.g. surfactant) and co-solvent (e.g. propylene glycol, ethanol) has been observed and established, but is not fully understood, nor has it been optimized, with respect to the most effective concentration(s) to be used. Regulatory acceptance must also be considered. Regulatory approval within the United States for an enhancer known as Azone proved to be extremely difficult because, as a *new* chemical developed specifically for skin permeation enhancement, it was subjected to an examination almost as detailed as that customary for a new therapeutic agent. Needless to say, this is an expensive path to follow for what is essentially a low-concentration excipient in a formulation and, as a result, the strategy now is to identify already-known and in-use materials (or combinations thereof) which have enhancing capabilities. These "generally regarded as safe" components offer a much easier regulatory path than that reserved for a new chemical entity.

8.6.2 Iontophoresis

Iontophoresis may be defined as the facilitation of (ionizable) drug delivery across the skin by an applied electrical potential. The driving force may be simply visualized as electrostatic repulsion. Practically speaking, the potential difference across the skin provides a force in addition to the passive flow of solute induced by the concentration gradient (Figure 8.10). The isoelectric point of human skin is around pH 4 which implies that skin, under normal physiological conditions, supports a net negative charge. Hence, the skin is permselective to the passage of positive ions and, as a result, more momentum is transferred to the solvent in the direction of cation flow. Thus, iontophoresis also induces a convective flow (called *electroosmosis*) whereby the flux of both charged and uncharged species can be significantly enhanced over passive levels. Thus, all things being equal, positively charged compounds are delivered more efficiently from the anode than negatively charged compounds from the cathode than neutral substances from the anode. Predictably, there appears to be an inverse dependence of iontophoretic permeability on molecular weight.

Whether there is an "upper limit" has not been determined, although delivery of quite large molecules (e.g. cytochrome c, molecular weight ~12 kDa) has been reported. In practical terms, this means that the viability of delivery as a function of increasing molecular weight is dependent upon a concomitant increase in pharmacological potency (i.e. big molecules are only realistic candidates if they are very potent and require very small doses). It should also be noted that, with respect to peptide transport, amino acid sequence and conformation are potentially important variables that can dramatically impact upon iontophoretic delivery.

From a practical standpoint, iontophoresis offers, under ideal circumstances, the singular advantage that it is an enhancement procedure which acts on the drug rather than on the skin (as is the case with chemical enhancers, for example). Typically, a constant or pulsed direct current is applied between the two electrodes placed on the skin surface. The current determines the charge flowing in the circuit, and hence the number of ions moving across the skin – if the current is doubled, the number of ions transferred across the skin is increased by a factor of two; if the current is turned off, ion flow through the membrane should return to the passive (i.e. negligible) level. Even though the drug may only carry a fraction of the total charge flowing (or may even be primarily transported by electroosmosis), its flux will be directly proportional to the applied current density, and hence highly controlled and controllable.

In iontophoresis, reversible electrodes (e.g. Ag/AgCl), which do not lead to the hydrolysis of water at the potentials used, are preferred. The passage of 0.5 mA cm^{-2} across human skin (typically believed to be the maximum acceptable current density) requires a voltage of ~1–10 V. Acceptable levels of current density and total current are dependent upon the treatment area and duration of current passage. The ionic composition of the delivery system should be selected so that there is minimum competition with the

Figure 8.10 Schematic diagram of an iontophoretic drug delivery device

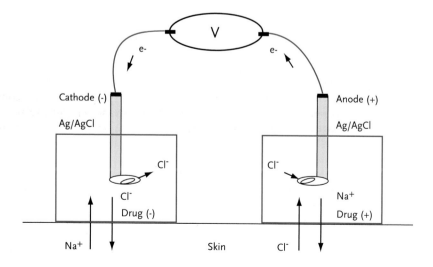

drug to carry charge across the skin (i.e. the idea is to maximize the fraction of charge carried by the drug across the skin). However, there must be sufficient electrolyte present to sustain current passage and to satisfy the electrochemical requirements of the electrodes. And, as mentioned above, in the case of larger compounds, for which electroosmosis may be the major mechanism of transport, different formulation strategies may be required.

Recently, in the US, the use of an existing iontophoretic device in conjunction with an approved solution (for injection) of lidocaine hydrochloride was accepted by the FDA for the induction of local anesthesia. Other, integrated products are known to be moving through the development pipeline; those furthest along are one containing fentanyl for analgesia, and another which is a more sophisticated device also containing lidocaine. Conservatively, one can expect these systems to reach the marketplace at the beginning of the 21st century. A number of other compounds have also been successfully delivered in limited *in vivo* trials, including peptidomimetics, leutinizing hormone releasing hormone (LHRH), somatostatin and calcitonin. Insulin, however, remains an unattained objective at this time. On a more positive note, an iontophoretic system (the GlucoWatch Biographer) for the noninvasive *extraction* and analysis of systemic glucose levels was approved by the FDA in early 2001. This device takes advantage of the symmetry of iontophoresis (i.e. the flow of current induces the movement of ions under both electrodes both into and out of the skin), and the phenomenon of electroosmosis, to sample blood sugar repeatedly, noninvasively and automatically.

8.6.3 Prodrugs

In the topical drug delivery area, especially in the design of more effective steroidal drugs, the prodrug approach has demonstrated success. In particular, it has been possible to create molecules with much better skin permeation properties from which the active species is subsequently "released", either enzymatically, or by simple hydrolysis, at the level of the viable epidermis. At the transdermal level, on the other hand, an equivalent strategy has not (at least, consciously) been used. That is, redesigning a molecule with good pharmacological effect when, for example, injected to enable its facile transdermal permeation and delivery. Why not? The answer is simply financial – such an approach creates in effect (insofar as the regulatory agencies are concerned) a new chemical entity which must be subjected to the same in-depth scrutiny as the "parent" compound. Under these circumstances, most pharmaceutical companies would prefer to invest in the search for a different, orally active analog.

8.6.4 Novel formulation approaches

8.6.4.1 *Colloidal systems*

There has been a reasonable amount of activity directed towards the use of different types of colloid as topical dosage forms. The microparticulate species employed include liposomes, niosomes and microemulsions (see chapter 5). Usually, the aim of this strategy is to improve, somehow, the delivery of lipophilic drugs, which have low inherent solubilities in most of the classical formulation excipients. While numerous and expensive liposomal and niosomal-based cosmetic products can be found on sale in every large department store, the use of this technology in pharmaceutical preparations has yet to make a significant impact. These systems are difficult to stabilize, use ingredients which are not cheap, and remain difficult to justify in terms of therapeutic benefit (relative to simpler, cheaper vehicles). Although progress of such formulaics for the parenteral route are showing considerable promise (see chapter 5), their efficient release into and through the skin is not guaranteed. Claims that such colloidal carriers can transport their "payloads" intact across the stratum corneum have not been substantiated. Given that the space between the corneocytes of the stratum corneum is on the order of 0.1 μm, and that this space is filled with lipid bilayers and the occasional desmosome, it is difficult to imagine how even the smallest unilamellar vesicle ($\sim$ 0.25 μm) might find a way across the barrier. Targeting of vesicles to specific appendageal structures, such as the hair follicle, has been discussed and illustrated qualitatively, but the practical utility (and efficiency) of such an effort is still a matter for investigation more than development.

8.6.4.2 *Supersaturation*

A thermodynamic option for increasing drug flux across the skin is the use of supersaturated formulations. In this approach, saturated solutions of drug in miscible cosolvent mixtures of different composition are combined to create a resulting formulation in which the drug is present at n-fold its saturation concentration. This thermodynamically unstable state persists normally for only a short time, before crystallization occurs, and must therefore be stabilized in some way (typically by the addition of a small amount of a polymer such as hydroxypropylmethylcellulose). With such systems, it has been shown that drug flux can be increased proportionately over that achievable using a simply saturated solution. Furthermore, it appears that this strategy can also induce supersaturation of the drug in the stratum corneum. The idea is attractive as it appears to be driven only by thermodynamics, without obvious perturbation of the barrier *per se*. Significant degrees of enhancement also appear possible (e.g. 8-fold with piroxicam). The principal concerns relate to stability and shelf life of a product based upon supersaturation; however, creative packaging (i.e. keeping the saturated solutions to be mixed separate until just before use), or the creation of a supersaturated state *in situ* upon application, are ideas under consideration to circumvent this problem.

8.7 CONCLUSIONS

In summary, it is useful to specify the "distinguishing features" of transdermal drug delivery. This route of administration involves a reproducibly adhesive and occlusive system, which covers post-application a specific, unchanging site of pre-determined area. The anatomic choices for administration are pre-set and identified on the approved labeling for the system. Usually, the drug is present in the patch throughout the application period at unit, or at least constant, thermodynamic activity, resulting most typically in a significant period of approximately zero-order drug delivery. Administration is possible from once-a-day to once-a-week; again, the application time is a key feature of the patch labeling. For the systems currently marketed, there is an established relationship between the plasma concentrations achieved and the therapeutic effect desired. Bioequivalency between different devices containing the same drug is based upon matching of plasma concentration versus time profiles. Transdermal drug delivery almost certainly results in local skin tissue levels of the drug which are significantly higher than those achieved by more conventional routes of administration. For this reason, particular attention must be paid to questions of skin irritation and sensitization.

Finally, it is important to note the beneficial contributions of transdermal drug delivery after nearly 20 years of commercialization. It has been possible to achieve blood level profiles of a drug quite distinct from those produced using other, more conventional dosage forms (e.g. oral tablets), and to avoid the large "peaks and troughs" associated with frequent multiple dosing. These distinct plasma concentration profiles have been obtained from patches of quite different design, from which drug is released by more than a single mechanism. The absolute blood level of a transdermally delivered drug can be manipulated in a linear fashion by changing the active surface area of the patch. Because the transdermal route of administration largely avoids the first-pass effect, ratios of metabolites different from those seen after oral dosing are produced (usually with beneficial reduction in side-effects). Transdermal delivery has found application in diverse therapeutic areas, and has demonstrated an ability to provide sustained drug input for periods of 0.5 to 7 days. Not infrequently, the drugs delivered transdermally have proven difficult to formulate for other routes of administration. And last, but not least, transdermal delivery has resulted in a significant improvement in the potential for better patient compliance and drug utilization. Thus, despite the challenges of moving drugs across the skin, transdermal administration has established itself as a successful and feasible route of absorption. Further advances in the technologies of enhancement, and the design and development of more potent therapeutic agents, can only increase the applications and usefulness of this unique and sophisticated technology.

8.8 FURTHER READING

Hadgraft, J. and Guy, R. (eds) (1989) *Transdermal drug delivery. Developmental issues and research initiatives.* Marcel Dekker, Inc., New York.

Bronaugh, R.L. and Maibach, H.I. (eds) (1989) *Percutaneous absorption. Mechanisms – Methodology – Drug delivery*. Marcel Dekker, Inc., New York.

Smith, E.W. and Maibach, H.I. (eds) (1995) *Percutaneous penetration enhancers*. CRC Press, Inc., Boca Raton.

Walters, K.A. and Hadgraft, J. (eds) (1993) *Pharmaceutical skin permeation enhancement*. Marcel Dekker, Inc. New York.

Potts, R.O. and Guy, R.H. (eds) (1997) *Mechanisms of transdermal drug delivery*. Marcel Dekker, Inc. New York.

Guy, R.H. (1996). Current status and future prospects of transdermal drug delivery. *Pharm. Res.*, 13:1765–1769.

Guy, R.H. (1992) Theme Editor Iontophoresis, *Advanced Drug Delivery Reviews*, 9 Issues 2/3.

Schaefer, H. and Redelmeier, T.E. (eds) (1996) *Skin barrier. Principles of percutaneous absorption*. Karger AG, Basel.

Cleary, G.W. (1993) Transdermal Delivery Systems: A Medical Rationale. In: *Topical Drug Bioavailability, Bioequivalence, and Penetration*. (Shah, V.P. and Maibach, H.I., eds). Plenum Press, New York, pp. 17–68.

Barry, B.W. (ed.) (1983) *Dermatological formulations. Percutaneous absorption*. Marcel Dekker, Inc., New York.

A full-text version of this chapter with supplementary information and illustrations can be found at: *http://pharma1.cur-archamps.fr/~guy/lecture.html*

8.9 SELF-ASSESSMENT QUESTIONS

1. Explain why the skin may initially appear as an unlikely route for drug delivery.

2. Describe the structure of the skin with reference to the key physiological features.

3. List the physiological factors which may affect transdermal bioavailability.

4. Describe the basic physical chemistry which may be used to model transdermal drug transport.

5. Describe the advantages and disadvantages of transdermal drug delivery over other routes of drug delivery.

6. Describe the three categories of conventional transdermal drug delivery systems.

7. Using appropriate examples, describe the importance of rate-control in transdermal delivery.

8. List five examples of commercially available drugs that are delivered by transdermal delivery systems.

9. List the criteria that have been proposed for successful penetration enhancers.

10. Using an appropriate diagram, outline the principle of iontophoresis.

Alison B. Lansley and Gary P. Martin

OBJECTIVES

On completion of this chapter the reader should be able to:

- Compare the nasal route with other absorptive sites for drugs in the body
- Give a general overview of the structure of the nasal cavity
- List the advantages and disadvantages of nasal drug delivery
- Give some examples of currently used nasal drug delivery systems
- Describe the various approaches to enhancing nasal drug delivery

9.1 INTRODUCTION

Certain drugs are delivered to the nasal cavity because this is their intended site of action; these are administered as nasal drops or sprays for a local effect. Such drugs in clinical use include decongestants, antibiotics and mucolytics. Due to its accessibility, the nasal cavity has also been used experimentally to investigate the safety and efficacy of gene delivery even though the gene used (the gene for the Cystic Fibrosis Transmembrane Receptor (CFTR) protein) is ultimately intended to be delivered to the lung. This is another example of local delivery since the lining of the nose was the intended site of action for the study.

The nasal cavity may also be exploited as a route of entry into the *systemic* circulation, either because the absorption profile of the drug is appropriate to its clinical application, e.g. a fast onset of action for the treatment of migraine with sumatriptan and/or for those compounds which cannot be given orally because they are destroyed in the gastrointestinal fluids, metabolized in the wall of the gastrointestinal tract or undergo extensive biotransformation by the liver during their first passage around the circulation. As well as some conventional drug molecules, these include the "new biotherapeutics" such as peptides, polypeptides and antisense DNA which, in the absence of an alternative non-invasive route of delivery, are usually given by injection. These molecules are unlikely to realize their full clinical potential unless the patient can easily and conveniently self-administer the drug and hence this goal has led to the investigation of various transmucosal routes for drug delivery including the buccal, pulmonary, rectal and nasal routes. So far, nasal delivery has been the most successful of these alternative routes, with nasal sprays for buserelin, desmopressin, oxytocin and calcitonin already available commercially.

Extensive research is currently being carried out in this area and the potential of the nasal route for systemic drug delivery comprises the focus of this chapter.

9.2 STRUCTURE AND PHYSIOLOGY OF THE NASAL CAVITY

The nasal cavity extends 12–14 cm, from the nostrils to the nasopharynx (throat) and is divided in two, laterally, by the nasal septum (Figure 9.1).

9.2.1 Physiological structure

The nasal vestibule has the smallest cross-sectional area in the respiratory tract (approximately 0.3 cm^2 on each side) and extends from the entrance of the nostrils, which are guarded by vibrissae (hairs), to the anterior ends of the inferior turbinates. The lining of the vestibule changes from skin at the entrance, to squamous epithelium and then to ciliated columnar secretory epithelium at the turbinates. The area from the anterior ends of the turbinates to the anterior portion of the

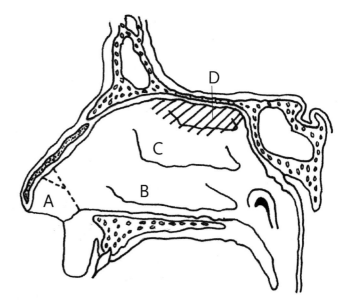

Figure 9.1 Lateral wall of the nasal cavity. A: nasal vestibule; B: inferior turbinate; C: middle turbinate; D: superior turbinate; Hatched area: the olfactory region

nasopharynx constitutes the main nasal passage. Here the walls of the nasal septum are folded to create the turbinates and meatuses (air spaces). The narrow width of the meatuses (0.5–1.0 mm) helps to maintain contact between the airstream and the epithelium lining the nasal passage. The olfactory region of the nose is located towards the roof of the nasal cavity and is lined with non-ciliated neuro-epithelium. The remainder of the main nasal passage is lined with pseudostratified columnar secretory epithelium consisting of basal cells, goblet cells and columnar cells which may be ciliated or unciliated (Figure 9.2). Microvilli are found on the columnar cells which increase the surface area available for absorption.

The nasal mucosa is highly vascular; superficial and deep layers of arterioles supply the lamina propria and between the venules and capillaries there are numerous sinuses or venous lakes which are linked to erectile tissue, particularly in the middle and inferior turbinates, which enable the airways to widen or narrow. This autonomically controlled vasculature of the nasal tissue, in combination with its rich supply of secretory cells, is of importance in the modification of inspired air.

9.2.2 Olfaction

One of the lesser functions of the nose in man is that of olfaction. The olfactory region of the nose, a small patch of tissue containing the smell receptors, is located towards the roof of the nasal cavity and is lined with non-ciliated neuro-epithelium. Approximately 20% of the air flowing through the nasal cavity is directed upwards to the olfactory region. Here, bipolar neurones react to inspired air and initiate impulses in the olfactory nerves.

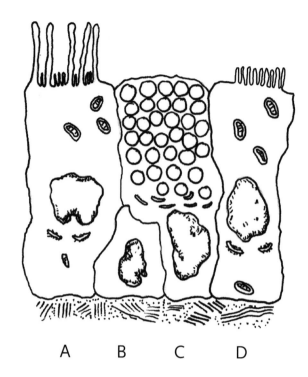

Figure 9.2 Diagram of the four cell types in the nasal respiratory epithelium. A: ciliated columnar cell covered by cilia and microvilli of uniform length; B: basal cell; C: goblet cell packed with mucus granules; D: non-ciliated columnar cell, covered by microvilli of uniform length. (Redrawn from Mygind, N., 1979 *Nasal Allergy*, 2nd edition. Blackwell Scientific Publications Oxford).

A   B   C   D

9.2.3 Modification of inspired air

The principal function of the nasal cavity in man is that of air-conditioning. The anatomy of the nose permits intimate contact between the inspired air and the mucosal surfaces enabling the air to be *warmed* and *humidified* by the vasculature and secretions of the epithelium. Inspired air of 23 °C and 40% relative humidity can be brought to 32 °C and 98% relative humidity upon inhalation via the nose.

An additional form of air-conditioning is concerned with the removal of particulates, such as dust, microorganisms and allergens, from the inspired air. The large cross-sectional area of the nasal cavity and relatively low air velocities are ideal for particle deposition, as is the turbulence caused beyond constrictions where changes in air flow direction occur. The efficiency of particle removal from the air-stream is dependent on a number of factors including the aerodynamic diameter of the inhaled particles:

- Particles greater than 10 μm are generally filtered out by the vibrissae at the nostrils.
- Smaller particles (approximately 5–10 μm) tend to deposit in the nasal passages and are subsequently cleared by the process of *mucociliary clearance* (discussed below).
- Particles less than 2 μm are not normally filtered out and may enter the lungs.

Chapter Nine

9.2.4 Mucociliary clearance

Mucociliary clearance contributes to the body's defense mechanisms by entrapping potentially hazardous substances, such as dust and microorganisms, within the viscoelastic mucus blanket lining the nasal passages. The mucus is then propelled by the claw-like tips of the cilia, beating in a co-ordinated manner within the periciliary fluid, towards the nasopharynx where the mucus and any entrapped particulates is either swallowed or expectorated. Electron micrographs of cilia beating beneath a mucus layer are shown in Figure 9.3. In the nasal cavity, mucus is moved by the cilia at a rate of approximately 10 cm min^{-1} and clearance of the bulk of the mucus from the nose to the nasopharynx occurs over 10–20 minutes.

Efficient mucociliary clearance depends on a successful relationship between the:

- cilia
- periciliary fluid
- mucus

which are discussed in detail below. Changes in any of these three parameters can alter the characteristics of clearance and those patients with compromised clearance, such as those afflicted with conditions such as cystic fibrosis or ciliary dyskinesia, appear to be more susceptible to chronic respiratory infections.

Figure 9.3 Electron micrographs showing cilia beating beneath a mucus layer. Courtesy of M.J. Sanderson, Department of Physiology, University of Massachusetts Medical School, Worcester, Mass, USA.

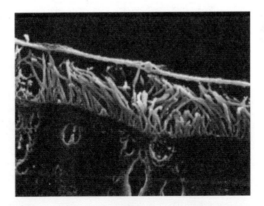

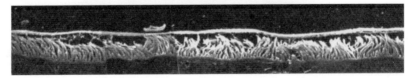

9.2.4.1 Periciliary fluid

Periciliary fluid is a watery, ionic solution, maintained by transepithelial ion transport, that provides an environment within which the cilia are able to beat. It also provides a reservoir of fluid for the humidification of inspired air. The depth of the periciliary fluid dictates whether the overlying mucus layer is at the ciliary tips and thus available for clearance:

- Should the periciliary fluid become too deep, it is hypothesized that the ciliary tips would be unable to reach the mucus layer and that clearance would therefore be compromised.
- If the periciliary fluid were too shallow, the cilia would become entangled in the mucus gel and mucus transport would again be compromised.

9.2.4.2 Mucus

The nasal epithelium, like many other epithelia in contact with the external environment, is covered by a mucus gel. The mucus plays a number of important physiological roles:

- It entraps substances entering the nasal cavity and participates in the removal of particulates via mucociliary clearance; this process protects the underlying mucosa.
- The capacity of mucus to hold water permits the humidification of the inspired air and also aids heat transfer, since water is a better conductor of heat than air.

Approximately 1.5–2 litres of mucus are secreted daily by goblet cells and serous glands within the nasal cavity. In addition, some contribu-

Table 9.1 The principal constituents of airway secretions

Constituent	Example
Glycoconjugates	mucus glycoproteins glycosaminoglycans
Proteins	albumin IgG secretory IgA lactoferrin lysozyme non-secretory IgA
Proteases	neutral endopeptidase aminopeptidase peroxidase carboxypeptidase N
Lipids	phospholipids triglycerides free fatty acids cholesterol
Nucleic acids	DNA/RNA

tion to nasal secretions is made by the lacrimal glands. Mucus is mainly composed of water (90–95%), salts (1–2%), lipids (about 30% of the non-aqueous secretion) and mucins (0.5–5%) which lend the substance its gel-like properties.

The composition of nasal secretion is given in Table 9.1. The protein content of nasal secretions includes:

- secretory IgA, which acts to prevent the attachment of microorganisms to the mucosa;
- lysozyme, which attacks the cell walls of susceptible microorganisms and acts optimally at acidic pH (the pH of nasal secretions is generally 5.5–6.5, but becomes more alkaline during bouts of the common cold);
- lactoferrin, which sequesters any free iron in secretions which might otherwise be used by iron-requiring microorganisms;
- various other enzymes.

Respiratory mucins are high molecular weight glycoproteins that are polydisperse in mass ($2–40 \times 10^6$ Da). They are long, linear, apparently flexible threads which vary in length from 0.5 to 10 μm. They are composed of sub-units (monomers) each about 500 nm in length. The monomers are joined end to end via disulfide bonds (Figure 9.4). Each monomer is comprised of a protein "backbone" core, with alternating oligosaccharide-rich regions (approximately 100 nm in length) and "naked" regions of folded protein stabilized by disulfide bonds.

The protein "backbone" cloaked by the oligosaccharides is rich in the amino acids serine, threonine and proline. The naked protein regions are characterized by a high cysteine content which provides the sulfur molecules for disulfide bonding. The wide range of sizes of respiratory mucins is believed to result from a variable number of sub-units forming the polymer.

A characteristic of mucins is their high carbohydrate content (up to 80% by mass), mainly in the form of short O-linked oligosaccharide chains. Serine and threonine provide the sites of O-glycan attachment via the linkage sugar N-acetylgalactosamine (GalNAc) and the oligosaccharide chains may also contain N-acetylglucosamine (GlcNac), galactose (Gal), fucose, sialic acids and sulfate. Twenty or more monosaccharides may be present in an oligosaccharide chain. Small amounts of N-linked oligosaccharide are also present in mucins, which seem to be important in the correct folding of the naked regions of the core protein.

The function of mucin oligosaccharides is not fully understood but, since certain bacteria bind specific oligosaccharide ligands, it is thought that oligosaccharides may aid bacterial attachment to respiratory mucus. The accessibility of such bacteria to the underlying epithelium is thus prevented or limited and the microorganisms are subsequently destroyed by enzymatic attack and/or removed from the nasal cavity by the action of mucociliary clearance. Mucin oligosaccharides also play an essential role in the hydration of mucus.

At least seven mucin genes (MUC1, 2, 3, 4, 5AC, 5B and 7) are expressed in the respiratory epithelium, but the contribution each

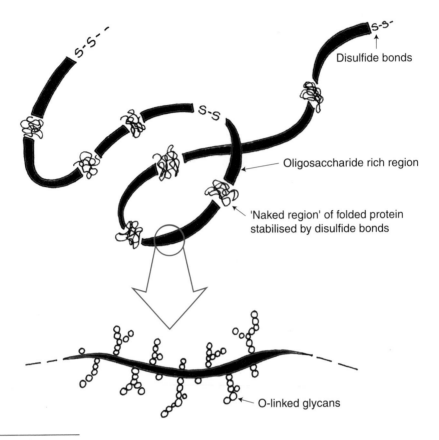

S-S--

Disulfide bonds

S-S

Oligosaccharide rich region

'Naked region' of folded protein
stabilised by disulfide bonds

O-linked glycans

Figure 9.4 Schematic representation of the macromolecular architecture of a large gel-forming respiratory mucin. Two mucin subunits, each about 500 nm in length, are joined end to end via disulfide bonds (S-S) and consist of oligosaccharide-rich regions (represented by the thickened line) and folded domains stabilized by disulfide bonds (represented by the knots). An expanded portion of one of the oligosaccharide-rich regions (not drawn to scale) shows the variety and density of the attached O-linked glycans

makes to the formation of a mucus gel is unclear. At the time of writing, only the products of MUC2 and MUC5AC have been shown to be of the large gel-forming type and MUC5AC mucin (and two as yet unidentified mucins, probably from MUC5B) appear to be present in normal secretions.

Mucus possesses both solid-like (elastic) and liquid-like (viscous) attributes simultaneously and is therefore termed a viscoelastic gel. The viscoelastic properties arise from the non-covalent interactions (entanglements) between the predominantly anionic mucin molecules, although weak hydrogen-bonding and ligand-like attractions between protein regions of adjacent molecules may also play a role. Gel properties are affected by:

- mucin size;
- mucin polydispersity;
- the type of mucins present.

It is widely held that mucus should possess specific rheological properties for clearance from the airway to occur. Any alteration in mucus rheology that compromises clearance can predispose the individual to airway disease and infection. Some agents capable of altering mucus rheology are listed in Table 9.2. In addition, the state of mucus hydration (or mucin concentration) will affect the properties of the gel. In

Table 9.2 Agents capable of altering the rheological properties of mucus	Mucolytics "mucus-thinning"	Mucospissics "mucus-thickening"
	N-acetylcysteine carbocysteine mercaptoethanesulfonate mercaptoethanol bile salts synthetic surfactants urea guanidinium chloride sodium thiocyanate monovalent cations DNase	DNA bacterial alginate tetracyclines chlorhexidine Congo Red trivalent metal ions tetraborate

patients with cystic fibrosis, dehydration of mucus is believed to contribute to the increased viscoelasticity of the secretion and its poor clearance. An increase in mucus viscoelasticity is also thought to occur in asthma, chronic bronchitis, chronic obstructive pulmonary disease and acute respiratory distress syndrome.

9.2.5 Cilia

The beat cycle of a respiratory tract cilium is composed of three phases:

Effective stroke

The cilium maximizes its height enabling the "ciliary crown" at its tip to interact with the under-surface of the mucus gel which is then propelled forward as the cilium moves through an almost planar arc (Figure 9.5).

Rest phase

At the end of the effective stroke the cilium disengages from the mucus gel and enters the rest phase where it lies parallel to the epithelium pointing in the direction of mucus flow. This position is believed to discourage any reversal of mucus movement.

Figure 9.5 Diagram showing the character of the effective stroke (a) and the recovery stroke (b) of a cilium. The mucus blanket (c) is always propelled in the same direction as the effective stroke (d)

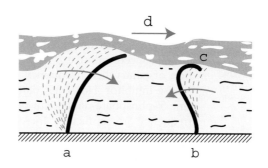

Recovery stroke

The cilium "unrolls" within the periciliary fluid ready for the next effective stroke. Undergoing the recovery stroke beneath the mucus layer prevents retrograde mucus transport (Figure 9.5).

There are approximately 200 cilia on each ciliated cell. They are packed at a density of 6–8 cilia per μm^2 and cannot move without affecting neighbouring cilia. In order to perform an unhindered beat cycle the movement of each cilium is slightly out of phase with that of its neighbor, leading to a phenomenon termed "ciliary metachrony". Metachrony results solely from hydrodynamic coupling between adjacent cilia and provides the necessary cooperation within a field of cilia to permit them to transport mucus.

Airway cilia are approximately 0.25 μm in diameter and 3–7 μm long, tending to be longer in the upper airways. Each cilium is bounded by an evagination of the plasma membrane and, as shown diagrammatically (Figure 9.6), contains a central core called the axoneme, composed of two single microtubules, arranged as a central pair surrounded by nine doublet microtubules. Each outer doublet microtubule consists of an A subfiber which is circular in cross-section, and an incomplete B subfiber, which is C-shaped in cross-section. The A subfiber bears "arms" consisting of the protein dynein. The inner and outer dynein arms of the A subfiber project towards the B subfiber of the adjacent microtubule. A nexin (NX) link joins adjacent doublets and radial spokes project from each A subfiber and associate, via the spoke head, with the projections of the central microtubules.

The ability of the microtubules to slide past each other, propelled by the ATP-dependent mechano-chemical cycling of the dynein arms, brings about ciliary motility. Since the microtubules are constrained at the ciliary tip, it is possible to imagine how the sliding of microtubules on one side of the cilium might cause the cilium to bend. How such sliding is translated into a full beat cycle is still the subject of extensive research.

A wide number of agents are able to alter the rate of ciliary beating; this can either be via a non-specific, toxic effect, e.g. certain preservatives and penetration enhancers, or by ligand–receptor interactions at the cell membrane, e.g. β-adrenergic agonists, adenosine, ATP. The latter interaction generally causes an increase or decrease in the intracellular concentration of a second messenger substance such as Ca^{2+} or cAMP which is responsible for altering ciliary beat frequency.

cAMP is believed to be involved in the control of ciliary beat frequency via phosphorylation since agents increasing intracellular cAMP concentration, e.g. isoprenaline (isoproterenol), cause an elevation of ciliary beat frequency which can be inhibited by a protein kinase inhibitor. However, data concerning the role of cyclic guanosine 5'-phosphate-dependent protein phosphorylation on ciliary beat frequency are conflicting. Increases in the intracellular concentration of Ca^{2+} ($[Ca^{2+}]_i$) increases ciliary beat frequency possibly via protein phosphorylation induced by calcium/calmodulin kinase.

Figure 9.6 Diagram showing the ultrastructure of an airway cilium. CM, central microtubules; NX, nexin link; RS, radial spoke; SH, spoke head; CP, projections of the central microtubules. (redrawn from Sanderson, M. J. (1997) Mechanisms controlling airway ciliary activity. In Rogers, D. F. and Lethem, M. I. (eds.) *Airway Mucus: Basic Mechanisms and Clinical Perspectives*. Birkhauser Verlag, Basel).

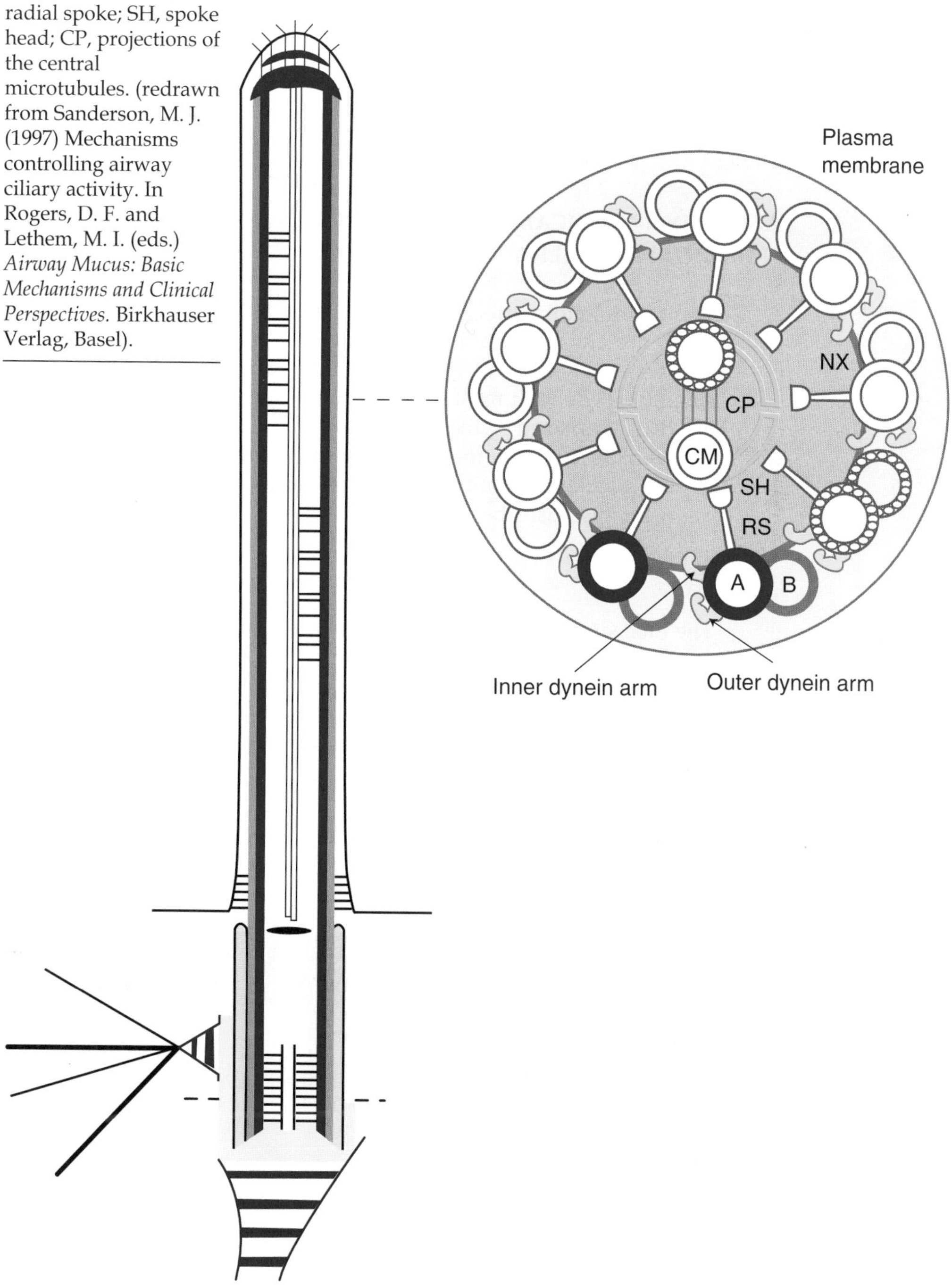

Ciliated cells also respond to mechanical stimulation by increasing their beat frequency, an effect which spreads to surrounding cells (5–7 cells in all directions) and is mediated by an increase in $[Ca^{2+}]_i$. It is believed that the second messenger, inositol trisphosphate (IP_3), is produced in the stimulated cell and diffuses through gap junctions to adjacent cells to cause the release of intracellular stores of Ca^{2+} via the IP_3 receptor. Such intercellular signaling provides the opportunity for cooperative cellular activity which would be advantageous to the ciliated epithelium in its efforts to transport mucus. Airway cilia may be able to upregulate their beat frequency in response to an increase in the mucus load.

9.3 PHYSIOLOGICAL FACTORS AFFECTING NASAL BIOAVAILABILITY

The main factors affecting the absorption of drugs from the nasal cavity are physiological in origin. Table 9.3 shows some physiological barriers which might affect the amount of drug reaching the systemic circulation. As with most sites of drug absorption, the bioavailability of a drug is affected by the *area* available for absorption, the *contact time* between the drug and the absorption site, *metabolism* of the drug prior to and during absorption and the *pathology* of the absorbing tissue. These are discussed below.

9.3.1 Area

The total surface area of both nasal cavities is about 160 cm^2. The area available for absorption is enhanced by:

- the convolutions of the turbinates, and
- the microvilli present on the surface of the ciliated and unciliated cells of the respiratory epithelium.

However, the *effective* surface area for absorption is influenced by the type of dosage form from which the drug is administered, as described below.

Table 9.3 Potential physiological barriers to the absorption of drugs via the nasal cavity (from Gizurarson, 1993)

Barriers	Small molecules (% loss)	High M. Wt. Molecules (% loss)
Degradation	0–15	0–5
Clearance [a]	0–30	20–50
Deposition (anterior loss)	10–20	10–20
Health status and environment	10–20	10–40
Membrane permeability [a,b]	0–30	20–50
Mucus layer	< 1	< 1

[a] depends on excipients
[b] depends on physicochemical characteristics of the drug, e.g. partition coefficient, charge, etc.

Chapter Nine

9.3.2 Blood supply

As discussed above, the nasal mucosa is highly vascular. This property facilitates its physiological role in heat exchange and also potentially, drug absorption. The rich blood supply means that drugs absorbed via the nasal route have a rapid onset of action, which can be exploited for therapeutic gain.

9.3.3 Contact time and mucociliary clearance

The length of time the drug is in contact with the absorbing tissue will influence how much drug crosses the mucosa. In the nasal cavity this is influenced by the rate at which the drug is cleared from the absorption site by mucociliary clearance and by metabolism.

While the mucociliary clearance of deposited particles is advantageous if the particles are likely to be hazardous, the clearance of a deposited drug is clearly not beneficial if it prevents absorption.

The *site of deposition* in the nasal cavity profoundly affects the rate of mucociliary clearance of a drug moiety:

- Particles deposited on ciliated regions (for example, the turbinates) of the mucosa are immediately available for clearance.
- Particles deposited on non-ciliated regions (for example, the anterior of the nasal cavity) will move more slowly (such particles will land on mucus which is being dragged through the cavity from ciliated areas).
- Particles which deposit on the nasopharyngeal regions will be swallowed immediately and are therefore not available for nasal absorption.

As described above, clearance of the bulk of the mucus from the nose to the nasopharynx occurs over 10–20 minutes. Clearance appears to be biphasic (Figure 9.7); 40% of a radiolabeled solution administered

Figure 9.7 Graph illustrating biphasic clearance of a radiolabeled solution delivered from a metered-dose spray. Deposition site; □ Turbinates; ▲ Nasopharynx ●

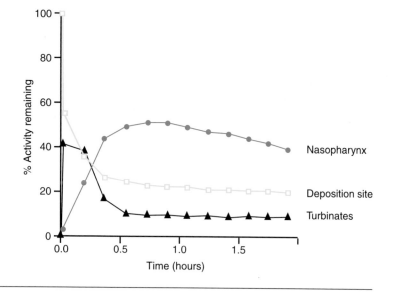

either as a nasal spray or as drops is cleared rapidly within 20 minutes, then a second slower phase of clearance follows when clearance of the nasal spray is slower than clearance of the drops. This is probably because most of the spray has deposited on non-ciliated regions of the nasal cavity.

The implications of this for drug absorption are that administration of a drug as drops may only be suitable if the drug molecule is rapidly absorbed. Those drug molecules which diffuse across the nasal epithelium more slowly will need a longer contact time and may be better administered as sprays. The absorption rate of certain drugs may be so slow that therapeutically active plasma levels are not attained.

A further consideration is that drug molecules which are cleared by the action of mucociliary clearance from the nasal cavity to the GI tract may be absorbed from the GI tract if they are not metabolized. This secondary absorption via the GI tract would be seen as a second peak in the plasma drug concentration profile.

9.3.4 Disease

The rate of mucociliary clearance can be affected by the pathophysiological condition of the nasal cavity and this will also affect the rate of clearance of administered drug. Such conditions include rhinitis, the common cold, hayfever, sinusitis, asthma, nasal polyposis, Sjogren's and Kartagener's syndromes. In addition, environmental factors such as humidity, temperature and pollution can also affect the rate of nasal clearance.

The common cold consists of two distinct phases: mucus hypersecretion, followed by nasal congestion. It has been shown that during the former phase, less than 10% of a dose administered as a nasal spray will remain in the nasal cavity after 25 minutes. In contrast, almost all the administered dose will still be present at the site of deposition up to 90 minutes after administration during the nasal congestion phase. This would clearly lead to unpredictable absorption of an administered drug which would be unacceptable for a potent drug with a narrow therapeutic window. The inclusion of a vasoconstrictor such as oxymetazoline in the formulation might relieve such symptoms and provide more reproducible drug absorption.

As well as affecting mucociliary clearance, many nasal diseases including hayfever induce inflammation in the nasal cavity and render the nasal epithelium "leakier" or more permeable than normal. This would be likely to affect drug absorption but not necessarily in a reproducible manner.

9.3.5 Enzymatic activity

The nasal secretions possess a wide range of enzymes (Table 9.1) and enzymes are also present in the epithelium of the nasal cavity. It has been suggested that the low bioavailabilities of some nasally administered peptides results from their enzymatic degradation in the nasal cavity. The nasal mucosa and fluids have been shown to possess a variety of exopeptidases and endopeptidases (see Section 1.6.1) but care should be exercised in interpreting studies of peptide stability, which are often carried out using homogenates of nasal tissue. In such studies peptides are exposed to both extra- and intracellular enzymes. The actions of intracellular enzymes will not be significant if the peptide is absorbed by the paracellular route (see Section 9.3.8.1), never coming into contact with the inside of the cell.

As described in Section 1.6.1 exopeptidases cleave at N- and C-termini and include aminopeptidases, carboxypeptidases and dipeptidyl peptidase, whereas endopeptidases cleave at an internal peptide bond and include enkephalinase and cathepsin B. Small peptides are relatively resistant to the action of endopeptidases but their activity is significant for large peptides.

Although enzymatic activity is present in the nasal cavity, this activity is generally lower than the enzymatic activity of the gastrointestinal tract, making this route an attractive alternative to the oral delivery of enzymatically labile drugs such as therapeutic peptides and proteins. However, the cytochrome P450 activity in the olfactory region of the nasal epithelium is actually higher than that in the liver, principally due to a three- to four-fold higher NADPH-cytochrome P450 reductase content. These enzymes are capable of metabolizing inhaled pollutants into reactive metabolites which may induce nasal tumors.

9.3.6 Immunological clearance

The immune system functions to recognize and eliminate foreign materials. Antibodies are secreted in the nasal cavity and may be found in high concentrations in the mucus layer where they are able to neutralize antigens presented to the nasal mucosa. Foreign proteins delivered to the body are capable of eliciting an immune response and indeed antibodies have been detected in nasal secretions in response to the intranasal administration of insulin. Clearly this situation is undesirable since the therapeutic molecule will undergo degradation and the patient is likely to suffer with symptoms associated with allergic diseases such as hayfever. It is possible that pharmaceutical excipients which cause inflammation of the nasal cavity might exacerbate such reactions.

9.3.7 Mucus barrier

In addition to its involvement in mucociliary clearance, mucus can also affect drug delivery by interacting directly with nasally administered drugs by:

- acting as a physical barrier to drug diffusion, and/or
- binding to drugs.

One method by which mucus protects the nasal epithelium is by acting as a physical barrier and respiratory mucus has been reported to retard the diffusion of water and a range of β-lactam antibiotics used to treat respiratory infections. The use of mucolytics, which alter the viscoelasticity of mucus, has been shown to increase the absorption of intranasally administered human growth hormone (hGH, M. Wt. = 22 kDa). However, other studies have shown that antibodies (150–970 kDa) are able to diffuse through cervical mucus relatively unimpeded; these latter studies tend to suggest that the diffusion barrier presented by mucus in the nasal cavity would be insignificant.

The binding of drugs to mucin can account for their limited diffusion. Positively charged drug molecules can bind to mucus glycoproteins via electrostatic interactions with the large number of negatively charged sialic acid and sulfate ester residues. Such residues have low pKa values and are thus ionized under most physiological conditions. Hydrogen-bonding is also possible, between drugs and the hydroxyl groups on the sugars and other O- and N-containing groups on the protein backbone. Hydrophobic interactions between drugs and a globular protein region of the glycoprotein molecule can also occur.

Tetracycline has been shown to bind to gastrointestinal mucus by hydrogen-bonding and via electrostatic and hydrophobic interactions. It has been suggested that cephaloridine and gentamicin bind intestinal mucin via ionic interactions. In addition, gentamicin has been shown to bind to sputum and tobramycin binds to glycoprotein- and DNA-rich fractions of sputum.

9.3.8   Transport routes and mechanisms

As discussed extensively in Chapter 1 (Section 1.3.3), the organization and architecture of epithelial mucosae restrict drug permeation across the epithelial barrier to two main routes (Figure 1.3):

- the paracellular route: *between* adjacent epithelial cells via the mechanisms of passive diffusion or solvent drag;
- the transcellular route: *across* the epithelial cells, which can occur by any of the following mechanisms: passive diffusion, carrier-mediated transport and via endocytic processes.

As has been stressed for all the transepithelial routes in this book, it is important to remember that although a drug molecule may be predominantly absorbed via one particular route/mechanism, it is also likely that sub-optimal transport will occur via alternative routes and mechanisms.

9.3.8.1   *The paracellular route*

The paracellular permeability of the nasal epithelium is approximately the same as that of the intestine, thus small hydrophilic molecules can passively diffuse between adjacent cells. Passive diffusion between the cells is driven by a concentration gradient, with the rate of absorption governed by Fick's first law of diffusion (see Section 1.3.3).

9.3.8.2   *The transcellular route*

Transcellular passive diffusion

For most conventional drug molecules, which tend to be small and lipophilic, absorption occurs transcellularly, by passive diffusion across the cells of the epithelium. Again, movement occurs down a concentration gradient, according to Fick's first law of diffusion (see Section 1.3.3). The degree of ionization of a drug species is an important property for absorption via passive transcellular diffusion (see Section 1.3.4.2) and is dependent on the pKa of the drug and the pH of the environment; the pH of nasal secretions is normally in the region 5.5–6.5.

Carrier-mediated processes

Active transport mechanisms for di- and tri-peptides, as well as L-amino acids, have been demonstrated in the nasal epithelium.

Endocytic processes

Most compounds of interest for nasal delivery have a molecular weight in excess of 1,000 Da and until recently were thought to cross the cells endocytically. However, a recent study in rats has shown the transport of fluoroscein isothiocyanate (FITC)-labeled dextran (M. Wt. = 3,000 Da) to be via the paracellular pathway, with only a proportion moving endocytically. Hardly any transport of FITC-labeled dextran with a molecular weight of 10,000 Da was observed unless a penetration enhancer was co-administered, but the penetration enhancer, sodium taurodihydrofusidate (STDHF), caused cell swelling and extrusion of mucus.

9.4 FORMULATION FACTORS AFFECTING NASAL BIOAVAILABILITY

9.4.1 Physicochemical factors associated with the drug

The physicochemical properties of a molecule which affect its absorption across the nasal epithelium are broadly the same as those affecting transepithelial absorption at any site and have been discussed extensively in Section 1.3.4. These factors influence the mechanism and rate of drug absorption through the nasal epithelium.

For nasal drug delivery, it has been suggested that two mechanisms of absorption exist, based on the physicochemical properties of the drug:

- a fast rate, which is dependent on the lipophilicity of the drug;
- a slower rate, which is dependent on molecular weight.

Thus, lipophilic drugs such as propanolol, progesterone, 17β-œstradiol, naloxone and testosterone are absorbed rapidly and completely from the nasal cavity. In contrast, their oral bioavailabilities range from 25% for propranolol to less than 1% for progesterone.

The slower rate of absorption (probably via the paracellular route and also sub-optimally via the transcellular route) is considered to provide adequate absorption of low molecular weight polar compounds in the window of opportunity provided by mucociliary clearance (approximately 10–20 minutes). Above a molecular weight of 1,000 Da the nasal absorption of compounds declines. Thus the absorption of hydrophilic drugs is more variable than that of lipophilic compounds and certain salts, for example sodium cromoglycate, are rapidly absorbed across the nasal mucosa, whereas the absorption of peptides and proteins varies from 100% for the pentapeptide, metkephamid (molecular weight 660 Da), to 1% for gonadorelin (GnRH, molecular weight 1,300 Da).

9.4.2 Concentration

As discussed above, in the majority of cases the absorption of the drug of interest across the nasal mucosa is via passive diffusion (paracellular or transcellular). As such, the rate of absorption will be affected by the concentration of drug in solution at the absorbing membrane. The higher the drug concentration, the steeper the concentration gradient driving the absorption process and the faster the drug will be absorbed. Therefore if the drug is formulated as a solution, the highest concentration possible should be chosen that is compatible with an accurate and reproducible dosing volume. However, care must be taken, as high local drug concentrations over extended periods of time may also cause severe local irritation or adverse tissue reactions.

9.4.3 Factors associated with the dosage form

Drugs to be administered to the nasal cavity are generally formulated as *nasal drops*, which deposit a film of drug solution, or *nasal sprays* which deposit an aerosol of particles, droplets or particles suspended in droplets. For absorption of aerosol formulations, deposition of the aerosol must occur followed by dissolution of solid particles if applicable.

The extent and site of deposition of an aerosol from a nasal spray will depend upon:

- the aerodynamic diameter of the particle (which is also a function of droplet size, shape and density);
- the particle charge (which might also depend on the drug, formulation excipients and method of aerosolization);
- the velocity at which the particle is moving (which depends on respiratory patterns).

In general, particles or droplets in the size range 5–10 μm tend to deposit in the nasal passages. Although the extent and site of particle deposition can be estimated from a knowledge of the aerodynamic size distribution of the aerosol, the situation can be complicated by the fact that the size of the particle can increase (and possibly its density decrease) as a result of water condensation, due to the humidity change upon entering the nasal cavity.

Deposition mechanisms in the nose include inertial impaction, sedimentation, diffusion, interception and electrostatic attraction. The structure and physiology of the nasal cavity, with the small cross-

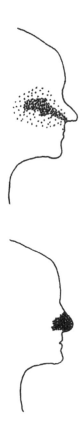

Figure 9.8 Deposition and clearance of nasal drops (upper panel: 4 minutes after administration) and a nasal spray (lower panel: 1 minute after administration) in a normal subject

section for airflow and sharp curves, suggests that *inertial impaction* is the most significant mechanism for drug deposition in the nasal cavity.

Studies using radiolabeled nasal drops and sprays show that (Figure 9.8):

- nasal drops disperse a drug solution throughout the length of the nasal cavity from atrium to nasopharynx, offering a relatively large area for immediate absorption;
- nasal sprays tend to deposit at the front of the nasal cavity with little of the dose reaching the turbinates.

The implications to nasal bioavailability of these deposition patterns from the different delivery devices is discussed further below (see Section 9.6).

9.4.4 Other formulation factors

Additional formulation factors which affect nasal drug delivery include the:

- density of the vehicle;
- viscosity of the vehicle;
- pH of the dosage form;
- tonicity of the dosage form;

- inclusion of formulation additives such as penetration enhancers, enzyme inhibitors, bioadhesives etc.

These factors are discussed below in Section 9.7.

9.5 ADVANTAGES AND DISADVANTAGES OF NASAL DRUG DELIVERY

A brief overview of both the advantages and disadvantages of nasal drug delivery is given below. These can depend on the nature of the drug being delivered.

9.5.1 Advantages

The general advantages of the nasal cavity for drug delivery include:

Large surface area

The nasal cavity offers a relatively large surface area (approximately 160 cm^2) for drug absorption.

Rich blood supply

The highly vascular surface of the nasal mucosa ensures rapid absorption and onset of action, as well as the maintenance of "sink" conditions (see Section 1.3.3.2).

Low metabolic activity

The metabolic activity of the nasal cavity towards peptides and proteins is less than that of the GI tract, making this route an attractive alternative to the oral delivery of these moieties. In contrast to the oral route, this route avoids degradation in the intestinal wall or the liver, prior to the drug reaching the systemic circulation.

Accessibility

The nasal cavity offers a readily accessible surface for drug delivery, obviating the need for complex delivery devices to enable the drug to reach its absorption site. Thus devices for nasal delivery are simpler in design than those intended to deliver drugs to, for instance, the alveolar region of the lung and are non-invasive, requiring the simple instillation of drops or sprays.

Ease of administration

Nasal devices, such as metered-dose nasal sprays, are simple for the patient to use and might be expected to be more acceptable to the patient than the use of pessaries or suppositories for the intravaginal and rectal delivery routes respectively.

Intestinal alternative

The nasal route may become a useful alternative to the intestinal route for drug absorption in situations where use of the gastrointestinal route is unfeasible. Examples include:

- patients with nausea and vomiting;
- patients with swallowing difficulties and/or children;
- drugs that are unstable in the gastrointestinal fluids;
- drugs that undergo extensive first-pass effects in the gut wall or liver.

9.5.2   Disadvantages

The disadvantages of the nasal cavity for drug delivery include:

Mucociliary clearance

Mucociliary clearance reduces the retention time of drugs within the nasal cavity and thus the opportunity for absorption. For drugs which are rapidly absorbed, mucociliary clearance is likely to be of little consequence, but for those compounds with physicochemical properties dictating slow absorption the effect of mucociliary clearance is likely to be profound.

Mucus barrier

Drug diffusion may be limited by the physical barrier of the mucus layer and the binding of drugs to mucins.

Metabolic activity

While the metabolic activity of the nasal cavity towards peptides and proteins is less than that of the GI tract, it should be recognized that the nasal mucosa and secretions do have the ability to degrade drugs and that measures may be necessary to overcome this.

Limited to potent molecules

For drugs of a high molecular weight (which are thus poorly absorbed), the route is limited only to potent drug molecules; typically those with effective plasma concentrations in the ng mL^{-1} (or lower) range.

Lack of reproducibility

The major problem associated with intranasal delivery is the question of whether it can provide *reliable* absorption. Diseases such as the common cold and hayfever are recognized to alter the condition of the nose, either increasing or decreasing mucociliary clearance, or altering the permeability of the absorbing mucosa. The frequency with which these diseases occur means that patients requiring chronic drug therapy will undergo periods when drug absorption might be expected to be higher or lower than "normal". For drugs with a narrow therapeutic index, such variations may be unacceptable.

Adverse reactions

Locally irritating or sensitizing drugs must be used with caution in this route. Nasal epithelia, and in particular the cilia, are highly sensitive and fragile. This contrasts with, for example, the buccal epithelium which is much more robust and less prone to irritation. The fragility of the tissue also means that this route is particularly sensitive to the adverse effects of penetration enhancers. Damage to the epithelium could result in compromised mucocilary clearance which is associated with respiratory disease.

9.6 CURRENT TECHNOLOGIES FOR NASAL DRUG DELIVERY

Current technologies for nasal drug delivery are concerned with:

- the local delivery of drugs such as decongestants, antibiotics and mucolytics, for treatment of conditions of the nasal cavity;
- the systemic delivery of low molecular weight drugs (< 500 Da), including therapeutic peptides. Some intranasally delivered drugs showing systemic absorption are given in Table 9.4.

Delivery devices currently in use include nasal sprays and drops:

9.6.1 Nasal sprays

Nasal sprays are available as squeeze bottles, which would not be expected to give reproducible dosing. They are also available as metered-dose devices, which would be expected to give more reproducible dosing, as a mechanical actuation delivers a pre-determined volume to the patient. Thus the dose of drug received by the patient will be dependent on the concentration of drug in the formulation. Commercial examples of metered-dose sprays include Syntaris, Beconase and Rhinocort which deliver flunisolide, beclomethasone and budesonide respectively.

As discussed above, nasal sprays tend to deposit at their impaction site, in the anterior, unciliated regions of the nasal cavity, where airflow associated with inspiration is high and mucociliary clearance is slow or erratic. Thus a drug moiety depositing in this region is cleared slowly and is transported over a large area *en route* to the pharynx. These factors promote drug absorption.

9.6.2 Nasal drops

Nasal drops rely upon the instillation of one or more drops of drug solution, either from a dropper with a flexible (rubber) teat, or directly from a "squeezable" plastic container into the nasal cavity.

As described above, nasal drops, if administered correctly, deposit drug throughout the nasal cavity (Figure 9.8), which offers a larger

Class	Drug
Analgesics	morphine; oxycodone
Anticholinesterases	neostigmine; tubocurarine
Antiemetics	metoclopramide
Antiinfectives	gentamicin; tobramicin; cephazolin; acyclovir
Antimigraine drugs	sumatripan; dihydroergotamine
Antimuscarinics	hyoscine (scopolamine); atropine; ipratropium
Cardiovascular drugs	propranolol; atenolol; timolol trinitroglycerine; hydralazine; nifedipine verapamil
CNS stimulants	cocaine; nicotine
Dopaminergic drugs	apomorphine; bromocriptine
Hormones and analogues	growth hormone; corticotrophin (ACTH); calcitonin; desmopressin (DDAVP); lypressin; oxytocin; buserelin; nafarelin; progesterone; norethisterone; 17β-estradiol; testosterone; insulin; Gonadorelin (Gonadotrophin-releasing hormone; GnRH; LH-RH)
Miscellaneous amino acids/peptides	interferon; metkephamid; l-tyrosine; angiopeptin; granulocyte-colony stimulating factor (G-CSF); glucagon; octreotide
Sedatives	midazolam; diazepam; temazepam; propiomazine
Vaccines	Influenza; Measles; Polio; Rhinovirus Type 13; Respiratory Synctial virus

Table 9.4 Some intranasally-delivered drugs showing systemic absorption

effective area for immediate absorption than if the drug is delivered in the form of a spray. However this also means that:

- some drug is inevitably deposited on ciliated regions of the mucosa and is therefore immediately available for clearance;
- a proportion of the dose actually deposits at the nasopharynx where it may be immediately swallowed and is therefore not available for nasal absorption.

To ensure a complete coating of the nasal mucosa from the atrium to the nasopharynx, the method depicted in Figure 9.9 is recommended. Since this is either unknown or inconvenient to most patients, variable drug absorption is likely to result, which would be unacceptable for drugs with a narrow therapeutic window.

9.6.3 Nasal sprays vs. nasal drops

With both drops and sprays, about 40% of the administered dose is cleared rapidly within 20 minutes, then a second, slower phase of clearance follows. In this second slower phase, clearance of the drops is much faster than clearance of the spray, probably because most of the spray deposits on non-ciliated regions. Due to this faster clearance,

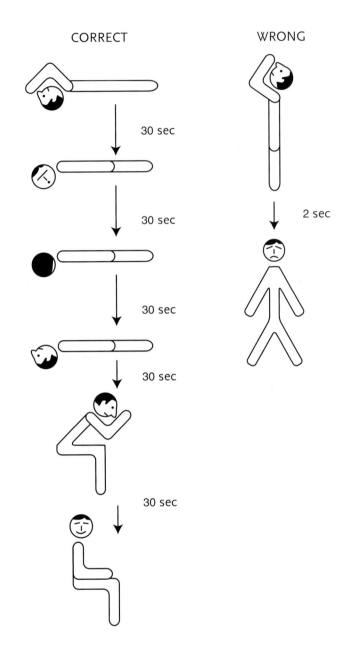

CORRECT   WRONG

30 sec

30 sec   2 sec

30 sec

30 sec

30 sec

Figure 9.9 Illustration of correct and incorrect administration from a nasal drop-bottle

nasal drops are more suitable for drug moieties which are rapidly absorbed.

Drug molecules which diffuse across the nasal epithelium relatively slowly will need a longer contact time and may therefore be better administered as sprays. The bioavailability of the peptide drug desmo-pressin is greater from a metered-dose nasal spray than from drops. The success of this dosage form in promoting nasal absorption is evidenced by the commercial availability of nasal sprays for the systemic delivery of various peptide drugs, including buserelin, desmopressin, oxytocin and calcitonin.

9.7   NEW TECHNOLOGIES IN NASAL DELIVERY

As can be seen from Table 9.4, many conventional drugs have been investigated for systemic delivery via the nasal cavity and these are of relatively low molecular weight (in most cases less than 500 Da). However, peptides and proteins generally have a molecular weight in excess of 1,000 Da and are therefore unlikely to be absorbed across the nasal mucosa in any appreciable amounts without pharmaceutical intervention. New technologies in nasal delivery are primarily concerned with strategies to increase drug absorption. These approaches are summarised in Table 9.5.

Strategies under development to promote drug absorption via the nasal cavity are detailed below.

9.7.1   Increasing the permeability of the nasal epithelium

A variety of molecules have been studied in an effort to find a compound which is able to increase the permeability of the nasal epithelium without causing harm (Table 9.5).

The mechanisms of absorption promotion proposed for the different compounds are numerous and it is likely that more than one mechanism is involved:

Alteration of mucus layer

Agents that decrease the viscoelasticity of mucus, for example anionic and cationic surfactants and bile salts, have been shown to increase absorption.

Alteration of tight junctions

Substances that sequester extracellular calcium ions, which are required to maintain tight junction integrity for example EDTA, bile salts, will cause the tight junctions to open. Thus, the paracellular route becomes leakier, permitting increased absorption of substances that use this route.

Reversed micelle formation

The differing adjuvant activities of various bile salt species relate to their differing capacities to penetrate and self-associate as reverse micelles within the membrane. In reverse micelles, the hydrophilic surfaces of the molecules face inward and the hydrophobic surfaces face outward from the lipid environment. The formation of reverse micelles within the cell membranes may create an aqueous pore, through which drug moieties can pass.

Extraction by co-micellization

Solubilization of cell membrane lipids, for example the removal of cholesterol by surfactants such as bile salts and polyoxyethylene ethers.

Chemical	Physical	Enzyme inhibitors
Surfactants Synthetic Surfactants – Laureth 9 (9 lauryl ether) – Brij (polyoxyethylene ether)	osmotic pressure pH	*Peptidase Inhibitors* amastatin bacitracin boroleucine
Naturally-occurring surfactants (i) Phospholipids Didecanoyl-L-α- phosphatidyl choline Lysophosphatidylcholine (ii) Bile salts Sodium cholate Sodium deoxycholate Sodium taurocholate (iii) Bile salt analogues Sodium taurodi- hydrofusidate (STDHF) (iv) Plant extracts Quillaja saponins	drug concentration viscosity e.g. methylcellulose bioadhesive systems e.g. some polymers and microspheres powder *vs.* solution microspheres e.g. starch, dextran, hyaluronan esters, carbomer oily suspension	bestatin diprotinin leupeptin aprotinin soyabean trypsin inhibitor camostat mesilate
Polymers Chitosan, poloxamer 407, methylcellulose, hyaluronan, carbomer, sodium carboxymethylcellulose	liposomes thermogelling systems e.g. ethyl(hydroxyethyl) cellulose, Pluronic F127	
Cyclodextrins dimethyl β cyclodextrin	posture	
Chelating agents ethylenediaminetetraacetic acid (EDTA)		
Preservatives e.g. parahydroxybenzoates, benzalkonium chloride		
Other compounds ascorbic acid, tartaric acid, glycofurol 75, acylcarnitines		

Erosion of mucosal surface

Cellular erosion, cell-cell separation, loss of cilia and formation of a dense mucus coat in response to injury can be caused by surfactants such as bile salts.

However, a serious drawback for the use of penetration enhancers may be their potential deleterious effect to the epithelial tissue, either directly, by perturbing vital cell structures and/or functions, or indirectly, by permeabilizing the epithelium and thus paving the way for inward penetration of toxic agents and organisms. For example, it is generally held that surface-active compounds only enhance penetration when the absorbing membrane has been damaged. Patients have experienced stinging and lacrimation when STDHF was used as a penetration enhancer at a concentration of 0.8% w/v.

This severely limits the clinical development of such compounds and some of the more recently published work has concentrated on illustrating this toxicity and employing strategies to mitigate it. For instance, the co-administration of cyclodextrins or phosphatidylcholine has been reported to reduce the toxicity of certain surfactants, the latter by the formation of mixed micelles.

In addition to exerting effects on the epithelium (i.e. true penetration-enhancing effects), penetration enhancers may also promote nasal delivery via solubility effects. For example, cyclodextrins are used to solubilize drugs and thus increase the concentration of drug driving diffusion at the absorption site; an added benefit of having the drug at a higher concentration is that the same dose can be achieved in a smaller volume of solution. For example, the addition of β-cyclodextrin to dihydroergotamine can enable the drug concentration to be increased from 4 mg mL^{-1} to 10 mg mL^{-1}. As a result, the volume usually administered to the nasal cavity (0.5 mL), which can result in spillage, can be reduced. Cyclodextrins are also capable of dissociating insulin hexamers into smaller aggregates which may provide an additional mechanism for absorption promotion. However, it should not be overlooked that a direct relationship has been reported between the extent of absorption enhancement by cyclodextrins and damage to the nasal membrane.

Penetration enhancers may also promote delivery by increasing drug stability, due to the enhancer decreasing the activity of enzymes which may degrade the drug. This property is discussed further below.

9.7.2 Increasing contact time at absorption site

Prolonging the contact time between the drug and its absorption site is likely to increase the bioavailability of the drug. Since drugs may be cleared from the nasal cavity by mucociliary clearance, swallowing and/or by metabolism, the inhibition or avoidance of these clearance mechanisms should result in increased absorption. Strategies being investigated include:

9.7.2.1 *Modifying the site of deposition*

Although it is assumed that the turbinates are the principal sites for the systemic absorption of intranasally delivered drugs, these are also an area of high mucociliary clearance, especially in the highly ciliated middle and posterior region. Thus drug deposited in the anterior region of the nasal cavity may be expected to clear less rapidly and have a greater opportunity to be absorbed. As already described, this explains why nasal sprays, which deposit anteriorly in the nasal cavity, offer improved bioavailability compared to nasal drops, which deposit throughout the nose.

Increasing the viscosity of solutions administered to the nasal cavity with, for example, methylcellulose, hyaluronan etc., has been shown to increase the time the formulation is retained in the nasal cavity and to enhance the absorption of certain drugs. It is thought that, up to an optimum viscosity, higher viscosity solutions give a more localized deposition in the anterior portion of the nose (i.e. low clearance site). As viscosity can affect droplet size by altering the surface tension of the solution, the more localized deposition in the anterior of the nose may be due to viscosity-related changes in the particle size of the delivered droplets.

The volume of drug solution delivered to the nose also seems to have an effect on the bioavailability of the drug. For example, the bioavailability of desmopressin was doubled when it was delivered as two 50 μl actuations from a metered nasal spray in comparison to the delivery of one 100 μl actuation. This may be attributed to prolonged retention of the dose at the administration site.

9.7.2.2 Use of bioadhesives

Bioadhesives (sometimes also termed mucoadhesives) adhere to biological substrates such as mucus or tissue. Bioadhesives are proposed to influence drug bioavailability by:

- decreasing the rate of clearance from the absorption site thereby increasing the time available for absorption;
- increasing the local drug concentration at the site of adhesion/absorption;
- protecting the drug from dilution and possible degradation by nasal secretions.

A number of different bioadhesive formulations are possible:

Bioadhesive solutions/suspensions

Many viscosity enhancers are also considered to be bioadhesive and putative bioadhesive polymer gels, including methylcellulose, sodium carboxymethylcellulose, chitosan, Carbopol 934P (one of the carbomers) and Pluronic F127, have been shown to decrease the rate of mucociliary clearance in the rat by 7–57%. By reducing or abolishing ciliary motility, the rate of clearance of the drug from the nasal cavity is reduced. A nasal solution formulation of chitosan has been shown to be less toxic to ciliated epithelia than STDHF and to yield an absolute bioavailability of 31% for the analgesic, morphine-6-glucuronide, in sheep. In addition, chitosan has been shown to enhance the nasal absorption of insulin (molecular weight 5.8 kDa) in rats and sheep. Some bioadhesives, such as carbomers, have also been shown to complex with mucus, increasing the viscoelasticity of the latter and reducing its clearance.

Certain polymers are termed "thermogelling" e.g. ethyl(hydroxyethyl)cellulose and Pluronic F127 (Poloxamer 407). In aqueous solution above a certain concentration, such systems are liquid at room temperature and below, but at physiological temperatures (32–37 °C), the viscosity of the solutions increases. Once in the nasal cavity, the viscosity of these solutions will increase, due to the increased temperature, and the contact time between the drug and the absorbing membrane should be extended compared to that of a simple solution. Such systems have also been investigated to enhance vaginal and ocular drug delivery (see Sections 11.7.6 and 12.3.3.4.2 respectively).

Dry powder bioadhesives

A slightly different approach is to deliver the active drug in a dry powder carrier system, for example microcrystalline cellulose, hydroxyethyl starch, cross-linked dextran, microcrystalline chitosan, carbomer, pectin, or alginic acid. The polymer absorbs water upon contact with the nasal mucosa and swells to become a viscous gel, often demonstrating bioadhesive properties. Such systems can remain in the nasal cavity for as long as six hours. For example, the bioavailability in rats of the somatostatin analogue, octreotide, was shown to be enhanced by the co-administration of alginic acid and cross-linked dextran as dry powders.

Certain carriers prolong the time during which therapeutic plasma concentrations of drug are maintained, effectively providing sustained release. This is believed to occur due to the rate and extent of water uptake being modified by the formulation, as well as to the type of gel formed by the excipients. As the polymers hydrate by withdrawing water from the secretions of the nasal epithelium, localized changes in mucociliary clearance occur, due to the presence of a hydrating polymer and potentially due to induced alterations in the viscoelasticity of the mucus gel.

Colloidal bioadhesives

Bioadhesive microspheres composed from a variety of materials such as starch, carbomer, hyaluronan esters, dextrans have been used to prolong the retention time of the drug within the nasal cavity. The clearance half-life of microspheres can be in the order of 3–4 hours, in comparison with 15 minutes for a simple solution. Improved bioavailabilities have been seen for gentamicin, insulin and desmopressin.

A temporary widening of the tight junctions of cultured cells, which coincided with an increase in the rate of absorption of the applied drug, insulin, has been observed in the presence of starch microspheres. It is likely that the dry starch microspheres took up water from the cells causing them to dehydrate and "shrink" resulting in a separation of the intercellular junctions. Should this be the case, it provides evidence for the paracellular absorption of insulin.

Liposomes (see Section 5.3.1) have also been used to encapsulate drugs presented to the nasal mucosa in order to achieve the sustained release of rapidly absorbed drugs, for example propranolol.

9.7.2.3 *Reducing rate of mucociliary clearance*

An alternative approach is to reduce the rate of mucociliary clearance and hence increase the retention time of the drug. This can be achieved by including an excipient in the formulation with a reversible ciliostatic effect; such agents include certain preservatives. However, it is important that the chosen strategy does not permanently compromise mucociliary clearance, which would adversely affect airway homeostasis and defense.

Many penetration enhancers cause irreversible ciliostasis, e.g. STDHF (0.3%), laureth 9 (0.3%), sodium deoxycholate (0.3%), or irreversibly halt mucociliary transport, e.g. STDHF (1%), laureth 9 (1%), sodium deoxycholate (1%). Others, such as sodium glycocholate, are well tolerated. However the long-term effects of even a temporary impediment to the mechanism of nasal clearance is unknown and such an approach should be used with caution.

9.7.3 Inhibition of enzymatic degradation

Another clearance mechanism at work within the nasal cavity is the enzymatic degradation of the active drug by the nasal secretions and mucosa. For instance, cytochrome P450-dependent monooxygenase metabolizes nasal decongestants, nicotine, cocaine and progesterone. With respect to the degradation of peptides and proteins, a variety of protease inhibitors have been studied including bestatin, diprotinin A and aprotinin, which inhibit leucine aminopeptidase, dipeptidyl peptidase and trypsin respectively (Table 9.5). Some inhibitors are active against more than one peptidase, for example leupeptin inhibits both cathepsin and trypsin. The choice of inhibitor depends upon the peptide, for instance inhibitors having a trypsin-inhibitory effect have been shown to enhance the nasal absorption of salmon calcitonin in rats.

Interestingly, compounds which have been investigated for their penetration-enhancing effect at the absorbing membrane have also been shown to decrease the metabolism of certain peptides. By denaturing leucine aminopeptidase and preventing enzyme–substrate complex formation, the bile salt sodium glycocholate has been shown to protect insulin from proteolysis in the rat nasal mucosa.

In addition to formulation additives, peptides can be chemically modified to improve their stability to proteases, as described in Chapter 1 (Section 1.6.1).

9.7.4 Miscellaneous methods of absorption enhancement

Miscellaneous methods of absorption enhancement include:

Altering the osmotic pressure (tonicity) of formulations

Deviations from isotonicity were shown to increase the absorption of salmon calcitonin (molecular weight 4.5 kDa) four- to five-fold by one group. However, altering the tonicity of the formulation had no effect on the absorption of human granulocyte colony-stimulating factor (molecular weight 19 kDa). In another study, decreasing the pH of the formulation was shown to enhance absorption. Alterations of osmotic pressure and pH beyond a certain range might be expected to result in damage to the epithelium and hence increase its permeability to xenobiotics.

Delivering the drug as a dry powder

A further approach has been to deliver drugs in the form of a powder (but without a bioadhesive carrier). For example, freeze-dried insulin has been shown to be better absorbed as a powder than in solution, although the absorption of glucagon and dihydroergotamine, when delivered from liquid or powder formulations, was equivalent.

9.8 CONCLUSIONS

The intra-nasal route possesses many advantages for the systemic delivery of drugs. However, problems which require resolving include developing absorption promoters with minimal toxicity and overcoming adverse nasal pathology to ensure accurate and reproducible dosing.

9.9 FURTHER READING

Gizurarson, S. (1993) The relevance of nasal physiology to the design of drug absorption studies. *Advanced Drug Delivery Reviews*, 11:329–347.

Lansley, A.B. (1993) Mucocilary clearance and drug delivery via the respiratory tract. *Advanced Drug Delivery Reviews*, 11:299–327.

Rogers, D.F. and Lethem, M.I. (eds.) (1997) *Airway Mucus: Basic Mechanisms and Clinical Perspectives*. Birkhauser Verlag, Basel.

Chien, Y.W. (ed.) (1985) *Transnasal Systemic Medications*. Elsevier, Amsterdam.

Chien, Y.W. and Chang, S.F. (1992) *Nasal Drug Delivery and Delivery Systems in Novel Drug Delivery Systems* (Chien, Y.W., (ed.). Marcel Dekker, New York, pp. 229–268.

Hardy, J.G., Lee, S.W. and Wilson, C.G. (1985) Intranasal drug delivery by spray and drops. *J. Pharm. Pharmacol.*, 37:294–297.

McMartin, C., Hutchinson, L.E.F., Hyde, R. and Peters, G.E. (1987) Analysis of structural requirements for the absorption of drugs and macromolecules from the nasal cavity. *J. Pharm. Sci.*, 76:535–540.

Sarkar, M.A. (1992) Drug metabolism in the nasal mucosa. *Pharm. Res.* 9:1–9.

9.10 SELF-ASSESSMENT QUESTIONS

1. Outline the structure and physiology of the nasal cavity.
2. Describe the process of mucocilary clearance.
3. List the physiological factors affecting nasal bioavailability.
4. Describe the formulation factors that may affect nasal bio-availability.
5. Outline the advantages and disadvantages of nasal drug delivery.
6. Describe the two current technologies used in nasal drug delivery. Indicate the relative merits of each technology.
7. List the mechanisms by which the permeability of the nasal epithelium may be increased to improve the efficacy of nasal drug delivery.
8. Describe the various types of bioadhesives used to enhance nasal drug delivery.

Pulmonary Drug Delivery

Glyn Taylor and Ian Kellaway

OBJECTIVES

On completion of this chapter the reader should be able to:

- Describe the structure and physiology of the lung
- Discuss the barriers to pulmonary drug delivery
- Outline the advantages and disadvantages of pulmonary drug delivery
- Describe the current pulmonary drug delivery technologies
- Outline the future directions of pulmonary drug delivery

10.1 INTRODUCTION

Pulmonary drug delivery is primarily used to treat conditions of the airways, delivering locally acting drugs directly to their site of action (Table 10.1). Delivery of anti-asthmatic and other locally acting drugs directly to their site of action reduces the dose needed to produce a pharmacological effect, while the low concentrations in the systemic circulation may also reduce side-effects.

The lung may additionally be employed as a route for delivery of drugs into the systemic circulation, and onward to an effect site located elsewhere in the body. A product containing ergotamine tartrate is available as an aerosolized dosage inhaler for the treatment of migraine. Volatile anesthetics, including, for example, halothane, are also given via the pulmonary route. In recent years, the possibility of utilizing the pulmonary route for the systemic delivery of peptides and other molecules which are not absorbed through the gastrointestinal tract has also been explored. Pulmonary drug delivery for both local and systemic effects will be discussed in this chapter.

10.2 STRUCTURE AND PHYSIOLOGY OF THE LUNGS

10.2.1 Lung regions

The respiratory tract starts at the nose and terminates deep in the lung at an alveolar sac. There are a number of schemes for categorizing the different regions of the respiratory tract. With respect to pulmonary drug delivery, division into the following three regions is useful (Figure 10.1):

Nasopharyngeal (NP) region

This is also referred to as the "upper airways", which includes the respiratory airways from the nose down to the larynx. This region has been described extensively in Chapter 9.

Tracheo-bronchial (TB) region

This is also referred to as the "central"or "conducting airways", which starts at the larynx, and extends via the trachea, bronchi, and bronchioles and ends at the terminal bronchioles.

Table 10.1 Drugs administered by inhalation for local action in the airways. COPD = chronic obstructive pulmonary disease; CF = cystic fibrosis

Drug Type	Disease	Examples
b_2-adrenoceptor agonists	asthma, COPD	salbutamol, terbutaline, fenoterol, salmeterol
corticosteroids	asthma, COPD	budesonide, beclomethasone
anticholinergics	asthma, COPD	ipratropium bromide
anti-inflammatory	asthma	nedocromil, cromoglycate
mucolytics	CF	N-acetylcysteine
antibiotics	respiratory infections (CF, AIDS)	pentamidine, aminoglycosides e.g. tobramycin

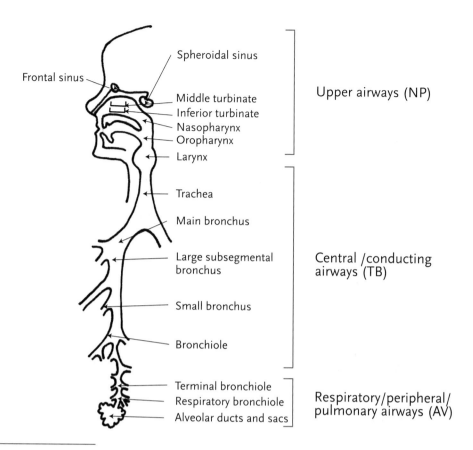

Spheroidal sinus

Frontal sinus

Middle turbinate
Inferior turbinate
Nasopharynx
Oropharynx
Larynx

Trachea

Main bronchus

Large subsegmental
bronchus

Small bronchus

Bronchiole

Terminal bronchiole
Respiratory bronchiole
Alveolar ducts and sacs

Upper airways (NP)

Central /conducting
airways (TB)

Respiratory/peripheral/
pulmonary airways (AV)

Figure 10.1 Different regions of the human respiratory tract

Alveolar (A) region

This is also referred to as the "respiratory airways", "peripheral airways" or "pulmonary region", comprising the respiratory bronchioles, alveolar ducts and alveoli.

The term "pulmonary" can be misleading since some authors use it with reference to the whole lung, while others restrict its use to the A region. In this chapter pulmonary refers to the whole lung. The use of "upper respiratory tract" (i.e. NP plus trachea) and "lower respiratory tract" (i.e. TB plus A) is also commonplace.

10.2.2 Architecture of the airways

The basic architecture of the tracheobronchial region is predominantly one of a symmetric series of dichotomous branches. Every branching of the tracheobronchial tree leads to a new "generation" of airways; for example, the trachea ("generation 0") bifurcates into two main bronchi ("generation 1") and then follows sequential branching into lobar bronchi ("generation 2"), segmental bronchi ("generation 3"), intrasegmental bronchi, bronchioles, secondary bronchioles and ultimately the terminal bronchioles ("generation 16"). The terminal bronchioles mark the limit of the tracheobronchial region, beyond which lies the alveolar region ("generations 17 to 23"). Progression from the trachea to the extremities of the tracheobronchial tree is characterized by decreases in both the diameter and length of the tubules with each branching, but the geometrically increasing number of airways results in dramatic increases in surface area.

This model of the human lung with a symmetric dichotomously branching system has been extensively used to simulate particle deposition under different conditions (e.g. inspiratory flow rate). It should be borne in mind, however, that in humans, the left and right lungs are not identical and each contains irregular dichotomous and trichotomous branching patterns. Additionally, while the average path length from trachea to terminal bronchioles is 16 branches, short paths of only 8 to 10 branches may also exist.

The terminal bronchioles mark the end of the tracheobronchial region. The alveolar region begins at the respiratory bronchioles, where alveoli begin to appear in the airway walls. Further branching of the respiratory bronchioles is associated with increasing frequency of alveoli appearing until the airway terminates at a respiratory unit, which contains alveolar ducts, atria and about 20 alveoli. The alveoli are packed tightly with adjacent alveoli separated by a common alveolar septum. In the whole lung there are several hundred million alveoli.

10.2.3 Pulmonary epithelium

The lung contains more than 40 different cell types, of which more than six line the airways (Figure 10.2). The diversity of pulmonary epithelia can be illustrated by examining its structure at three principal levels (Figure 10.3):

The bronchi

These are lined predominantly with ciliated and goblet cells. Some serous cells, brush cells and Clara cells are also present with few Kulchitsky cells.

The bronchioles

These are primarily lined with ciliated cuboidal cells. The frequency of goblet and serous cells decreases with progression along the airways while the number of Clara cells increases. The epithelium is much thinner and there is less mucus in this region.

The alveolar region

This is devoid of mucus and has a much flatter epithelium, which becomes the simple squamous type, 0.1–0.5 μm thick. Two principal epithelial cell types are present:

- Type-I pneumocytes: thin cells offering a very short airways–blood path length for the diffusion of gases and drug molecules. Type-I pneumocytes occupy about 93% of the surface area of the alveolar sacs, despite being only half as abundant as type-II cells.

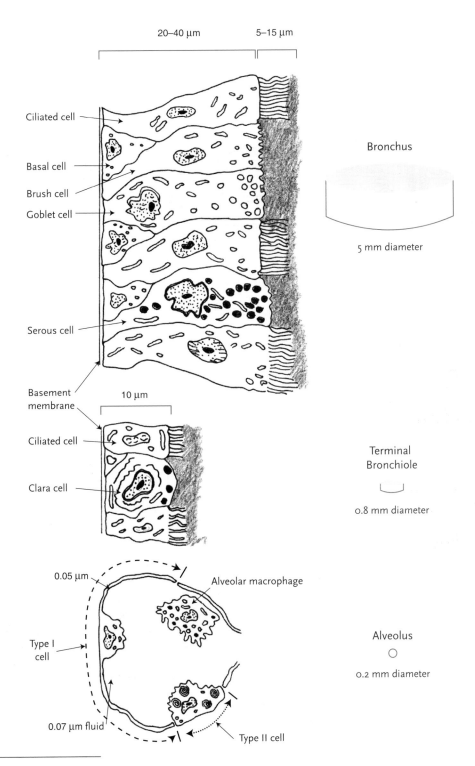

20–40 μm   5–15 μm

Ciliated cell

Basal cell

Brush cell

Goblet cell

Serous cell

Basement membrane

10 μm

Ciliated cell

Clara cell

Bronchus

5 mm diameter

Terminal Bronchiole

0.8 mm diameter

0.05 μm

Alveolar macrophage

Type I cell

Alveolus

0.2 mm diameter

0.07 μm fluid

Type II cell

Figure 10.2
Pulmonary epithelial cells

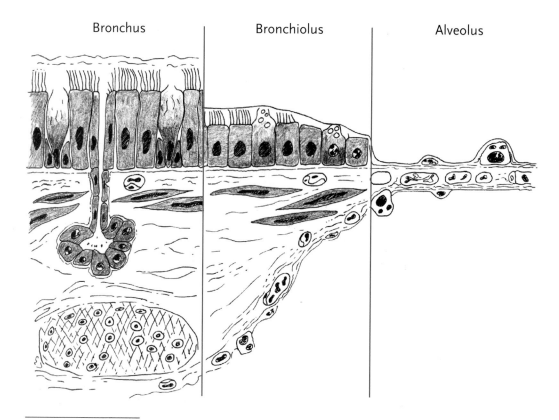

| Bronchus | Bronchiolus | Alveolus |

- Type-II pneumocytes: cuboidal cells that store and secrete pulmonary surfactant.

Alveolar macrophages account for ~ 3% of cells in the A region. These phagocytic cells scavenge and transport particulate matter to the lymph nodes and the mucociliary escalator (see below).

10.2.4 Ciliated cells

In the tracheobronchial region, a high proportion of the epithelial cells are ciliated such that there is a near complete covering of the central airways by cilia (Figure 10.2). Towards the periphery of the tracheobronchial region, the cilia are less abundant and are absent in the alveolar region. The ciliated cells each have about 200 cilia with numerous interspersed microvilli, of about 1–2 μm in length.

The cilia are hair-like projections about 0.25 μm in diameter and 5 μm in length. They are bathed in an epithelial lining fluid, secreted mainly from the serous cells in the submucosal glands. The tips of the cilia project through the epithelial lining fluid into a layer of mucus secreted from goblet cells. The cilia beat in an organized fashion to propel mucus along the airways to the throat, as discussed below (see Section 10.3.4.2).

10.2.5 Mucus

Mucus does not exist in the alveolar region, but is present as a viscoelastic layer in the tracheobronchial region. The mucus largely originates from the vagally innervated submucosal glands, with a smaller contribution from goblet cells. As discusssed in detail in Chapter 9 (Section 9.2.4.2), respiratory mucus is a complex mixture with includes glycoproteins, proteins and lipids. Its composition is also highly variable in disease states, with infections being accompanied by high levels of DNA.

10.2.6 Lung surfactant

Epithelial type-II cells constantly secrete and reutilize lung surfactant. It consists of lipid-rich lipoproteins with the lipid composition dominated by phosphatidylcholine with a high dipalmitoyl content. About 85–90% of isolated surfactant is lipid of which 95% is phosphoglycerols with cholesterol as the main neutral component. A number of proteins are also present and, in addition to albumin, which might be a contaminant, consists of four non-serum apoproteins (SP-A, SP-B, SP-C and SP-D). Multiple functions are ascribed to these apoproteins including metabolic control of lung surfactant synthesis, recycling by alveolar type-II cells and immediate enhancement of the spreading of phospholipids.

Lung surfactant decreases the surface tension and thereby maintains the morphology and function critical for respiration. Deficiency of surfactant in the newborn infant is a condition known as respiratory distress syndrome (RDS) and in adults as adult respiratory distress syndrome (ARDS). A number of commercial artificial surfactants, e.g. Exosurf and ALEC, together with natural surfactant preparations, e.g. Surventa and Curosurf, are currently available to treat these conditions.

10.3 FACTORS AFFECTING PULMONARY DRUG DELIVERY

10.3.1 Mechanisms of particle deposition in the airways

The adult human lung is exposed to more than 10,000 litres of air each day. Thus with each intake of air, the lung receives a high burden of dusts, fumes, pollens, microbes and other contaminants. Efficient defense mechanisms have evolved to minimize the burden of foreign particles entering the airways, and clearing those that succeed in being deposited.

All devices employed for drug delivery to the airways of the lung generate an aerosol. Therapeutic aerosols are two-phase colloidal systems in which the drug is contained in a dispersed phase which may be a liquid, solid or combination of the two, depending upon the formulation and method of aerosol generation (see Section 10.5). Clearly for successful therapy, the drug must be presented to the lung in aerosol droplets or particles that deposit in the appropriate lung region and in sufficient quantity to be effective.

Once the aerosol particle or droplet has deposited in the lung, there are a number of further barriers which must be overcome before the drug exerts its pharmacological effect. The respiratory defense mechanisms of mucociliary clearance and phagocytosis by macrophages may act upon undissolved particles. Aerosol particle dissolution may be slow and the drug may then subsequently be subject to enzymatic degradation before it reaches its site of pharmacological action.

The factors influencing the deposition and fate of pulmonary delivered drugs will be discussed in this section.

Aerosols for pulmonary drug delivery are delivered via the mouth. Three principal deposition mechanisms operate within the lower respiratory tract (Figure 10.4):

Inertial impaction

This is the dominant deposition mechanism for particles >1 μm in the upper tracheobronchial regions. A particle with a large momentum may be unable to follow the changing direction of the inspired air as it passes the bifurcations and as a result will collide with the airway walls as it continues on its original course. Impaction therefore usually occurs near the bifurcations, indeed the impaction of particles from tobacco smoke on the bifurcations may be one reason why these sites are often the foci for lung tumors. The probability of inertial impaction will be dependent upon particle momentum (the product of mass and velocity), thus particles with larger diameters or higher densities and those travelling in airstreams of higher velocity will show greater impaction. Airflow velocities in the main bronchi are estimated to be 100-fold higher than in the terminal bronchioles and 1,000-fold higher than in the A region (Figure 10.5).

Figure 10.4
Description of particle deposition mechanisms at an airway branching site

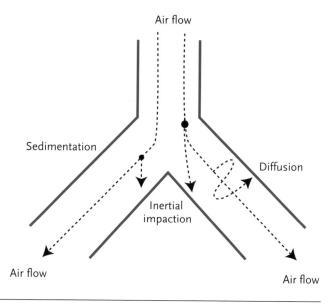

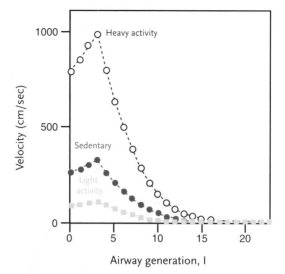

Figure 10.5 Air velocity profiles within the lung as a function of subject activity level of ventilation

Sedimentation

This is particle deposition resulting from settling under gravity. It becomes increasingly important for particles that reach airways where the airstream velocity is relatively low, e.g the bronchioles and alveolar region. The fraction of particles depositing by this mechanism will be dependent upon the time the particles spend in these regions.

Brownian diffusion

This is of little significance for particles >1 μm. Particles below this size are displaced by a random bombardment of gas molecules, which results in particle collision with the airway walls. The probability of particle deposition by diffusion increases as the particle size decreases. Brownian diffusion is also more prevalent in regions where airflow is very low or absent, e.g. in the alveoli.

Another method of deposition, that of interception, is of importance for fibers but is not of importance for drug delivery.

As a consequence of these physical forces acting on the aerosol particle, its deposition in the lung is highly dependent on diameter. Generally:

- Particles larger than 10 μm will impact in the upper airways and are rapidly removed by coughing, swallowing and mucociliary processes. An 8 μm particle inhaled at 30 L min^{-1} has approximately a 50% chance of impacting on the throat.
- Smaller particles in the size range 0.5–5 μm may escape impaction in the upper airways and will deposit by impaction and sedimentation in the lower TB and A regions. If the aerosol particle size is between about 3 and 5 μm then deposition will predominantly occur in the TB region. If the particles are less than about 3 μm then appreciable deposition in the A region is likely to occur.

- Submicron particles may not be deposited since some will be removed from the lung on the exhaled airstream before sedimentation can occur.

Thus only aerosols < ~5 μm in diameter show efficient penetration into the lungs. The "respirable fraction" of a therapeutic aerosol is often quoted as the percentage of drug present in aerosol particles less than 5 μm in size.

10.3.2 Physiological factors affecting particle deposition in the airways

10.3.2.1 Lung morphology

As described in Section 10.2, each successive generation of the tracheo-bronchial tree produces airways of decreasing diameter and length. Each bifurcation results in an increased probability for impaction and the decrease in airway diameter is associated with a smaller displacement required for a particle to contact a surface. Thus to travel down the airways, the drug particles must pass through a successive series of branching tubes of constantly decreasing size. The aerosol particles must constantly change direction in order to remain airborne. Thus lobes of the lung which have the shortest average pathlength will show greatest peripheral deposition.

10.3.2.2 Oral vs. nasal breathing

During normal nose breathing the majority of inhaled environmental particles are deposited in the nose and pharynx, as described in Chapter 9 (Section 9.2). Hence for pulmonary drug delivery, the aerosols are inhaled via the mouth.

10.3.2.3 Inspiratory flow rate

Increasing the inspiratory flow rate (IFR) will enhance deposition by impaction in the first few generations of the TB region. The increase in flow will not only increase particle momentum but will also result in an increase in turbulence, particularly in the larynx and trachea, which itself will enhance impaction in the proximal TB region. As illustrated in Figure 10.5, airflow is highest in the bronchi, rapidly decreasing in the bronchioles and alveolar region. Airflow velocity is also dependent upon physical activity and estimated airflow velocities resulting from sedentary (IFR of 14 L min^{-1}), light (IFR of 40 L min^{-1}) and heavy (IFR of 120 L min^{-1}) activities are shown in Figure 10.5. A similar range of IFRs are observed if untrained subjects use inhalation devices. The effects of IFR on deposition from devices which use the energy of inspiration to generate the drug aerosol (e.g. most DPIs) are more complex, since an increase in IFR will in most cases lead to the production of an aerosol of smaller particle size.

10.3.2.4 Co-ordination of aerosol generation with inspiration

The momentum of aerosol particles generated from pressurized metered-dose inhalers (pMDIs, see Section 10.5) is largely governed by the pMDI formulation rather than the subject's IFR. pMDI aerosol droplets will be travelling at velocities of 2,500–3,000 cm s^{-1}. A failure to co-ordinate actuation of the pMDI during the early phase of the inspiratory maneuver will result in near total particle impaction in the oropharnygeal region. Deposition from pMDIs may be increased at higher IFRs as a result of better aerosol entrainment and lower deposition in the throat.

10.3.2.5 *Tidal volume*

An increased IFR will usually be associated with an increase in the volume of air inhaled in one breath, the tidal volume. Clearly an increase in tidal volume will result in penetration of aerosol particles deeper into the TB and A regions and a greater chance for deposition within these regions.

10.3.2.6 *Breath holding*

Increasing the time between the end of inspiration and the start of exhalation increases the time for sedimentation to occur. Breath-holding is commonly used to optimize pulmonary drug delivery. For maximum effect, breath-holding for a period of 5–10 seconds post-inspiration is recommended. Under idealized conditions a 5 μm particle will settle a few mm during a 5-second breath hold.

10.3.2.7 *Disease states*

Bronchial obstruction as seen in a variety of pulmonary disorders will be associated with greater local airflows and turbulence and this will result in localized deposition in the larger airways of the TB region. The bronchoconstriction of asthma has a greater influence on exhalation than inhalation and thus deposition by sedimentation may be greater than normal.

10.3.3 Pharmaceutical factors affecting aerosol deposition

The technologies used to generate pharmaceutical aerosols are described in Section 10.5.

10.3.3.1 *Aerosol velocity*

The aerosols produced by nebulizers and dry powder inhalers (DPIs) are transported into the lung by entrainment on the inspired air and thus their velocity is determined by the inspiratory maneuver and lung physiology, as discussed above. In contrast, pMDIs generate aerosol droplets with velocities greater than the inspiratory airflow and consequently the aerosol will have a greater tendency to impact in the oropharyngeal region.

10.3.3.2 *Size*

Commercial devices do not lead to monodispersed particles and often the size distribution is wide and the particles may exhibit varying shapes. Therefore a number of terms are used to adequately characterize an aerosol sample:

- Particle size is conventionally defined as the *aerodynamic diameter*, which is the diameter of a spherical particle with unit density that settles at the same rate as the particle in question.
- The mass median aerodynamic diameter (MMAD) is defined as the aerodynamic diameter which divides the aerosol mass size distribution in half.
- The geometric standard deviation (GSD) is defined as the size ratio at 84.2% on the cumulative frequency curve to the median diameter. This assumes that the distribution of particle sizes is log-normal. A monodisperse, i.e. ideal aerosol, has a GSD of 1, although in practice an aerosol with a GSD of <1.22 is described as monodisperse while those aerosols with a GSD >1.22 are referred to as polydispersed or heterodispersed.

The MMAD and GSD of aerosols are therefore critical factors in determining the deposition patterns within the lung. Aerosols with larger MMADs will deposit higher in the respiratory tract since the aerosol particles will have greater momentum. A polydisperse aerosol is also likely to show greater deposition in the TB region than a monodisperse aerosol of the same MMAD.

10.3.3.3 *Shape*

Particles which are non-spherical will have at least one physical dimension which is greater than the aerodynamic diameter. Environmental fibers 50 μm in length can reach the A region because they align with the inspired airflow. Such materials then impact in the airways by a process of interception with the airway walls.

10.3.3.4 *Density*

Particles with densities less than 1 g cm^{-3} (unit density) will have a mean physical diameter greater than the aerodynamic parameter. Most micronized drugs for inhalation will have particle densities around 1, although materials produced by freeze-drying or spray-drying methods are likely to be significantly less dense. Large porous particles with physical diameters of 20 μm and densities of 0.4 g cm^{-3} are efficiently deposited in the lungs.

10.3.3.5 *Physical stability*

Therapeutic aerosols are often inherently physically unstable since they have a high concentration of particles and their close proximity may lead to mutual repulsion or other inter-particulate reactions. Aerosol particles generated by DPIs may be hygroscopic and, during their passage through the high humidity environments of the airways, may increase in size and thus have a greater chance of being prematurely deposited. It should not be assumed, however, that the uptake of water vapor will always occur. Aerosol droplets generated from pMDIs will rapidly decrease in size due to solvent evaporation. Similarly droplets from nebulizers will tend to decrease in size. The changes in particle size are therefore complex and thus deposition in the lung may be very different from that predicted on the basis of particle size analyses conducted at ambient RH.

10.3.4 The fate of particles in the airways

10.3.4.1 *Mucus barrier*

The first barrier which is encountered before the drug can reach its site of action is the mucus, present as a viscoelastic layer in the TB region. If the drug is given as an aerosolized powder then the drug first needs to dissolve in the mucus layer. Although mucus has a very high water content, varying between approximately 90–95%, its viscosity may result in a slow dissolution of drugs. Thus dissolution may be a rate determining step, especially for poorly soluble drugs, such as some of the corticosteroids which are delivered as dry powder aerosols. Improvement of drug penetration into mucus has been attempted using mucolytic drugs such as N-acetylcysteine, which act to reduce mucus viscosity. Highly water-soluble drugs, given as dry powder aerosols, may dissolve at the very high relative humidity (>99%) present in the airways air and impact as solution droplets.

Once in solution, the drug will diffuse through the mucus layer and enter the aqueous environment of the epithelial lining fluid. The rate of diffusion through the mucus will be dependent upon such factors as:

- the thickness of the mucus layer;
- mucus viscosity – although it should be appreciated that it is the viscosity of the mucus gel intersticies (i.e. the microviscosity) that is critical to drug penetration and not the macroviscosity of the whole gel;
- molecular size of the drug – for drugs not interacting with mucus glycoproteins, the diffusional resistance is only significant for molecules of mass > 1 KDa;
- any interactions which may occur between the drug and mucus – such interactions include the binding of positively charged drug molecules to mucus glycoproteins via electrostatic interactions with the negatively charged sialic acid residues, as well as hydrogen bonding and hydrophobic interactions.

In the TB region the mucus layer thickness is usually 0.5–5 μm but some reports suggests that this may increase to 50 μm in disease states. Mucus secretion may be stimulated as a response to "assault" by what the lung perceives as foreign bodies such as microorganisms and dusts or irritants such as cigarette smoke. Airways disease states such as bronchitis, cystic fibrosis and asthma are often associated with a hypersecretion of mucus. Clearly this presents a far greater barrier than is seen in the normal healthy lung.

Many studies have been performed with a variety of antibiotics delivered by aerosol for the treatment of chronic lung infections. The studies have produced mixed results with delivery to the lung from the bloodstream (after oral or parenteral dosing) often producing better clinical response. A number of factors, including the efficiency of drug delivery, may be responsible for these observations, but the overproduction of mucus in these disease states also seems likely to play a major role in preventing the drug reaching its target microorganism.

A detailed discussion of the structure and properties of mucus and respiratory mucins is given in Chapter 9 (Section 9.2.4.2).

10.3.4.2 *Mucociliary clearance*

In the healthy lung, the mucus layer does not exist as a stagnant layer but is constantly being propelled along the TB airways by the rhythmic beating of cilia on epithelial cells to the central bronchi, trachea and then to the throat, where the mucus and any entrapped particles are swallowed. In the TB region a high proportion of the epithelial cells are ciliated such that there is a near complete covering of the central airways by cilia. Towards the periphery of the TB region the cilia are less abundant and they are absent from the A region. Thus the end of the mucociliary escalator lies at the terminal bronchioles. The cilia beat at approximately 1,000 beats min^{-1} in an organized fashion and the ciliary movement may be conceived as a form of rhythmic waving which enables hook-like structures at the ciliary tips to propel mucus along the airways to the throat (see Section 9.2.5).

Particles and dissolved drugs entrapped in the mucus will be removed from the TB region via mucociliary clearance within a few hours after being deposited. This provides an efficient self-cleansing mechanism.

Mucociliary clearance is an organized, complex process which is highly dependent upon the composition and depth of the epithelial lining fluid and the viscoelastic properties of the mucus. In many airways diseases there is hypersecretion of mucus. This may cause an overloading of the ciliary transport process, resulting in a debilitated mucociliary clearance and the build-up of mucus as a thick, highly viscous layer. In these circumstances the mucus may only be removed by coughing. Thus while the mucociliary clearance of particles takes hours under normal circumstances, induced coughing may result in rapid removal of mucus and any associated drug within minutes. It should be remembered, however, that aerosolized drug deposition is likely to occur over a large surface area in the healthy and mild to moderate airways diseased lung. Coughing will remove mucus from a few localized areas where build-up has occurred and thus the fraction of the deposited dose removed by coughing is likely to be small. In cases of severe lung disease, drug deposition is likely to be highly localized and the situation may be different. For example, in cystic fibrosis patients, high levels of gentamicin, representing significant proportions of the deposited dose, were found in the sputum, when the aerosolized drug was deposited in the central airways.

10.3.4.3 *Alveolar clearance*

In the A region, deposited particles may be engulfed by alveolar macrophages which are then cleared from the lung by a number of different routes. The main route is via the mucociliary escalator, although transport from the A region to the start of the mucociliary escalator is a very slow process and may involve transport through interstitium and lymphatic tissues in addition to a transfer by random movement by macrophages. Macrophages may also be transported via lymphatic systems to lymph nodes and the bloodstream. The uptake of particles by macrophages is a fairly rapid process but the subsequent clearance of particle-laden macrophages only occurs over days or weeks.

10.3.5 Factors affecting the absorption and metabolism of drugs in the airways

It is important to consider the absorption and metabolism of drugs administered to lungs whether they are given to elicit a local or systemic effects. Absorption is clearly important for systemically-acting drugs since it is one element of the events leading to delivery of drug to its site of action. Absorption is equally important for locally-acting drugs since for these compounds it represents removal of drug from its site of action. Metabolism of drugs is also an important consideration since it may lead to drug inactivation or the production of active or toxic metabolites.

10.3.5.1 *Area*

The architecture of the lung is designed for the highly efficient exchange of gases. These same features also offer great potential for the delivery of systemically-acting compounds. The surface area of the airways is approximately 140 m^2, slightly larger than that of the small intestine. More importantly, however, a well-designed aerosol system can rapidly deliver drug to a high proportion of this surface area, whereas an orally delivered drug will have its access to the small intestine delayed by gastric emptying.

10.3.5.2 *Absorption barrier thickness*

The thickness of the absorption barrier is much smaller than for most other routes of drug delivery. In some parts of the alveolar region the airways to blood pathlength is less than 0.5 μm, an order of magnitude thinner than typical mucosal or epithelial membranes. This property facilitates very rapid transfer of gases, vapors and other small molecules. Drug absorption from this region is usually more rapid than from any other epithelial route of delivery. The absorption barrier thickness in the TB region of the lung is much thicker than in the A region but the absorption of drugs from this region is still likely to be much quicker than from any other mucosal route of delivery.

10.3.5.3 *Blood supply*

The lung receives 100% of the cardiac output via a network of fine capillaries. This rich blood supply which promotes rapid gaseous exchange is also beneficial for systemic drug delivery. Drugs absorbed from the lung pass directly to the heart avoiding first-pass metabolism in the liver, although some drugs will be subject to first-pass metabolism during absorption in the lung.

10.3.5.4 *The importance of regional differences*

The TB and A regions have a number of distinct physiological characteristics, which are relevant to a consideration of the delivery and fate of drugs within the lung:

- The surface area of the TB region is approximately 10-fold lower than in the A region.
- The airways-to-blood pathlength is more than 10-fold higher in the TB region.
- Blood flow is approximately 10-fold lower in the TB region.
- The capillary network is less extensive in the TB region.
- Mucociliary clearance is only present in the TB region.

These regional differences play an important role in the absorption of drugs into the systemic circulation, which is likely to occur more efficiently from the A region. Thus delivery systems designed for systemically-acting drugs should target the A region. As a general rule absorption from the A region occurs at rates more than twice those seen from the TB region.

Locally-acting drugs clearly need to be targeted to the region containing their site of action, which is generally the TB region. However, the situation is ambiguous for many drugs acting locally in the lung. Bronchodilator drugs act upon the smooth muscle of conducting airways and we might expect that a more central deposition of these drugs would give a greater pharmacodynamic response. However, there is currently no equivocal evidence of this.

Targeting locally-acting anti-inflammatory drugs is complex since there is dispute as to whether inflammation in the central airways is less or more important than that in peripheral airways. The situation is further complicated by possible redistribution of drugs within the lung, which seems likely to occur after deposition.

10.3.5.5 Membrane permeability

The main permeability barrier in the airways to blood pathway lies with the epithelium of the lung airway rather than the intersitium or endothelial lining of the capillaries. The epithelial permeability towards hydrophilic solutes is at least 10-fold lower than that of the endothelium. The epithelium of the lung is much more permeable than that of other mucosal routes. For example, less than 3% of an oral dose of sodium cromoglycate reaches the circulation whereas more than 70% is absorbed from the lung into the bloodstream after inhalation.

In the A region the tight junction gap between type-I alveolar cells is reported as 1 nm. Other pores with equivalent radii of about 10 nm have also been identified. Consequently the permeability of the paracellular route is much greater than seen with other membranes. Large molecules up to 150 kDa are reported to be absorbed to a small extent into the bloodstream after pulmonary administration.

10.3.5.6 Factors affecting membrane permeability

Lung permeability in the newborn is very high since proteins from the fluid-filled lungs need to be absorbed into the circulation. Permeability then decreases during the first few weeks of life and then shows no further age-related changes.

An increase in permeability of the alveolar membrane is seen in a number of pulmonary disease states including adult respiratory distress syndrome and fibrosis. Conversely, asthma does not appear to alter alveolar membrane permeability. Increased permeability will be seen in association with inflammatory reactions, where there is an influx of polymorphs and other cells into the airways. Inhalation of toxicants, such as smoke and industrial dusts, is associated with increased permeability.

Hyperinflation of the lung by vigorous exercise or repeatedly performing lung function tests may also lead to increased membrane permeability, possibly resulting from a disturbance of the intercellular junctions.

10.3.5.7 *Transport routes*

The routes of drug absorption into the bloodstream can be classified as:

- paracellular: occurring between epithelial, interstitial and endothelial cells.
- transcellular: occurring through the above cells.

Lipid-soluble drugs are usually absorbed transcellularly, since they partition into the lipid membranes of the epithelial cells and then diffuse through the cells, down a concentration gradient according to Fick's Law (see Section 1.3.3.2). Lung absorption rate constants correlate with the lipid/buffer distribution coefficients for a number of compounds. Highly lipophilic drugs show very rapid absorption, for example morphine shows peak blood levels within 5 minutes after inhalation.

Compounds which are poorly lipid-soluble may be absorbed via the paracellular route, the drug absorption rate being inversely related to their molecular size. The absorption of these hydrophilic drugs will generally be slower than that of lipophilic drugs but will still occur more rapidly than from other mucosal routes including intestinal, rectal, nasal and buccal (see Chapters 6, 7 and 9).

Saturable carrier-transport mechanisms have also been identified for organic anions such as sodium cromoglycate but the contribution of these mechanisms to the overall absorption of these compounds after therapeutic dosing is not known.

Large molecular weight drugs may be absorbed by the process of transcytosis, in which the macromolecule is carried in vesicles from one side of a cell to the other (see Section 1.3.3.2). Endocytosis may occur via phagocytosis by alveolar macrophages or via pinocytosis by type-I and type-II cells which involves flask-shaped invaginations called caveolae. Transcytotic mechanisms occur in type-I cells for albumin and pulmonary delivered macromolecules may be transported by similar routes. Pinocytosis mechanisms in type-II cells are responsible for the recycling of pulmonary surfactant. The role of these mechanisms in the absorption of drugs into the bloodstream has not been quantified and for some drugs, more than one route of absorption exists.

Absorption from the gastrointestinal tract may also occur, either because of direct swallowing of a portion of the inhaled dose, or because of secondary swallowing following mucociliary clearance.

10.3.5.8 *Enzymatic activity*

The endothelial cells of the lung play an important role in the metabolism of certain endogenous compounds and most of the drug metabolizing enzyme systems found in the liver occur in lung tissues. Many isozymes of the cytochrome P-450 family have been identified in the respiratory tract with the highest concentrations of these occurring in the nasal and smaller airways with lower levels in the trachea and main bronchi. In the lung these isozymes are most concentrated in Clara cells, type-II cells and to a lesser extent in alveolar macrophages.

Non-cytochrome P-450 dependent enzyme systems, including esterases, peptidases, flavin-containing monooxygenase, catechol-O-methyl transferase, UDP-glucuronosyl transferases, sulphotranferases and glutathione-S-transferase, are also present in the lung. Their distribution tends to be more widespread and their activities much higher than is seen with the P-450 systems.

Locally-acting inhaled drugs may be inactivated by these enzyme systems, for example isoprenaline and rimiterol are metabolized by catechol-O-methyl transferase. The inhaled steroid beclomethasone dipropionate is hydrolysed by esterases, firstly to an active metabolite, beclomethasone monopropionate, and then to an inactive metabolite, beclomethasone.

Inhaled drugs intended for systemic action are likely to be subjected to some first-pass metabolism during their absorption from the lung. The extent of this pre-systemic first-pass metabolism in the lung has not been fully quantified for many drugs but is estimated to be far less than that seen in the gastrointestinal tract and liver after oral dosing (see Section 6.3.3).

10.4 ADVANTAGES AND DISADVANTAGES OF PULMONARY DRUG DELIVERY

Pulmonary drug delivery offers several advantages, but also disadvantages, as drug delivery systems depending on the nature of the drug being delivered. A brief overview of both the advantages and disadvantages of pulmonary drug delivery is given below.

10.4.1 Locally-acting drugs

The delivery of anti-asthmatic and other locally-acting drugs directly to their site of action in the lungs is associated with a number of advantages:

- the dose needed to produce a pharmacological effect can be reduced (cf. oral dosing);
- low concentrations in the systemic circulation are associated with reduced systemic side-effects;
- rapid onset of action;

- avoidance of gastrointestinal upset;
- avoidance of intestinal and hepatic first-pass metabolism.

Local administration is also associated with some disadvantages for these drugs:

- oropharyngeal deposition may give local side-effects;
- patients may have difficulty using the delivery devices correctly.

10.4.2 Systemically acting drugs

For the delivery of systemically-acting drugs not suitable for delivery via the oral route (for example, insulin), the lungs also offer a number of potential advantages:

- The lungs offer a very large surface area for drug absorption.
- The permeability of the lung membranes towards many compounds is higher than that of the small intestine and other mucosal routes.
- The highly vascular surface of the A region promotes rapid absorption and onset of action.
- The lung offers a much less hostile environment than the oral route to most drugs, including proteins and peptides.

The disadvantages of the lungs for delivery of systemically-acting drugs include:

- The lungs are not readily accessible surfaces for drug delivery. Complex delivery devices are required to target drugs to the airways and these devices may be inefficient.
- Aerosol devices can be difficult to use; for example, it has been estimated that approximately 50% or more adult patients have difficulty using conventional metered-dose inhalers efficiently, even after careful training. Dexterity is also required, which may be lacking in the very young and elderly populations.
- Various factors affect the reproducibility of drug delivery to the lungs, including physiological (respiratory maneuver) and pharmaceutical (device, formulation) variables. For the systemic delivery of drugs with a narrow therapeutic index, such variations may be unacceptable.
- Drug absorption may be limited by the physical barrier of the mucus layer and the interactions of drugs with mucus.
- Mucociliary clearance reduces the retention time of drugs within the lungs. Efficient drug delivery of slowly absorbed drugs must overcome the ability of the lung to remove drug particles by mucociliary transport.

The significance of drug absorption and mucociliary clearance will diminish as devices and formulations are developed which will achieve high-efficiency targeting of the A region.

10.5 CURRENT TECHNOLOGIES FOR PULMONARY DRUG DELIVERY

Current technologies for pulmonary drug delivery are primarily concerned with the local delivery of drugs such as anti-asthmatics directly to their site of action. In order to deliver drugs to the lung, a therapeutic aerosol must be generated for inhalation. An aerosol can be considered as a colloidal, relatively stable two-phase system, consisting of finely divided condensed matter in a gaseous continuum. The dispersed phase may be liquid, solid or a combination of the two. Atomization is the process by which an aerosol is produced and can be electrically, pneumatically or mechanically powered. Currently there are three principal categories of aerosol generator employed in inhalation therapy:

- nebulizer;
- pressurized metered-dose inhaler (pMDI);
- dry powder inhaler (DPI).

The mechanism, advantages, disadvantages and the potential strategies for improvement of the devices used for aerosol generation are summarized in Table 10.2.

Table 10.2 Features of the devices currently used for aerosol generation

Device	Mechanism	Advantages	Disadvantages	Improvements
Nebulizer	jet nebulization ultrasonic nebulization.	Generates small particles with higher delivery capacities than pMDIs and DPIs; no coordination required.	Inconvenient; long inhalation times; poor dose control; lack of portability; expensive.	More compact and portable devices; breath enhanced nebulizers; dosimetric nebulizers.
pMDI	Drug suspension or solution in volatile propellant.	Unit dosing; inexpensive.	CFC's; aerosol velocity; coordination difficulties.	HFA's; breath-actuated inhalers; spacers/reservoirs.
DPI	Dry powder insufflation.	Avoids coordination problems; lower drug loss by impaction and no propellant problems associated with pMDIs.	High inspiratory effort may be required; coughing reflex; may be less convenient then pMDI.	More sophisticated multiple dose devices.

10.5.1 Nebulizers

Nebulizers are devices for converting aqueous solutions or micronized suspensions of drug into an aerosol for inhalation, although the drug formulations are, wherever possible, aqueous solutions. Selection of appropriate salts and pH adjustment will usually permit the desired concentration to be achieved. If this is not feasible, then the use of co-solvents such as ethanol and/or propylene glycol can be considered. However, such solvents change both the surface tension and viscosity of the solvent system which in turn influence aerosol output and droplet size. Water insoluble drugs can be formulated either by micellar solubilization, or by forming a micronized suspension.

Nebulizer solutions are often presented as concentrated solutions from which aliquots are withdrawn for dilution before administration. Such solutions require the addition of preservatives, e.g. benzalkonium chloride, and antioxidants (e.g. sulphites). Both excipient types have been implicated with paradoxical bronchospasm and hence the current tendency to use small unit-dose solutions that are isotonic and free from preservatives and antioxidants.

Atomization is the process by which sprays are produced by converting a liquid into aerosolized liquid particles. The large increase in the liquid–air interface, together with the transportation of the drops, requires energy input. The forces governing the process of converting a liquid into aerosolized liquid particles are:

- surface tension – serves to resist the increase in the liquid-air interface;
- viscosity – resists change in shape of the drops as they are produced;
- aerodynamic forces – cause disruption of the interface by acting on the bulk liquid.

The primary drops may be further dispersed into even smaller drops or coalescence may occur.

Nebulizers are specialized atomizers which permit recycling of the liquid. They have in-built baffles to ensure that large primary drops are returned to the reservoir and thus the aerosol emitted from the device has a size distribution which will aid airway penetration.

Nebulizers generate aerosols by one of two principal mechanisms:

- high velocity airstream dispersion (air-jet or Venturi nebulizers);
- ultrasonic energy dispersion (ultrasonic nebulizers).

10.5.1.1 *Air-jet nebulizers*

The principal design features of this type of nebulizer are illustrated in Figure 10.6. Drug solution is drawn from the reservoir up the capillary as a result of the region of negative pressure created by the compressed air passing over the open end of the capillary (Venturi effect). The resulting high shear forces convert the liquid into a polydispersed aerosol. The larger drops are removed by the various baffles and internal surfaces and return to the reservoir. The smaller respirable drops are carried on

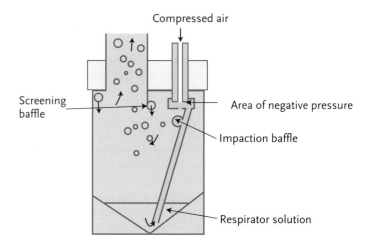

Figure 10.6 Principles of operation of an air-jet nebulizer

Compressed air

Screening baffle

Area of negative pressure

Impaction baffle

Respirator solution

♀ Large droplets for recirculation

the airstream out of the nebulizer and via either a mouthpiece or face mask into the airways of the patient. However, generally less than 1% of entrained liquid is released from the nebulizer.

There are many commercially available nebulizers with differing mass output rates and aerosol size distributions which will be a function of operating conditions, such as compressed air flow rate. As described above, for maximum efficacy, the drug-loaded droplets need to be less than 5 μm. In the treatment or prophylaxis of *P.carinii* pneumonia with nebulized pentamidine where the target is the alveolar space it is preferable to use nebulizers capable of generating droplets of less than 2 μm.

Output is often assessed by weighing the device before and after the nebulization period. Output is usually expressed as volume/unit time (mL min^{-1}) or volume per unit airflow (mL L^{-1} air) although density of solutions is not always considered. Such measurements of mass output do not, however, provide information on drug delivery rates.

During nebulization from air jet nebulizers, cooling of the reservoir solution occurs which, together with vapor loss, results in concentration of the drug solution. This in turn produces an aerosol output in which the drug concentration increases with time. Concentration of the drug solution in the reservoir can lead to drug recrystallization with subsequent blockage within the device or variation in aerosol particle size.

The compressed gas source is from either cylinders or air compressors and hence air-jet nebulizers tend to be more frequently encountered in hospitals than in the domiciliary environment.

10.5.1.2 *Ultrasonic nebulizers*

These nebulizers rely on a transducer made from a piezo-electric crystal which produces high frequency sound waves in the liquid in the nebulizing unit. The waves give rise to vertical capillaries of liquid ("fountains") which, when the amplitude of the energy applied is sufficient, break up to provide an aerosol.

Ultrasonic nebulization results in a rise in solution temperature and a decrease in aerosol MMAD with time. The increase in temperature may eliminate the use of this type of nebulizer for the administration of thermolabile drugs to the lung.

Although they are compact units and hence easily portable, the dense aerosol plume produced often has a population of drops with a higher MMAD and GSD in comparison to air-jet nebulizers and hence ultrasonic nebulizers tend to be less widely used.

10.5.1.3 *Improvements in nebulizer design*

Both the air-jet and ultrasonic nebulizer previously described produce an aerosol at a constant rate, irrespective of whether the patient is inhaling, exhaling or in breath-hold. This means that up to two-thirds of the aerosol will be lost to the environment during the exhalation and breath-holding phases of the respiratory cycle. Strategies to overcome this limitation include the use of:

- breath-enhanced nebulizers – which direct the patient's inhaled air within the nebulizer, to produce an enhanced volume of aerosol during the inhalation phase;
- dosimetric nebulizers – which release aerosol only during the inhalation phase. The AER_x and Respinal are two recent examples of dosimetric spray nebulization device.

10.5.2 Pressurized metered-dose inhalers (pMDIs)

Introduced in the 1950s, pMDIs have remained the most popular means for achieving domiciliary inhalation therapy. The pMDI provides for multiple dosing by utilizing a metering valve in conjunction with a propellant. A typical unit (Figure 10.7) comprises:

Figure 10.7 Diagram of a metered-dose inhaler

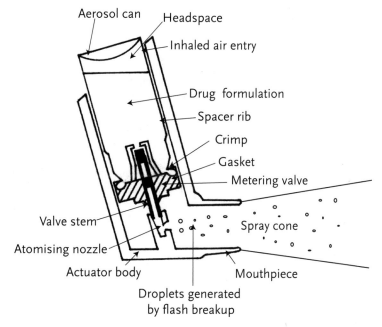

Container (10 mL)

This must be chemically inert and is often fabricated by extrusion of aluminum to avoid seams. This ensures mechanical strength so that the container can withstand internal pressures of >400 kPa. An alternative to aluminum is plastic-coated glass vials; however, these are only suitable for use with propellants generating lower internal pressures.

Metering valve

This hermetically seals the container and is designed to release a fixed volume of the product during each actuation. Valve volumes are typically in the range of 25 to 100 μl.

An elastomer seal

This is critical to the valve performance as it controls propellant leakage and metering reproducibility. Chemical constituent extraction from the seals by the propellants should be tightly controlled.

The actuator

This permits easy actuation of the valve, provides an orifice through which the spray is discharged and directs the spray into the patient's mouth. Orifice size can vary: large orifices in combination with large-volume metering valves permit the administration of concentrated, i.e. higher dose, suspensions with reduced tendency for blockage. However, smaller orifices are generally preferred since for low volume, dilute suspensions, a small drop size is produced, with the potential for greater penetration of the airways.

Traditionally, propellants have consisted of chlorofluorocarbon (CFC) blends (Table 10.3) which have ensured low pulmonary toxicity, high chemical stability and compatibility with packaging materials. The three most widely used CFCs are:

- trichlorofluoromethane, CFC 11;
- dichlorofluoromethane, CFC 12;
- 1,2-dichlorotetrafluoromethane, CFC 114.

	CFC 11	CFC 12	CFC 114	HFA 134a	HFA 227
Formula	$CFCl_3$	CCl_2F_2	$CClF_2CClF_2$	CF_3CH_2F	CF_3CHFCF_3
Mol. Wt. (Da)	137.4	120.9	170.9	102.0	170.0
Vapour Pressure (psig @ 20°C)	−1.8	67.6	11.9	81.0	43.0
Boiling Point (°C)	24	−30	4	−27	−17
Liquid density (g ml^{-1} @ 20°C)	1.49	1.33	1.47	1.21	1.41

Table 10.3 Physicochemical properties of propellants

The propellant blends used in pMDIs have a high vapor pressure of 350–450 kPa at room temperature, but because the device is sealed, only a small fraction of the propellant exists as a gas. Depression of the actuator opens the valve and the metered volume is discharged through the orifice as a result of the internal pressure within the aerosol canister. The rapid reduction in pressure to atmospheric induces extremely rapid evaporation, or flashing, of the propellant. It is the latent heat of evaporation of the volatile propellant that provides the energy for atomization. The energy disrupts the liquid into large drops moving at a velocity of approximately 30 m s^{-1}. Flashing is an adiabatic process and the residual propellant becomes supercooled. Evaporation therefore proceeds much more slowly and requires energy from the surrounding atmosphere. The drops decelerate rapidly due to air resistance and evaporation of propellant continues such that at 5 s post-actuation, the aerosol MMAD approaches that of the original drug particles.

A number of properties associated with the propellants are critical to pMDI formulation:

Vapor pressure

This determines both the MMAD and the drop velocity within the emitted aerosol. The higher the vapor pressure, the greater the velocity and generally higher oropharyngeal deposition will occur. Lowering the vapor pressure will reduce the oropharyngeal deposition but will almost certainly produce larger, more slowly evaporating propellant drops which will subsequently deposit high in the bronchial tree.

Solvency

Since most drugs are insoluble in the propellants, they are usually presented as suspensions. Micronized drug is dispersed with the aid of a surfactant such as oleic acid, sorbitan trioleate or lecithin. At concentrations up to 2% w/w the surfactant stabilizes the suspended particles by adsorption at the drug propellant interface and in addition serves as a valve lubricant. The tendency is to use minimum surfactant concentrations to reduce drug solubility within the propellant by solubilization (to reduce Ostwald ripening during the shelf life of the pMDI). Low surfactant concentrations will also avoid substantial reductions in the propellant evaporation rates from aerosolized drops.

Density

Differences in density between drug particles and the propellant will determine sedimentation rates (either sinking or floating). This becomes important if a delay occurs between shaking and actuating the pMDI. Deflocculation of the suspension by judicious surfactant selection may minimize the effect which can give rise to variable dosing during the life of the pressurized pack.

By blending CFCs, it is possible to achieve appropriate vapor pressure, solvency and liquid density. However, CFCs have been linked with the depletion of the stratospheric ozone layer and will be phased out in accordance with the "Montreal Protocol on Substances that Deplete the Ozone Layer". Current substitutes are the hydrofluoroalkanes (HFAs), e.g. 1,1,1,2-tetrafluoroethane (HFA-134a) and 1,1,2,3,3,3-heptafluoropropane (HFA 227) (Table 10.3).

In the switch from CFC to the more polar HFA propellants, one of the major problems has been inadequate solubility of the surfactants (used to stabilize the micronized drug particles) in the HFA. Solubility can be adjusted within the CFC propellant, e.g. CFC 12 is a far better solvent than CFC 11. However, for HFAs, blends do not exist and so solvency can only be addressed by using a cosolvent such as ethanol. It must be remembered that changing the solvency of the propellant will almost certainly affect the all-important vapor pressure and thus the MMAD, the particle velocity and the deposition site. Alternative stabilizers have been investigated and include PVP, fluorinated surfactants and Poloxamers. In addition to solubility effects, difficulties associated with the use of HFAs also include incompatibility with elastomer components in the metering valves.

A disadvantage of pMDIs is that droplets leaving the actuator orifice can be too large and can have extremely high velocities, leading to extensive impaction in the oropharyngeal region. The so-called "cold-freon" effect may result in patients stopping their inhalations immediately after actuating the pMDI.

In order to be effective, metered-dose aerosols should be triggered during the course of a deep, slow (>5 seconds) inhalation, followed by 5–10 seconds of breath holding. The breath-holding period is intended to maximize particle deposition by sedimentation and diffusion mechanisms (see Section 10.3.1). Patients can experience problems in developing an adequate inhaler technique and coordinating actuation with inspiration. Studies have shown that 50% or more adult patients have difficulty using conventional metered-dose inhalers efficiently, even after careful training. Coordination difficulties are even more common in children.

In order to overcome these limitations, spacer devices can be used. These are essentially extension tubes which effectively increase the distance between the orifice and the patient's oropharynx. This allows for deceleration of the particles and hence reduces oropharyngeal deposition. They also slightly reduce the importance of the patient coordinating pMDI actuation and inhalation. Holding chambers or reservoirs are larger diameter tubes often of conical or pear-shaped geometry and are designed to permit pMDI actuation prior to inhalation and to reduce drug loss on the interior wall. In-built flow restrictors have been introduced in attempts to control patients' inhalation rate. For patient convenience, spacers and reservoirs have been designed as collapsible or concertina-like structures.

An alternative approach to achieving patient coordination between actuation and inhalation is a breath actuated device such as the Autohaler. This device uses a mechanical vane to detect the appropriate inhalation rate for automatic firing of the pMDI.

10.5.3 Dry powder inhalers (DPIs)

These devices permit the drug to be delivered to the airways as a dry powder aerosol. All currently available DPIs are breath-actuated, thus the respirable cloud is produced in response to the patient's effort. DPIs therefore have the following advantages over pMDIs:

- They do not require a propellant – which has undoubtedly been the driving force behind the introduction of a large number of novel devices in recent years.
- They eliminate the need for patient coordination of actuation and inhalation associated with pMDIs.
- The particles are travelling at a slower rate, thus excessive drug loss due to impaction in the throat is avoided.

Every DPI device will exhibit an internal resistance which will determine the inhaled flow rate that a patient can achieve when using the device. As flow rate will inevitably be linked with inhaler performance, it is essential such factors be considered in any *in vitro* comparative testing of DPIs.

Every successful DPI requires development on two integrated fronts: powder technology and device design.

10.5.3.1 *Powder technology*

In addition to the drug powder, other powder excipients may be necessary. As described above (Section 10.3.1), successful delivery of drug particles into the lung requires that particle size should be controlled to <5 μm MMAD. Conventionally, this has been achieved by micronization, although more recently spray-drying and supercritical fluid technologies have been employed. However, particles of such small sizes exhibit exceptionally high surface energies, so that:

- particle aggregation readily occurs, making redispersion a difficult process;
- the formulation has poor flow and entrainment properties.

The most frequently employed approach to overcoming the problems associated with particle size is to use a carrier particle such as lactose. When the micronized drug is blended with a carrier of much larger size range (usually 20–100 μm), many of the drug particles become loosely associated with the lactose surface. When air is forced through such a powder bed by the patient inhaling, the bed dilates. The turbulent airflow within the device detaches the drug particles from the carrier particles within the device itself; the drug particles are then carried on the airstream into the lungs. Those carrier particles that escape from the device are largely deposited in the oropharynx of the patient.

Although high levels of turbulence will facilitate stripping of the drug particles from the carrier particles within the device, this course of action will also lead to an increase in resistance of the inhaler to airflow and thus to difficulties in inhaling through the device at a flow rate which produces optimum drug delivery. One way to provide high levels of turbulence without imposing large increases in airflow resistance is the judicious use and placement of grids of varying mesh sizes. It is observations such as these which emphasize the need for parallel development of device design and powder technology. More recently ternary powder blends have been claimed to provide a higher fine particle fraction of the drug when subjected to an aerosolization process.

10.5.3.2 *Device design*

Examination of a DPI design features will reveal the following principal mechanisms:

- dose metering
- aerosolization
- deaggregation
- aerosol direction into the patient's mouth.

Early dry powder inhaler devices were all unit-dose systems and depended on loading and triggering procedures. The Spinhaler and Rotahaler are two early examples of DPI technology. Both utilize pre-metered doses packed into hard gelatin capsules although different mechanisms of powder delivery are employed:

- The Spinhaler contains pins for perforating the capsule, the cap of which fits into an impeller which rotates as the patient inhales through the device. Particles are thus dispersed into the airstream.
- The Rotahaler has a blade which cuts the capsule in two: the body containing the powder falls into the inhaler while the cap is retained in the capsule loading port. The powder mass empties from the capsule body by the forces imparted by the inhaled airsteam and the drug particles subsequently enter the airways of the lung.

The tendency is to move to multiple-dosing reservoir devices. The first device employing a multidose reservoir was the Turbuhaler, designed to deliver 200×1 mg doses of terbutaline sulphate devoid of any carrier (Figure 10.8). The dose is metered into conical cavities by rotating the base of the inhaler. The inhaled airstream dislodges the drug from the cavities and dispersion continues in the inhalation channels which are helical to induce turbulent flow. A desiccant is employed to ensure that the powder reservoir remains dry during the shelf life of the inhaler.

The Diskhaler, also a multi-dose system, employs individual doses contained within blisters on a disk. On actuation, a needle pierces the upper and lower surfaces of one of the blisters. As the patient inhales, the contents of the blister are dispersed into the airstream, the drug particles dissociate from the carrier and a fraction is delivered to the lung. On re-priming the device, the disk rotates to expose the next blister to the piercing needle.

New DPI designs are numerous, with the novelty often associated with the technique for achieving powder aerosolization. Some of the recent patented devices incorporate an additional energy source to

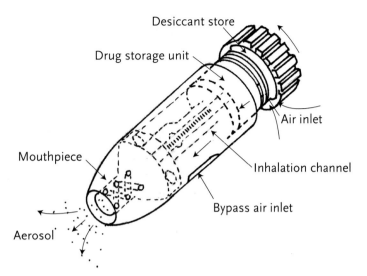

Desiccant store

Drug storage unit

Air inlet

Mouthpiece

Inhalation channel

Bypass air inlet

Aerosol

Figure 10.8 The essential components of a Turbuhaler

supplement the inspiratory force of the patient, in order to aerosolize the drug particles into the inhaled airstream. However, unless the addition energy source is breath activated (e.g. as in Spiros), such devices will be limited by the coordination difficulties typical of the pMDIs.

10.6 New technologies for pulmonary drug delivery

New technologies for pulmonary drug delivery are progressing along a number of fronts, including:

10.6.1 Device advances

Efforts are being directed towards improving the various devices currently used for aerosol generation. As described above, such efforts include the development of more portable nebulizers, replacing the use of CFCs in pMDIs with HFAs and the development of more sophisticated multiple dose DPIs, etc. (Table 10.2).

10.6.2 Delivery of the "new biotherapeutics"

New technologies are also addressing the pulmonary delivery of the "new biotherapeutics", i.e. the products of biotechnology and molecular biology such as peptides, proteins and gene therapies which have been described in detail in Chapter 1 (Section 1.6). Biopharmaceuticals under investigation for potential pulmonary delivery include those for local, and systemic, effects (Table 10.4).

A number of pharmaceutical companies are developing delivery systems for the delivery of macromolecules such as insulin. For example, The Inhale device system effectively disperses fine particles (which require a dispersion force far stronger than can be generated by a patient's inspiration); it also creates a stationary cloud to

Table 10.4
Biotherapeutics
investigated for
pulmonary delivery.

Local Delivery		Systemic Delivery	
Protein/Gene	*Potential Use*	*Peptide/Protein*	*Potential Use*
DNase	CF	insulin	insulin dependant diabetes
Alpha interferon	lung cancer, influenza	leuprolide	endometriosis, prostate cancer
Alpha-1-antitrypsin	emphysema, CF	oxytocin	hormone replacement
CFTR gene	gene therapy – CF	calcitonin	osteoporosis, Paget's disease
Alpha-1-antitrypsin gene	gene therapy – alpha-1-antitrypsin deficiency	growth hormone	pituitary dwarfism
		thyroid stimulating hormone	hypothyroidism
		DAVP	enuresis

enable efficient, reproducible deep lung deposition. Preliminary results for the systemic delivery of insulin using this device have been reported.

10.6.3 Novel drug delivery systems

Much effort is also currently being expended on the development of novel drug delivery systems for pulmonary drug delivery. By employing a colloidal carrier in which drug is dispersed, it is possible to control:

- the duration of local drug activity, or
- the plasma levels of systemically active agents.

A number of novel drug delivery systems have been identified as potential systems for controlling drug-release within the lung and include:

- liposomes;
- bioerodible microspheres composed of polymers such as polyesters (e.g. polylactic-co-glycolic acid) and polyanhydrides or naturally derived macromolecules such as albumin;
- drug-carrier conjugates, e.g. drug-cyclodextrin inclusion complexes and covalently linked drug-dextrans.

Further details of some of these systems have been provided in Chapter 5.

Tracheobronchial deposition of such carriers may not be desirable as clearance on the mucociliary escalator will occur in a relatively short time providing insufficient time for release from these controlled-release systems. Alveolar deposition will, in contrast, result in extended clearance times which are dependent on the nature of the carrier particle and may therefore be a better option for the effective use of such carrier systems for pulmonary drug delivery.

The rate of liposome accumulation in alveolar type-II cells is dependent on lipid composition. It is therefore possible to select liposome compositions displaying minimal interaction with these cells and thereby function as controlled-release systems for entrapped solutes. For example, liposomes composed of dipalmitoylphosphatidylcholine and cholesterol and containing entrapped sodium cromoglycate will provide sustained delivery of the drug for over 24 hours. Conversely other liposome compositions could be utilized for enhanced epithelial interaction and transport of the drug (e.g. cationic lipids for the cellular delivery of the CFTR gene).

Alveolar accumulation of carriers is an important toxicological consideration, although for liposomes, type-II cells will utilize administered phospholipids in the production of lung surfactant.

Delivery of novel colloids to the lung has largely focused on nebulization procedures, primarily because DPIs and pMDIs are typically incapable of depositing a large percentage of the emitted dose in the peripheral lung. For liposomes, size and composition are important in maintaining liposome integrity and hence entrapped drug during the nebulization process. There is some evidence to suggest that liposomes, as well as microspheres, may be administered in powder form utilizing DPIs.

10.6.4 Penetration enhancers

Penetration enhancers have been investigated for most mucosal and epithelial routes (see Sections 6.7.4, 8.5.3 and 9.7.1 for further details). The major challenge that remains is to find enhancers that will reversibly increase membrane permeability without causing toxicity during long-term use. Various surfactants and protease inhibitors have been reported to increase the pulmonary absorption of peptides and proteins on an experimental basis but their clinical use is not established and the current general consensus seems to be against their inclusion in pulmonary formulations.

10.7 CONCLUSIONS

Currently, pulmonary drug delivery is a widely used route for locally-acting drugs. The future will undoubtedly see products for inhalation on the market which contain systemically-acting drugs. Based on the published literature, it is likely that we will witness new designs in devices and formulations to achieve greater bioavailability and control in the pulmonary delivery of both conventional drugs (small organic molecules) and the increasing number of proteins, nucleotides and biotechnology compounds which require a mucosal transport route to the systemic circulation.

10.8 FURTHER READING

Hickey, A.J. (ed.) (1996) *Inhalation Aerosols: Physical and Biological Basis for Therapy*. Marcel Dekker, New York.

Byron, P.R. (ed.) (1990) *Respiratory Drug Delivery*. CRC Press, Boca Raton, FL.

Adjei, A.L. and Gupta, P.K. (eds) (1997) *Inhalation Delivery of Therapeutic Peptides and Proteins*. Marcel Dekker, New York.

Yu, J. and Chien, Y.W. (1997) Pulmonary Drug Delivery: Physiological and Mechanistic Aspects. *Crit. Rev. in Therapeut. Drug Carrier Sys.*, 14:395–453.

Niven, R.W. (1995) Delivery of Biotherapeutics by Inhalational Aerosol *Crit. Rev. in Therapeut. Drug Carrier Sys.*, 12:151–231.

Li W-I and Edwards, D.A. (1997) Aerosol Particle Transport and Deaggregation Phenomena in the Mouth and Throat. *Adv. Drug Del. Rev.*, 26:41–49.

10.9 SELF-ASSESSMENT QUESTIONS

1. Outline the structure and physiology of the lung.

2. Describe the key features of the pulmonary epithelium.

3. Describe the mechanisms of particle deposition in the airways.

4. List the physiological factors affecting particle deposition in the lung.

5. Describe the pharmaceutical factors affecting aerosol deposition in the lung.

6. Describe the factors affecting the absorption and metabolism of drugs in the airways.

7. List the advantages and disadvantages of pulmonary drug delivery.

8. Describe the three principal categories of aerosol generator employed in inhalation therapy.

9. Outline the rationale for the development of "new technologies" for pulmonary drug delivery.

Vaginal Drug Delivery

Hiroaki Okada and Anya M. Hillery

OBJECTIVES

On completion of this chapter the reader should be able to:

- Compare the vagina with other absorptive sites for drugs in the body
- Give a general overview of the structure of the vagina
- List the advantages and disadvantages of vaginal drug delivery
- Give some examples of vaginal drug delivery systems
- Describe approaches for enhancing vaginal drug delivery

11.1 INTRODUCTION

Until recently, vaginal preparations on the market were restricted to those that were topically effective for localized treatment of a variety of conditions. Preparations for local delivery include:

Anti-infectives

These include antibacterial, antifungal, antiprotozoal, antichlamydial and antiviral agents. Vaginitis is responsible for a large proportion of outpatient gynecologic visits. Symptoms include vaginal discharge, offensive odor, itching, and vaginal irritation. Three etiologies account for over 90% of the cases: trichomonas (25%), candida (*Candida albicans*, yeast) (25%), and bacterial vaginosis (40%). Metronidazole and other 5-nitroimidazoles (tinidazole, ornidazole) are used in the treatment of trichomonas. Vaginal yeast infections (candida) are treated primarily with antifungal imidazole drugs (clotrimazole, econazole, isoconazole and miconazole).

The preparations, which are available over the counter, generally comprise pessaries or creams inserted high into the vagina. Oral or intravaginal metronidazole is effective in the treatment of bacterial vaginosis. Intravaginal administration of metronidazole results in much lower systemic levels than oral administration, thus side-effects such as nausea, alcohol intolerance and peripheral neuropathy, as well as the risk of possible teratogenic effects, are reduced with vaginal treatment.

Estrogens

At the onset of menopause, at approximately 50 years of age, there is a decline in circulating estrogen, which worsens over the next 7–8 years. A related physiological event associated with a decline in estrogen levels is a substantial reduction in vaginal blood flow, with concomitant drying of vaginal tissue. Symptoms of dry vagina include discomfort with tight fitting clothing, burning sensation, purulent discharge, postcoital bleeding, lack of lubrication with sexual arousal, and dyspareunia. There is also a substantial rise in vaginal pH to as high as 7, which increases the incidence of vaginal infections.

Vaginal estrogen creams are highly effective in the treatment of atrophic vaginitis. A very low dose is recommended in order to minimize absorption of the estrogen and therefore combat endometrial stimulation. Modified vaginal release estrogen tablets and an estrogen impregnated vaginal ring are also available to treat vaginal dryness.

Spermicidal agents

These include nonoxynol-9, octoxinol and *p*-di-isobutylphenoxypoly(ethoxyethanol). Spermicidal contraceptives are useful additional safeguards but do not give adequate contraceptive protection if used alone; they are suitable for use with barrier methods. They have two components: a spermicide and a vehicle which itself may have some inhibiting effects on sperm activity. Vehicles commonly used include foams, gels, creams and pessaries.

The systemic absorption of these drugs had previously been considered only from the standpoint of toxicity. However, in addition to local delivery, there has recently been considerable interest in the possibility of vaginal delivery for the systemic delivery of drugs, via the mucous membranes of the vagina.

Current technologies in vaginal drug delivery are concerned with the systemic delivery of drugs such as estrogens, progesterones and prostaglandins. New technologies are exploring the systemic delivery of, for example, therapeutic peptides and proteins, via the vaginal route. This chapter reviews the structure and physiology of the vagina and the present and future utilization of the vagina for drug delivery.

11.2 STRUCTURE AND PHYSIOLOGY OF THE VAGINA

The vaginal tract in the adult female is about 2 cm in width and consists of an anterior wall of about 8 cm in length and a posterior wall, about 11 cm in length (Figure 11.1).

It is normally collapsed on itself and can hold between 2–3 g of fluid or gel without leakage to the outside. Microscopically, the vaginal wall consists of:

- the epithelial layer, with underlying basement membrane;
- the lamina propria (connective tissue);
- the muscular layer;
- the tunica adventitia (the vaginal fascia, which consists of loose connective tissue).

Figure 11.1 Sagittal section of the female pelvis

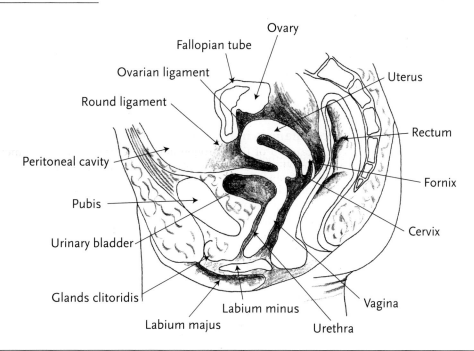

11.2.1 The vaginal epithelium

The human vaginal epithelium is composed of noncornified, stratified squamous cells, similar to those of the buccal mucosa (see Section 7.2.1) and somewhat similar to the skin epithelium (see Section 8.2.1). The vaginal epithelium is composed of five different cell layers:

- superficial (about 10 rows of cells): large polygonal cells with a high degree of proliferation,
- transitional (about 10 rows of cells),
- intermediate (about 10 rows of cells),
- parabasal (2 rows of cells),
- basal (single row of cells).

An important aspect of the epithelium is an elaborate system of channels between the cells. These intercellular channels are capable of changing width as the hormone levels change during the menstrual cycle. The channels can accommodate rapid movement of leukocytes and large proteins such as IgG and albumin; they are an important pathway of watery secretion from the blood network to the tissue.

11.2.2 The lamina propria

The lamina propria is composed of dense connective tissue, consisting of collagen fibers, ground substance, and cells such as fibroblasts, macrophages, mast cells, lymphocytes, Langerhans cells, plasma cells, neutrophils, and eosinophils. The lamina propria contains a blood supply, a lymphatic drainage system, and a network of nerve fibers. It is through the blood vessels in the lamina propria that drugs can gain entry to the systemic circulation. Lymph drainage from the vagina takes place to the iliac sacral, gluteal, rectal, and inguinal lymphatic nodes.

11.3 PHYSIOLOGICAL FACTORS AFFECTING VAGINAL DRUG DELIVERY

Physiological factors affecting vaginal drug delivery include:

11.3.1 Cyclical changes in the vaginal epithelium

The vaginal epithelium undergoes cyclical changes, directly controlled by hormones such as estrogens, progesterones, luteinizing hormone (LH) and follicle-stimulating hormone (FSH). The changes are associated with aging (neonate, juvenile, adult and senescence), biphasic sexual cycling (follicular and luteal phases) and pregnancy.

The superficial, transitional and intermediate layers are strongly affected by the cyclical changes, which have profound effects on epithelial thickness and epithelial porosity as described below:

Follicular phase

During the late follicular phase, estrogen stimulates mitosis in the basal and parabasal layers. This proliferation of cells leads to an increase in

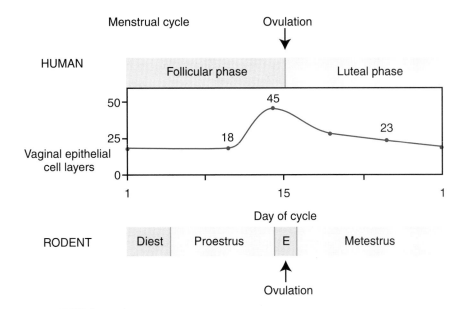

Figure 11.2 Variation in the number of epithelial cell layers during the menstrual cycle (~28 days) and timing of the rodent estrous cycle (4–5 days)

epithelial thickness, as well as in the number of layers (Figure 11.2). A parallel increase in the number of intercellular junctions renders the epithelium more cohesive. The number of desmosomes increases approximately 10-fold from the early to late follicular phase. The intercellular channels are narrow during the late follicular phase. Thus in this phase, the epithelium is thick, tight and cohesive.

Luteal phase

During the luteal phase, desquamation (shedding) occurs on the superficial epithelial layer, extending as far as the intermediate cells. The vaginal surface loses its intact structure and the epithelium becomes loose and porous. This cyclic desquamation is preceded by loosening of intercellular grooves, as well as a pore-like widening of the intercellular channels. Thus in this phase, the epithelium is thin, loose and porous.

Rodents have an estrous cycle characterized by diestrous (Diest), proestrous, estrous (E) and metestrous phases (Figure 11.2). The cyclical changes in the epithelium of rodents are similar to the changes in human, i.e.

- proestrus and estrus: the epithelium is thick, tight and cohesive;
- metestrus and diestrus: the epithelium is thin, loose and porous – the apparent porosity during metestrus and diestrus is presumed to be more than 10 times that during proestrus and estrus.

Postmenopause

In postmenopausal women, the incidence of mitosis in the basal and parabasal layers and the number of small blood vessels decreases. The vaginal epithelium becomes extremely thin, cell boundaries in the surface are less distinct, the micro-ridges of the cells are dramatically reduced, and the vagina is often invaded with leukocytes. Naturally, this thinning of the epithelium leads to a substantial increase in the permeability of this tissue.

Pregnancy

During pregnancy the most marked change occurring in the vagina is increased vascularity and venous stasis, and the epithelial layer is greatly thickened. Following delivery, the vagina requires several weeks to reestablish its prepregnancy appearance.

11.3.2 The vaginal fluids

Although the vaginal epithelium is relatively aglandular (in comparison with other possible delivery sites such as the GI tract), it is usually covered with a surface film of moisture, "the vaginal fluids". The vaginal fluid is composed of cervical fluid (the vagina receives approximately 2 g of mucus/day from the cervix) and also small amounts of the secretion from Bartholin's glands in the vaginal wall. However, the bulk of fluid to the tissue, and the lumen of the tissue, comes via transudation of fluid (via the intercellular channels) from the very extensive vascular bed in the tissue. During the normal menstrual cycle, the amount of fluid increases at ovulation, by mixing with the uterine fluid, oviductal fluid, follicular fluid, and even peritoneal fluid. The vaginal secretions, which serve as a protective barrier for infections, contain a variety of antimicrobial substances including lysozyme, lactoferrin, fibronectin, polyamines such as spermine and secretory IgA. The fluids also contain carbohydrate from the epithelial glycogen, amino acids, aliphatic acids and proteins.

The bioavailability of drugs administered via the vaginal route is dependent on both the effective dissolution of solid drug particles (if present) in the vaginal fluids prior to absorption and the degree of deactivation by enzymes present in the fluids. The physiological cyclical changes in the amount of vaginal fluids present in the vaginal cavity means that fluctuations in vaginal bioavailability can occur.

11.3.3 Vaginal pH

The pH in the vaginal lumen is controlled primarily by lactic acid produced from cellular glycogen, or by carbohydrates produced by the action of the normal vaginal microflora. Vaginal pH in an adult female varies between 4.0 and 5.0, depending on the particular stage of the menstrual cycle. The lowest values are found at mid-cycle and the highest during menstruation. This acidity plays a clinically important role in preventing the proliferation of pathogenic bacteria and there is a correlation between the pH of the vaginal secretions and the inhibition of chlamydial infections. During pregnancy, the pH is lowest and varies between 3.8 and 4.4 (due to an increase in cellular glycogen content); in the postmenopausal state or after ovariectomy, the pH increases to 7.0–7.4 (owing to a decrease in cellular glycogen content).

Vaginal pH affects the degree of ionization of drugs, which can affect their absorption properties (see Section 1.3.4.2). Physiological changes in the pH of the vaginal fluids can also result in fluctuations in vaginal bioavailability.

11.3.4 Enzyme activity

Lower enzymatic activity is thought to exist in the vaginal epithelium than in the gastrointestinal tract. For example, using casein as a substrate, the proteolytic activity determined in a 10% homogenate of rat vaginal membrane was found to be less than that in the small intestine.

The influence of the ovarian cycle on protease activity in the vagina has also been demonstrated. For example, the trypsin-like activity in rat vaginal smears was found to be maximal at proestrus. The activity of β-glucuronidase, acid phosphatase, alkaline phosphatase, and esterase all vary in the vaginal tissue of premenopausal and postmenopausal women.

11.3.5 Transport routes and mechanisms and the effect of cyclical changes on vaginal absorption mechanisms

As discussed in Chapter 1 (Section 1.3.3), drug permeation across the epithelial barrier is via two main routes (Figure 1.3):

- the paracellular route: between adjacent epithelial cells;
- the transcellular route: across the epithelial cells, which can occur by any of the following mechanisms: passive diffusion, carrier-mediated transport and via endocytic processes.

As described in general terms for the transepithelial absorption of drugs at any site (Section 1.3.3.1), hydrophilic compounds may be absorbed via the paracellular route, with drug absorption rates being inversely related to their molecular size. In contrast, lipid-soluble drugs are usually absorbed transcellularly, by passive diffusion through the epithelium, down a concentration gradient according to Fick's Law (Section 1.3.3.2). Drug diffusion rates correlate with their lipid/water diffusion coefficients and are inversely related to their molecular size (Section 1.3.4.3).

However, these general observations do not take into account the cyclical changes in the vaginal epithelium, which exert profound effects on vaginal absorption, especially for hydrophilic compounds. The permeability coefficient for the vaginal membrane (P_m) is equal to the sum of the permeability coefficient through the lipid pathway (P_l) and the pore pathway (P_p):

$$P_m = P_l + P_p$$

For lipophilic drugs, the contribution of the pore pathway to transport is negligible and drug absorption occurs transcellularly, via passive diffusion through the epithelial cells. Drug diffusion rates correlate with their lipid/water diffusion coefficients. For example, it has been shown that increasing the chain length (increasing the lipophilicity) of aliphatic alcohols and carboxylic acids results in an increased rate of vaginal absorption.

In contrast, for hydrophilic drugs, the pore pathway constitutes the major absorption pathway and this pathway is influenced by the physiological changes in the thickness of the vaginal epithelium and also in the number of intercellular pores and aqueous channels. As described earlier, in rodents, during proestrus and estrus, the epithelium is thick, tightly cohesive and contains a large number of intercellular junctions. However, the metestrous and diestrous phases are characterized by a thinning of the epithelium and a pore-like widening of the intercellular channels. As the vaginal epithelial membrane barrier becomes thin, loose and porous, the permeability is enhanced, particularly to hydrophilic substances. Thus even high molecular weight hydrophilic drugs can be absorbed by the intercellular route during the metestrous and diestrous phases. Several examples of this phenomena are described below:

Salicylic acid

Vaginal absorption of salicylic acid in different pH buffers has been investigated in rats during proestrus and diestrus. For the unionized, lipophilic form of the drug, the rate of vaginal absorption is rapid and similar for both stages. The unionized, lipophilic form is absorbed via transcellular passive diffusion and thus not affected by the stage of the estrous cycle. However, for the ionized, water-soluble form, a significant difference in the degree of absorption is observed:

- proestrus (tight epithelium) = 29% absorbed;
- diestrus (porous epithelium) = 66% absorbed.

The hydrophilic form is absorbed mainly through pore-like pathways such as the intercellular channels and thus is highly dependent on the stage of the cycle, with greater absorption occuring when the interceullular channels are wide and porous.

Insulin, phenol red and leuprorelin

The profound effects of the estrous cycle on the vaginal absorption of water-soluble compounds insulin, phenol red and leuprorelin (a potent GnRH analog) have been demonstrated (Figure 11.3). Vaginal administration of porcine insulin at a dose of 20 U/rat in an oleaginous suppository containing 10% citric acid (an absorption enhancer) resulted in large decreases in blood glucose levels (ΔAUC) during metestrus and diestrus, with smaller decreases in blood glucose during proestrus and estrus. These levels should correlate with vaginal absorption of insulin. The percentage of the dose of phenol red excreted in the urine increased more than an order of magnitude from the proestrous phase (2.4% absorbed) through to the diestrous phase

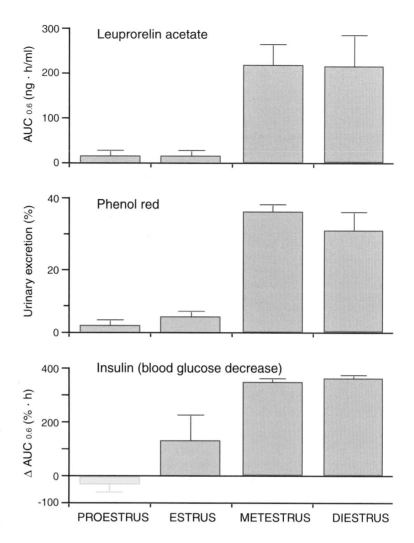

Figure 11.3 Effects of the estrous cycle on vaginal absorption of leuprorelin acetate, phenol red and insulin in rats

(31.4% absorbed). Leuprorelin showed similar enhanced absorption during the permeable phase of the estrous cycle (Figure 11.3).

Penicillin

In humans high blood levels of penicillin, sufficient to be therapeutic, were demonstrated following insertion of a vaginal suppository near the end of the menstrual cycle and during menopause. In contrast, absorption was shown to be somewhat diminished during estrus and late pregnancy.

Vidaribine

The permeability coefficients of the hydrophilic antiviral compound vidaribine are 5 to 100 times higher during early diestrus or diestrus than during estrus.

These results confirm that the cyclic changes in the reproductive system have profound implications for vaginal drug delivery as:

- the vaginal permeability to hydrophilic substances is enhanced during the metestrous and diestrous stages of the estrous cycle, corresponding to the late luteal and early follicular phases of the menstrual cycle;
- large fluctuations in absorption occur, depending on the particular stage of the menstrual cycle.

Other transcellular mechanisms of absorption include carrier-mediated transport and endocytic processes. Although it is well known that carrier-mediated transport systems exist for di- and tripeptides in the intestine, there is still no evidence for carrier-mediated transport of peptides across the vaginal mucosa, although prostaglandins have been demonstrated to utilize such a mechanism. Although there must be some type of endocytic transport of endogenous peptides into the epithelial cells in order to regulate proliferation, no receptor-mediated or bulk-fluid mechanisms have been reported.

11.4 FORMULATION FACTORS AFFECTING VAGINAL DRUG DELIVERY

11.4.1 Physicochemical factors associated with the drug

Drug properties which affect vaginal drug delivery are broadly the same as those affecting transepithelial absorption at any site and have been discussed extensively in Chapter 1 (Section 1.3.4).

Hydrophilic compounds may be absorbed via the paracellular route, moving between the epithelial cells via passive diffusion whereas lipid soluble drugs are usually absorbed transcellularly, at rates which correlate with their lipid/water diffusion coefficients. Macromolecules may be absorbed via endocytic processes.

However, in the vagina these factors must be considered in conjunction with the cyclical changes in the vaginal epithelium. Thus hydrophilic compounds show enhanced absorption during metestrus and diestrus, when the vaginal barrier becomes thin, loose and porous. In addition to physicochemical properties of the drug such as size, pKa, chemical stability etc., the charge of the membrane surface, pore size, and the drug must also be considered. Furthermore, peptides and proteins are susceptible to self-association, aggregation or polymerization in the medium due to changes in pH, ionic strength of the medium, or concentration of the substance. It is anticipated that the monomer, oligomer, or aggregated complex may each have a characteristic diffusion and permeation coefficient.

Further physicochemical factors associated with the drug which influence vaginal drug delivery include the solubility and stability of the drug in the vaginal fluids. Poorly soluble drugs may demonstrate rate-limiting dissolution in the vaginal fluids. For example, the vaginal absorption of metronidazole is limited not only by the drug permeability across the vaginal epithelium, but also by its dissolution into the small volume of fluid within the vaginal cavity. Furthermore, labile drugs may undergo enzymatic deactivation prior to absorption.

11.4.2 Factors associated with the dosage form

Conventional vaginal preparations are available in a wide variety of dosage forms, including pessaries, creams, aerosol foams, gels, tablets, inserts, diaphragms, sponges and vaginal rings. Such formulations are administered with the aid of an appropriate applicator into the vagina and have different characteristics with respect to ease of administration, drug release profile, sanitary aspects etc. Desirable attributes of all vaginal preparations include:

- no adverse reactions, such as tissue irritation;
- ease of application;
- even distribution of the drug throughout the vagina, rather than being concentrated in one spot;
- retention of the drug in the vagina, even when the patient is standing and walking;
- absence of an offensive odor;
- absence of staining of clothes or skin;
- compatibility with other forms of medication and contraception;
- minimal interference in sexual activity.

These factors become particularly important for preparations intended for long-term vaginal administration. Formulation factors which affect vaginal drug delivery which are common to the various types of vaginal dosage forms include:

Drug release

As discussed above, there is a relatively small volume of fluid within the vaginal cavity. Thus the rate-limiting step for systemic absorption of drugs from intravaginal creams, inserts and tablets is often dissolution within the vaginal fluid, particularly for poorly soluble drugs. Obviously, the type of dosage form affects the rate of dissolution; for example, a drug which is already dissolved in an aqueous vaginal gel will be more rapidly absorbed than a drug which is in solid form within a vaginal tablet preparation.

The effective area of contact

Although the area of the vaginal cavity is approximately 60 cm^2, the formulation will influence the size of the area over which the drug is deposited. The vehicle should facilitate even distribution of the drug throughout the vagina, rather than concentrating it in one spot. Factors such as the hydrophilicity and viscosity of the vehicle will determine how well it spreads through the vagina.

Contact time

The formulation will also influence the extent of the contact time the drug has with the absorbing surface of the vaginal epithelium. Drug delivery to the vagina is limited by residence time at the site. Typical delivery systems such as foams, gels and tablets are removed in a relatively short period of time by the self-cleansing action of the vaginal tract. New bioadhesive gel delivery systems are being developed to prolong contact time with the absorbing surface and are described below.

Concentration

The rate of absorption via passive diffusion processes (transcellular and paracellular) can be increased by increasing the drug concentration in solution at the absorbing surface (see Section 1.3.3.1). For systems intended for prolonged administration, a highly saturated formulation will also ensure that sufficient drug is present to ensure sustained drug delivery throughout the intended time of application. However, care must be taken, as high local drug concentrations over extended periods of time may also cause severe local irritation or adverse tissue reactions.

11.5 ADVANTAGES AND DISADVANTAGES OF VAGINAL DELIVERY

Vaginal drug delivery offers several advantages, but also disadvantages, as drug delivery systems, depending on the nature of the drug being delivered. A brief overview of both the advantages and disadvantages of vaginal drug delivery is given below.

11.5.1 Advantages

The advantages of vaginal drug delivery include:

Large surface area

The vagina offers a relatively large surface area (approximately $60 \, \text{cm}^2$) for drug absorption. However, it is much smaller than that offered by the nasal ($150 \, \text{cm}^3$), rectal ($200–400 \, \text{m}^2$), pulmonary ($75–700 \, \text{m}^2$) and intestinal ($200 \, \text{m}^2$) routes.

Rich blood supply

The highly vascular surface of the vaginal mucosa ensures relatively rapid absorption and onset of action, as well as the maintenance of sink conditions.

Low metabolic activity

The metabolic activity of the vagina towards peptides and proteins is less than that of the GI tract, making this route an attractive alternative to the oral delivery of these moieties. In contrast to the oral route, this route also avoids degradation in the intestinal wall or the liver, prior to the drug reaching the systemic circulation. Reduced first-pass effects after vaginal application of estrogens, progestogens and prostaglandins have all been reported in a number of studies.

Permeability

The vagina demonstrates a relatively high permeability to many drugs, particularly during the late luteal and early follicular phases of the menstrual cycle.

Ease of administration

Intravaginal dosage forms are relatively easy to administer and offer the feasibility of self-administration. Patient compliance is generally good, particularly if no leakage or staining occurs.

Prolonged retention

Prolonged retention of the drug is possible, if the appropriate delivery system such as vaginal silicone ring is used, thereby allowing a reduction in the dosing frequency.

Alternative when the oral route is unfeasible

The vaginal route may be appropriate in certain situations where the oral route is unfeasible, such as:

- patients with nausea and vomiting;
- patients with swallowing difficulties;
- drugs that cause gastric irritation;
- drugs that are unstable in the gastrointestinal fluids;
- drugs that undergo extensive first-pass effects in the gut wall or liver.

Zero-order controlled release

Vaginal drug delivery offers the potential to achieve zero-order controlled release over a controlled period. As described in Chapter 1 (see Section 1.5.1), controlled release offers the further advantages of:

- avoiding the peaks (risk of toxicity) and troughs (risk of ineffectiveness) of conventional therapy;
- reducing the dosing frequency;
- increasing patient compliance.

11.5.2 Disadvantages

The disadvantages of vaginal drug delivery include:

Limited to potent molecules

For drugs of a high molecular weight (which thus are poorly absorbed), the route is limited only to potent drug molecules, typically those with effective plasma concentrations in the ng/mL (or lower) range.

Adverse effects

The relatively low amount of fluids bathing the vaginal mucous membranes means the tissue is prone to adverse reactions, such as local irritation, caused by vaginal devices. Similarly, locally irritating or sensitizing drugs must be used with caution in this route. Furthermore, materials used in vaginal preparations should be sterilized and not act as a growth medium for the proliferation of pathogenic microorganisms, bacteria, fungi, and protozoa.

Hormone-dependent changes

Cyclic changes in the reproductive system mean that large fluctuations in vaginal bioavilability can occur. Cyclical changes in the vaginal epithelium include changes in the thickness and porosity of the vaginal epithelium, the amount and pH of the vaginal fluids and the degree of enzymatic activity present. Furthermore, estrogen therapy and steroidal contraceptives influence the vaginal fluid, epithelial thickness and vascularity, which also contributes to a lack of reproducibility in the vaginal absorption of drugs. Age-related changes, as well as changes during pregnancy, also occur. This lack of reproducibility constitutes a major problem associated with vaginal drug delivery and, for drugs with a narrow therapeutic index, such variations may be unacceptable.

Leakage

The bulbocavernosus muscles which surround the orifice of the vagina are not usually strong enough to retain vaginal preparations in the same way as the anal sphincter retains rectal suppositories. Slipping-out or leakage may occur, particularly in the case of preparations involving a relatively large volume of liquid or semisolid. This problem may be alleviated by using a vaginal preparation at night.

Life-cycle constraints

The vagina is the final part of the internal female genitalia, the parturient canal, and also serves as a passage for the outflow of cervical fluids and the menstrual flow. Menstruation, intercourse, pregnancy and delivery, and other anatomical or physiological changes in the life cycle of women must also be taken into account when the timing and effectiveness of drug application are being considered.

Applicability constraints

No matter what degree of optimization can actually be achieved via this route, it must be remembered that vaginal delivery is only applicable to approximately 50% of the population. Thus it may be that the true potential of this route lies in the treatment of female-specific conditions, such as in the treatment of climacteric symptoms of the menopause etc., rather than more general applications such as insulin/peptide delivery.

11.6 CURRENT TECHNOLOGIES IN VAGINAL DRUG DELIVERY

As described above, until recently vaginal preparations on the market were restricted exclusively to those that were topically effective and the issue of systemic absorption was a toxicological rather than therapeutic concern. However more recently, the vaginal delivery of estrogens, progesterones and prostaglandins has been considered in term of their systemic, as opposed to merely local, delivery. Current technologies in vaginal drug delivery are increasingly concerned with the systemic delivery of these agents and commercial preparations are now available:

11.6.1 Vaginal delivery of estrogens and progesterones

When used alone, estrogen replacement therapy increases the risk of endometrial cancer. This risk can be eliminated by treatment with a progestational agent for up to 14 days a month. However, the oral administration of natural progesterone has associated limitations:

- low oral bioavailability due to extensive first-pass metabolism and rapid clearance from the peripheral circulation;
- lack of efficacy: the endometrium is not converted to a fully secretory state (which protects against endometrial cancer);
- the high levels of metabolites (5α-pregnanolone and 5β-pregnanolone) generated by first-pass effects in the intestine and the liver often result in CNS toxicity, including hypnotic, anxiolytic or anti-epileptic effects.

These limitations can be overcome by the vaginal administration (tablets, suppositories, gels) of progesterone. Vaginal administration gives higher plasma levels than the oral route and levels are sustained for a longer time (Figure 11.4(a)). In addition to enhanced bioavailability, the vaginal route of progesterone delivery has also been shown to produce very low levels of the CNS toxic metabolites, 5α-pregnanolone and 5β-pregnanolone, thus CNS side-effects are minimized.

Estrogens are also subject to extensive first-pass effects (it has been shown that these first-pass effects occur predominantly in the intestinal wall, rather than in the liver) after oral administration. Again, vaginal administration of estradiol results in higher bioavailability than via the oral route (Figure 11.4(b)).

Because of the beneficial effects of the vaginal delivery of estrogens and progesterone in comparison to their oral delivery, various vaginal preparations (tablets, suppositories, gels, rings) of these agents are now available, for use:

- as contraceptives;
- in hormone replacement therapy(HRT);

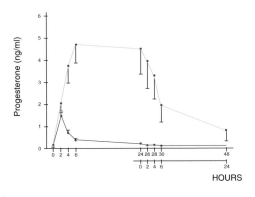

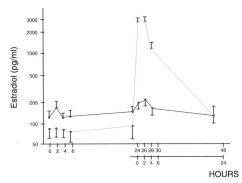

Figure 11.4 Plasma levels of progesterone and estradiol in women after vaginal (yellow) or oral (blue) administration of progesterone 100 mg, or estradiol 0.5 mg. For full experimental details see Nahoul, K. *et al*, Maturitas, 16: 185–202.

- in *in-vitro* fertilization programs (in the establishment of an in-phase endometrium in women undergoing donor oocyte programs).

A number of different types of vaginal rings containing various progesterones and estrogens have been investigated as a steroidal contraceptive since the mid-1970s, the most successful being a Silastic toroidal-shaped ring. This is designed for insertion into the vagina and positioned around the cervix for 21 days, in order to achieve a constant plasma progestin level and cyclic intravaginal contraception. Levonorgestrel, an extremely potent progestogen analog, is released from the device at about 20 μg/day, with a near zero-order release rate. Although the device is successful in achieving the prolonged release of levonorgestrel, irregular bleeding is a major drawback associated with its use.

In 1997, a new intravaginal formulation, Silastic silicone ring (Estring) was launched in the US for treating postmenopausal women with symptoms of urogenital aging, which is effective both topically and also systemically without first-pass metabolism. The ring is designed to provide a constant release of estradiol (6.5–9.5 μg/24 h) over a 3-month period. In postmenopausal women with symptoms of urogenital aging, the vaginal ring gives significantly better, or equal, improvements of vaginal mucosal maturation value and restoration of vaginal pH levels than estradiol--containing vaginal pessaries or conjugated estrogen vaginal creams and is significantly more acceptable.

Vaginal administration of progesterone is associated with a "first-uterine-pass effect", i.e. direct preferential vagina-to-uterus transport. Using a human *ex vivo* uterine perfusion model, the vaginal administration of radioactive progesterone was shown to result in the progressive migration of [^{3}H]progesterone into the uterus, where it reached high concentrations in both the endometrium and the myometrium.

Furthermore, vaginal administration of micronized progesterone has been shown to enhance progesterone delivery to the uterus by about 10-fold in comparison to im injection, despite the markedly higher (about 7-fold) circulating drug concentration achieved with im injection. Uterine selectivity after vaginal administration has further been observed for both danazol and the β-agonist terbutaline and the vaginal-to-uterine delivery of misoprostol is currently being investigated for the reliable termination of early pregnancy (see below).

Hence considerable evidence has accumulated demonstrating that the vaginal route permits targeted drug delivery to the uterus. This phenomenon opens new therapeutic options for the administration of compounds whose primary site of action is the uterus, thereby maximizing the desired effects, while minimizing the potential for adverse systemic effects.

11.6.2 Vaginal delivery of prostaglandins

Prostaglandin E$_2$ (PGE$_2$)

Prostaglandin E$_2$ (PGE$_2$) is an agent used to ripen the cervix for the induction of labor (it is also used for second-trimester abortion) and shows various beneficial effects:

- reduced time to onset of labor;
- reduced need for oxytocin during labor;
- shortened time to vaginal delivery;
- reduced need for Caesarean operative delivery.

Vaginal PGE$_2$ preparations include a controlled-release hydrogel polymer pessary, an oleaginous suppository, and various gels (triacetin, methylcellulose, starch-based gel). Vaginal PGE$_2$ preparations are easier to administer than intracervical preparations; intravaginal administration can be carried out by midwives and a speculum examination is not required.

Cernidil Vaginal Insert is a controlled-release pessary and insert containing 10 mg dinoprostone, which has been developed for cervical ripening in the induction of labor and has been recently introduced in the US. The insert ($0.8 \times 9.5 \times 29$ mm) is made of a cross-linked polymer hydrogel that swells in the vaginal fluid and releases PGE$_2$ from a 10 mg reservoir at a controlled rate of approximately 0.3 mg/h *in vivo*. The retrieval system comprises a Dacron polyester net which proximally surrounds the insert and has a long ribbon end. The total length of the net plus the ribbon is 31 cm.

The insert is placed in the posterior fornix of the vagina; insertion is performed digitally, thereby obviating the need for speculum examination. The system is effective in producing cervical ripening at term by releasing a small amount of the drug over a prolonged period. Furthermore, the system allows the obstetrician to control the dose administered and to terminate drug delivery by removal of the device, if uterine hyperstimulation or abnormal fetal heart rate changes should occur during the ripening process. Thus the system offers particular advantages in cases where there is concern about fetal condition or a risk of uterine over-activity.

Misoprostol

The most widely used medical method of terminating second-trimester pregnancy for fetal malformations or previous fetal death is the intravaginal use of prostaglandins; in particular, clinical interest is growing in the use of a synthetic prostaglandin E_1 analog, misoprostol. Intravaginal administration of misoprostol at a dose of 100–200 μg every 12 h is at least as effective as PGE_2 for termination of second-trimester pregnancy but it is less costly (about 1/300), is easier to administer (because it is placed in the vagina, not the cervix) and is associated with fewer adverse effects such as pyrexia, vomiting, diarrhea.

The bioavailability of vaginally administered misoprostol is 3 times higher than that of orally administered misoprostol, which may explain why intravaginal misoprostol has been reported to be more effective than oral misoprostol for medical abortion.

11.7 NEW TECHNOLOGIES IN VAGINAL DRUG DELIVERY

New technologies in vaginal drug delivery which are demonstrating considerable potential include:

11.7.1 Therapeutic peptide delivery

The first evidence of peptide absorption through the vaginal epithelium was reported in the early 1920s, when insulin administered vaginally to depancreatized dogs caused a rapid reduction in blood sugar levels. Recently, there has been renewed interest in the possibility of delivering therapeutic peptides and proteins via the vaginal epithelium. Large molecular weight peptides, including insulin, TSH, calcitonin, GnRH (gonadotropin releasing hormone) analogs, and various antigens have all demonstrated systemic absorption via the vaginal route. Specific examples of therapeutic peptide delivery are described below.

GnRH analogs

Vaginal application of GnRH and its synthetic analogs has been shown to induce a greater elevation of serum LH and FSH levels than oral administration of the same doses. In one study using immature rats, the bioavailability of GnRH analogs relative to the subcutaneous route

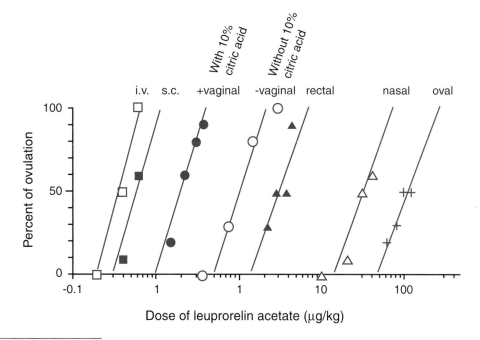

Figure 11.5 Ovulation induction by leuprorelin in diestrous rats after iv, sc, rectal, nasal, oral, and vaginal routes of administration. (Note: nasal absorption may have been underestimated in this study, due to drainage of the test solution. For example, nasal bioavailability has been determined as 18.7% in rats, in a study in which the nasal cavity was closed at the orifice and outlet)

was shown to be approximately 1–2% via the vaginal route and only 0.1% via the oral route.

In a human study, the synthetic GnRH analog leuprorelin was shown to be absorbed from the vagina and it elevated the plasma levels of the gonadotrophins (LH and FSH) and estrogen. A more prolonged LH release response was obtained using the vaginal route in comparison to the sc route, however the response was approximately half that obtained by sc injection. However, in this investigation, the analog was applied selectively at the early and mid-follicular phases, when the vaginal epithelium is thick and cohesive; greater bioavailability is to be expected during the luteal phase of the cycle, when the epithelium is porous and thin.

The uptake of leuprorelin via a variety of routes (iv, sc, rectal, nasal, oral, and vaginal) has been compared in diestrous rats. The bioavailability (as measured by a pharmacological effect, i.e. ovulation-inducing activity) for the vaginal route was relatively large, 3.8% from oleaginous and aqueous gel bases without the aid of an absorption promoter. In contrast, the bioavailability by the oral route was found to be about 0.4%. As can be seen from Figure 11.5, a much larger dose was needed by the oral and other routes in comparison to the vaginal route, in order to achieve ovulation induction.

Insulin

Rapid dose-related changes in the plasma glucose and insulin levels have been demonstrated in alloxan-induced diabetic rats and rabbits, after vaginal administration of insulin suspended in a poly(acrylate) aqueous gel (0.1%, pH 6.5).

Co-administration of insulin with the nonionic surface active agent, Cetomacrogol 1,000, in a PEG 400 base has been shown to lower blood glucose when administered vaginally to female rats with streptozocin-induced diabetes. However, the hypoglycemic effect was less than that achieved using the rectal route in the same base, or using the ip route.

11.7.2 Penetration enhancers

Although, as described above, the vagina is permeable to many peptides and proteins, in most cases the bioavailability is insufficient for systemic therapy and is also highly variable. Penetration enhancers may be used to promote peptide absorption across the vaginal epithelium. However, less extensive investigations on the use of penetration enhancers for the vaginal route have been carried out in comparison to other routes, such as intranasal and transdermal (see Sections 9.7.1 and 8.6.1).

Carboxylic acids

The absolute bioavailablilty in diestrous rats of the GnRH analog, leuprorelin, was increased from about 4% to about 20%, by adding polybasic carboxylic acids such as citric, succinic, tartaric and glycocholic acid. Various other studies have also shown that citric acid is able to promote the vaginal absorption of biologically active peptides and proteins, including:

- GnRH (as measured by ovulation-inducing activity);
- leuprorelin (as measured by regression of hormone-dependent mammary tumors);
- insulin (as measured by a reduction in plasma glucose levels).

The mechanism of enhancement of vaginal absorption of peptides by organic acids has been attributed to their acidifying and chelating abilities. In the case of the peptide leuprorelin, it seems that the effect of lowering the pH causes self-association or conformational changes of the peptide resulting in changes in the charge of leuprorelin and the epithelial surface. Since the pH of the vaginal lumen is normally 3.5 to 5.0, an acidic preparation of pH 3 to 4 should not disturb the normal ecology of the vagina.

The chelating activity of organic acids upsets epithelial cell–cell adhesion. Removal of Ca^{2+} from the tight junctions of the epithelial cells by the chelators results in opening of the junctions, thereby creating a leaky epithelium and enhancing drug delivery via the paracellular route. The chelating effects are reversible, for example changes in the vaginal epithelium produced by citric acid were rapidly reversed after the epithelium was washed with physiological saline solution. Substances with a strong chelating ability, such as EDTA, can cause pronounced absorption. Ultrastructual observations have shown that after daily treatment with EDTA, the desmosomes in the human vaginal epithelium open and the size of the intercellular spaces increase dramatically; again, these changes are reversible, but it does raise toxicological issues (see below).

α-Cyclodextrin

α-Cyclodextrin is found to facilitate the vaginal absorption of leuprorelin in rats approximately 6-fold, just as it does in the nasal absorption of leuprorelin and insulin in rats and dogs. Cyclodextrins can be used to solubilize drugs and thus potentially increase the concentration gradient driving passive diffusion across membranes. New research suggests that their enhancing effect may also be partly due to the removal of fatty acids, such as palmitic and oleic acids, which are minor membrane components.

Toxic effects

A major disadvantage associated with the use of penetration enhancers is their potential deleterious effect on the epithelial tissue. The damaging effects of various absorption enhancers have been investigated in vaginal absorption studies of gentamicin using ovariectomized rats. It was found that the penetration enhancers laureth-9 and lysophosphatidylcholine caused severe desquamation of the epithelium, whereas citric acid and palmitoylcarnitine were able to enhance absorption while causing only minor epithelial damage.

The vaginal absorption of insulin was studied in ovariectomized rats and in the absence of any enhancer, no decrease in blood glucose was observed. Co-administration of various absorption enhancers was able to significantly increase the degree of hypoglycemia. The histological changes in the vaginal epithelium after treatment with the enhancer systems were variable and often severe:

- palmitoylcarnitine chloride exhibited the greatest local toxicity including reduction of epithelial thickness and cell death.
- laureth-9 causes widespread epithelial cell loss, from which recovery is unlikely.
- a novel enhancer, lysophosphatidylglycerol, showed no epithelial disruption or desquamation.

11.7.3 Antiviral vaginal delivery

Antiviral vaginal gel

The development of topical vaginal virucidal agents would be useful in attempting to reduce the risk of HIV transmission among heterosexuals. Dextrin sulfate (DS) is a sulfated polysaccharide with an average molecular weight of 30 kD. It is a potent inhibitor of the growth of diverse laboratory strains of HIV-1 in a variety of human cell lines and peripheral blood lymphocytes. It has a high therapeutic index ($>10^4$) and is non-toxic in cell culture. DS and related polysaccharides act by blocking viral entry into host cells, in part because of their high molecular weight and charge, although specific binding to CD4, the viral envelop glycoprotein 120, and basic proteins on the cell surface, have also been reported.

Phase I studies suggest that DS vaginal gel used at doses of up to 100 μg/ml does not exert an adverse effect on vaginal epithelium, or on vaginal bacterial ecology. However, no conclusions can be drawn at this stage about the likely tolerability, safety and efficacy of the gel in the context of sexual intercourse.

Antiviral vaginal devices

Nonoxynol-9 is an approved spermicide with strong antiviral activity. A vaginal device which facilitates the controlled release of nonoxynol-9 has been developed for contraceptive and anti-STD purposes. The device, available as a diaphragm or a disk pessary, is fabricated from silicone elastomer matrix system. The drug release profile demonstrates square root time kinetics ($M \propto t^{1/2}$) (see Section 4.4.2).

While the spermicide-containing reusable diaphragms currently on the market are relatively effective when used in combination with a spermicidal formulation, they require careful fitting, insertion and maintenance. Moreover, adverse reactions, such as urinary tract infections, alterations in vaginal flora and occurrence of toxic shock syndrome, have been associated with their use. In contrast the silicone-based device described above has been reported to be stable, non-irritating and non-toxic.

Sodium cholate also exhibits strong spermicidal and antiviral activity; it was recently found to be useful in the selective destruction of HIV-infected cells as well as in the inhibition of HIV-1 itself. A vaginal sponge has also been recently developed comprising a soft poly(urethane) sponge impregnated with a gel containing 1% benzalkonium chloride, 0.5% nonoxynol-9, 0.5% sodium cholate, poly(dimethylsiloxane) (dispersing agent) and methylcellulose. The sponge therefore combines the actions of:

- a physical barrier that blocks the cervix;
- a material that absorbs the ejaculate;
- a spermicide;
- an antiviral agent.

Antiviral liposomal preparations

Intramuscular injection of α interferon was shown to be fairly efficacious in the treatment of genital warts; however, this route was associated with a number of side-effects including fever, myalgia, headache, nausea and fatigue. A liposomal preparation of α interferon for topical vaginal delivery has been developed, which offers the advantage of treating latent human papillomavirus infections as well as visible genital warts. The liposomal preparation can be self-administered intravaginally, without the need for multiple painful local, or im, injections. Preliminary investigations on the efficacy of this system are highly encouraging.

11.7.4 Vaginal mucosal vaccines

Absorption of bacterial antigens through the vaginal epithelium plays a fundamentally important role in the local production of antibodies to prevent bacterial infection of the genital organs.

As discussed in detail with respect to oral vaccines (see Section 6.7.7), mucosal surfaces are linked by a common mucosal immune system (CMIS). In the vagina, mucosal immune responses are initiated by the uptake of antigens from the vaginal surfaces (Figure 11.6). Whereas the gastrointestinal tract has identifiable aggregates of lymphoid tissue within the epithelium known as the Peyer's patches (see Section 6.2.2), and similar aggregates have been identified in the nasal cavity and the bronchial tract, the vagina does not appear to have discrete lymphoid aggregates. Instead antigens are taken up by antigen-presenting cells (APCs) in the vaginal membrane; the APCs move through the lymphatic vessels to the genital lymph node, where an immune response is initiated. Antigen-specific effector lymphocytes (B cells and T cells) migrate through the lymphatics and exit via the thoracic duct into the bloodstream. The primed B and T cells home to various mucosal sites including the genital mucosa, where they undergo maturation and secretion.

A vaginal vaccine has been developed for the treatment of recurrent urinary tract infections. The multi-strain vaccine, composed of 10 heat-killed bacterial uropathogenic strains, has been shown to be efficacious against cystitis in non-human primates when administered by the vaginal route. Bladder infections were significantly reduced and both systemic and local immune responses were generated.

Figure 11.6 Probable route of cellular traffic following vaginal exposure to vaccine antigen or to HIV or SIV infections

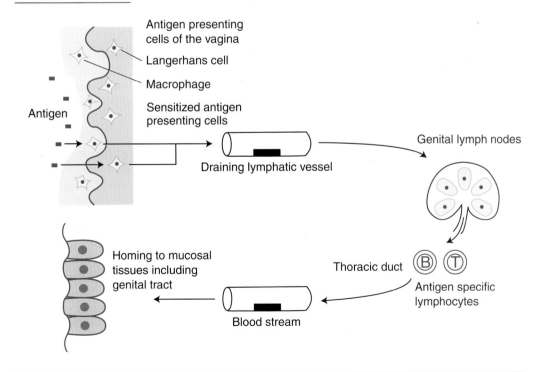

A cholera vaccine, comprising killed *Vibrio cholerae* cells and the recombinant cholera toxin B (CTB) subunit (the CTB subunit is used extensively as an adjuvant in mucosal immunization protocols, as it enhances binding of the vaccine to receptors on epithelial surfaces), significantly increased immune responses (both specific IgA and specific IgG) in both the cervix and the vagina, after vaginal immunization. In addition, local production of CTB-specific IgG in the genital tract could be demonstrated in vaginally immunized women. It was determined that vaginal immunization resulted in two different types of immune responses in mice: high and low. High responders to the immunizations had been immunized in the diestrous phase of the cycle. As explained above, the vaginal epithelium is thin and porous during this phase, which facilitates vaccine uptake.

Interestingly, vaginal immunization did not generate antibodies in the rectum. Similarly, rectal immunization induced high levels of specific IgA and IgG in rectal secretions, but not in female genital tract secretions. Thus, generation of optimal immune responses to sexually transmitted organisms in both the rectal and the genital mucosa of women may require local immunization at both of these sites.

Association of an antigen with an appropriate microparticulate carrier may enhance antigen uptake by vaginal antigen-presenting cells. This strategy for vaginal vaccine delivery is described below (Section 11.7.5).

11.7.5 Microparticulate systems

Microparticulate systems are being investigated for both vaginal drug and vaccine delivery:

Starch microspheres

Biodegradable starch microspheres, 40 μm in diameter, were shown to be capable of enhancing the vaginal absorption of insulin. The effect was further enhanced when the penetration enhancer lysophosphatidylcholine was used.

Hyaluronan ester microspheres

Hyaluronan is a naturally occurring mucopolysaccharide, consisting of repeating disaccharide units of D-glucuronic acid and N-acetyl-D-glucosamine. By esterification of the carboxyl groups of the glucuronic acid residue with alcohols, modified biopolymers can be produced which are biocompatible, mucoadhesive and biodegradable. The degradation rate can be controlled by the degree of esterification and by the type of alcohol substituent. Hyaluronan ester (HYAFF) microspheres (7 μm in diameter) can be prepared by a solvent extraction method. Experiments using radio-labeled microspheres have shown that after vaginal administration the microspheres are dispersed along the length of the vagina for prolonged periods, thereby demonstrating their potential as a long-acting intravaginal delivery system.

A vaginal pessary containing the microspheres dispersed in a Suppocire base have been investigated for the delivery of the polypeptide salmon calcitonin (sCT). Suppocire, a mixture of semi-synthetic polyethylene triglycerides, melts at 35–37 °C. After administration of the pessary, the formulation forms a fine emulsion on contact with the aqueous environment of the vagina, thus encouraging the dispersion of microspheres throughout the vaginal cavity.

It has been proposed that the bioadhesive microspheres may induce transient widening of intercellular junctions when applied nasally, or added to Caco-2 cell monolayers. It is thought that drug microspheres take up water from the cells, causing the cells to dehydrate and "shrink", thereby inducing the transient widening of the intercellular junctions and increased drug transport. In postmenopausal female volunteers, a vaginal pessary containing HYAFF/sCT microspheres was well tolerated and the relative bioavailability of sCT compared to sc injection was estimated to be approximately 30%, compared to 7.9% for nasal formulation.

Microparticulate vaccine delivery systems

A number of reasons may account for the adjuvant effects of microparticulate formulations for vaginal immunization:

- protection of antigens against degradative enzymatic activity;
- improved presentation to the APCs in the vaginal epithelium: "passive targeting";
- microparticulate-associated membrane-modifying properties which facilitate antigen transfer across normally poorly permeable barrier.

Work in this field has concentrated on the use of poly(lactide-co-glycolide) microparticles, which have the advantages of being biocompatible, biodegradable and well tolerated in humans. Promising results have also been obtained with the use of biodegradable starch microspheres in conjunction with the absorption enhancer lysophosphatidylcholine.

However, in general, only low levels of antibodies have been induced by intravaginal immunizations and the antibodies generated have been predominantly localized in the genital tract, even in the presence of potent antigen delivery systems.

11.7.6 Bioadhesives

Traditionally, pharmaceutical formulations for intravaginal use comprise creams, foams, pessaries and jellies. Such formulations are prone to leakage, which can result in:

- low efficacy, due to limited contact time with the absorbing surface;
- poor compliance.

Bioadhesive polymers can be used to prolong the contact of a drug with a mucosal surface, without inducing adverse local effects on the epithelium. Other beneficial effects conferred by the use of bioadhesive polymers include:

- increasing the local drug concentration at the site of adhesion/absorption;
- protecting the drug from dilution and possible degradation by vaginal secretions;
- prolonging the contact time of the dosage form near the absorbing surface.

Thus such polymers have attracted considerable interest as a means of improving drug delivery at mucosal sites, including the vagina. Reference has already been made to the promising results obtained using bioadhesive hyaluronane ester microspheres for vaginal drug delivery. Other bioadhesive polymers under investigation include:

Polycarbophil

Polycarbophil, a poly(acrylic acid) lightly cross-linked with divinyl glycol, can remain on vaginal tissue for extended periods and has demonstrated many potential clinical applications:

Dry vagina: the bioadhesive gel can hydrate vaginal tissue for 3–4 days after a single application. Tissue hydration is caused by an increased blood flow, thus increasing transudation of vaginal fluid though the intercellular channels of the vaginal epithelium.

Bacterial vaginosis: the acidic polymer (pKa 4.5) can dramatically lower pH. Clinical assessment of local tissue pH in postmenopausal women shows a reduction in pH from about 7 to 4 and maintenance of this acidic pH for about 3–4 days. This acidic pH is an unfavorable environment for pathogens, thereby protecting against bacterial vaginosis.

Spermicide-antiviral: the polymer appears to be an effective delivery system for the spermicidal/antiviral agent nonoxynol-9. By its ability to adhere to vaginal tissue while retaining nonoxynol-9 in its gel structure, it is an excellent extended effect spermicide. As an antiviral, nonoxynol-9 can only kill free HIV and is not noticeably active when the virus is within a lymphocyte. In contrast, the bioadhesive gel containing nonoxynol-9 attaches to lymphocytes and maintains sufficient contact time to allow the nonoxynol-9 surfactant to disrupt the cell wall, thus eliminating the lymphocyte and killing the virus within. This suggests that the polymer may be useful in the prophylaxis of AIDS and the treatment of other sexually transmitted diseases.

Progesterone delivery: as described above, estrogen replacement therapy increases the risk of endometrial cancer when used alone. This risk can be eliminated by treatment with a progestational agent for up to 14 days a month. The vaginal delivery of a polycarbophil gel loaded with progesterone has been shown to allow the extended vaginal delivery of the drug for 2–3 days from a single dose and protect the endometrium against cancer. Low serum levels of progesterone were detected after vaginal delivery, which corresponds to fewer side-effects. A commercial progesterone-loaded polycarbophil gel preparation for intravaginal delivery, Crinone, has recently been launched.

Peptide delivery: It has also been reported that a polycarbophil hydrogel formulation increased the vaginal membrane permeability of

GnRH, in comparison to a solution, in rats. Co-administration of the GnRH loaded gel with various enzyme inhibitors (EDTA, sodium taurodihydrofusidate and sodium laurate) resulted in ovulation-inducing activity comparable with that of a sc injection.

Smart hydrogel

Smart hydrogel preparations, comprising poly(acrylic acid) and a poloxamer (see Section 16.3.2.1), are administered into the vaginal cavity, where they coat the vaginal walls effectively. The temperature-dependent gelling of the system helps to prevent leak-back and provides sustained release properties. Smart hydrogel preparations containing estradiol have shown similar bioavailability to a commercial vaginal cream and suppository, even though the gel contained only 20% of the relative estradiol dose.

11.8 CONCLUSIONS

The vagina is a possible site for the systemic administration of various drugs. However, the low and erratic bioavailability of biopharmaceuticals via this route necessitates the use of absorption enhancers. Until safe, non-toxic absorption enhancers can be found, the route is of limited potential. A further major limitation of this route is the lack of reproducibility resulting from cyclic changes in the reproductive system. Finally, no matter what degree of optimization can be achieved via this route, it can only ever benefit approximately 50% of the population!

11.9 FURTHER READING

Hafez E.S.E. and Evans T.N. (eds) (1978) *The Human Vagina.* Elsevier/North-Holland Biomedical Press, Amsterdam.

Okada, H. (1991) Vaginal route of peptide and protein drug delivery. In: *Peptide and Protein Drug Delivery* (V.H.L. Lee, ed.). Marcel Dekker, New York, pp. 633–666.

Lee, V.H.L. Yamamoto, A. and Kompella U.B. (1991). Mucosal penetration enhancers for facilitation of peptide and protein drug absorption. *Crit. Rev. Ther. Drug Carr. Syst.,* 8:91–192.

Chien, Y.W. (1992) Intravaginal controlled-release drug administration. In: *Novel Drug Delivery Systems* (Chien, Y.W., ed.). Marcel Dekker, New York, pp. 529–558.

Richardson, J.L. and Illum, L. (1992) The vaginal route of peptide and protein drug delivery. *Adv. Drug Del. Rev.,* 8:341–366.

Muranishi, S., Yamamoto, A. and Okada, H. (1993) Rectal and vaginal absorption of peptides and proteins. In: *Biological Barriers to Protein Delivery.* (Audus K.L. and Raub T.J., eds). Plenum Press, New York, pp. 199–227.

Zhou, X.H. (1994) Overcoming enzymatic and absorption barrier to non-parenterally administered protein and peptide drug. *J. Contr. Rel.* 29:239–252.

Hochman, J. and Artursson, P. (1994) Mechanisms of absorption enhancement and tight junction regulation. *J. Contr. Rel.* 29:253–267.

Kiyono, H., Miller, C.J., Lu, Y., Lehner T. *et al.* (1995).The common mucosal immune system for the reproductive tract: basic principles applied toward an AIDS vaccine. *Adv. Drug Del. Rev.*, 18:23–51.

Sayani A.P. and Chien Y.W. (1996) Systemic delivery of peptides and proteins across absorptive mucosae. *Crit. Rev. Ther. Drug Carr. Syst.*, 13:85–184.

11.10 SELF-ASSESSMENT QUESTIONS

1. Give examples of the classes of the pharmaceutical agents which are presently marketed as topical formulations for vaginal administration.

2. Which other epithelial membrane has a structure most similar to that of the vaginal epithelium?

3. During which phase of the menstrual cycle is the vaginal epithelia thickest and the epithelial tight junctions most cohesive, thereby reducing the absorption of hydrophilic compounds via the paracellular route?

4. Which of the following do not leak through the intercellular channels of vaginal epithelium at the late luteal phase and early follicular phase? (a) erythrocytes, (b) IgG, (c) albumin, (d) leukocytes.

5. What factor controls the pH in the vaginal lumen at between pH 4 and pH 5, preventing the proliferation of pathogenic bacteria?

6. List the disadvantages of the vaginal route for drug delivery.

7. Describe the types of absorption enhancers under development for use in vaginal route.

8. Describe the possible reasons for enhanced vaginal vaccination using microparticulate systems.

9. Describe how bioadhesive gels enhance the vaginal absorption of drugs.

12 Ophthalmic Drug Delivery

Clive G. Wilson, Y.P. Zhu, P. Kurmala, L.S. Rao and B. Dhillon

OBJECTIVES

On completion of this chapter the reader should be able to:

- Describe the structure and physiology of the eye
- Describe the barriers to ocular drug delivery
- Describe the approaches used to optimize topical ocular delivery
- Describe the approaches used in intraocular drug delivery
- Discuss the limitations of ocular drug delivery

12.1 Introduction

As discussed in Chapter 1 (Section 1.1) certain drugs (including peptides, proteins and nucleic acid therapeutics) are unsuitable for oral delivery and must be given intravenously. Research has recently been directed towards the development of alternatives to the parenteral route, such as the transdermal, nasal and other routes thus far discussed in this book, for the systemic delivery of such drugs.

However, unlike the other routes described in this text, ophthalmic drug delivery is used only for the treatment of *local* conditions of the eye and cannot be used as a portal of drug entry to the *systemic* circulation. Nevertheless, this route warrants study within the general context of drug delivery and targeting, as the local delivery of drugs to their site of action represents a form of drug targeting, reducing the dose needed to produce a pharmacological effect and also minimizing side-effects. Furthermore, significant advances have been made to optimize the localized delivery of medication to the eye, so that the route is now associated with highly sophisticated drug delivery technologies; some of these technologies are unique to the eye and many are also found in the other delivery routes.

The eye is a sensory organ, prone to a wide variety of diseases which may be of a systemic origin, such as diabetes or hypertension, or peculiar to the eye, such as glaucoma, cataract and macular degeneration. Furthermore, since the eye is located on the surface of the body, it is also easily injured and infected.

According to the location of diseases, ocular disorders are grouped as periocular and intraocular conditions. Periocular diseases include:

Blepharitis

An infection of the lid structures (usually by *Staphylococcus aureus*) with concomitant seborrhea, rosacea, a dry eye and abnormalities of the meibomein glands and their lipid secretions.

Conjunctivitis

The condition when redness of the eye and the presence of a foreign-body sensation are evident. There are many causes of conjunctivitis, but the great majority are the result of acute infection or allergy. Bacterial conjunctivitis is the most common ocular infection.

Keratitis

The condition in which patients have a decreased vision, ocular pain, red eye, and often a cloudy/opaque cornea. Keratitis is mainly caused by bacteria, viruses, fungi, protozoa and parasites.

Trachoma

This is caused by the organism *Chalmydia trachomatis*; it is the most common cause of blindness in North Africa and the Middle East.

Dry eye

If for any reason the composition of tears is changed, or an inadequate volume of tears is produced, the symptom of dry eye will result. Dry eye conditions are not just a cause for ocular discomfort, but can also result in corneal damage.

Periocular diseases such as these are relatively easily treated using topical formulations. Intraocular conditions are more difficult to manage and include intraocular infections: i.e. infections in the inner eye, including the aqueous humor, iris, vitreous humor and retina. They occur commonly after ocular surgery, trauma or due to endogenous causes. Such infections carry a high risk for damage to the eye and also afford the possibility of spread of infection from the eye into the brain. A common intraocular disease is glaucoma, considered to be one of the major ophthalmic clinical problems in the world. More than 2% of the population over the age of 40 have this disease, in which an increased intraocular pressure (IOP) greater than 22 mm Hg ultimately compromises blood flow to the retina and thus causes death of the peripheral optic nerves. This process results in visual field loss and ultimately blindness. Recently, physicians have become more familiar with the condition known as normotensive glaucoma. About 20% of glaucoma patients have near normal intraocular pressures and in these patients the disease may result from spasm of the arterial supply.

Disorders of the posterior segment of the eye are particularly difficult to treat. The efficient clearance mechanisms at the front of the eye reduce the concentrations of drug able to diffuse to the back of the eye. Futhermore, many of these disorders are chronic conditions, requiring continuous therapy. The diseases of the back of the eye include: Cytomeaglovirus retinits (CMVR), Proliferative vitreoretinopathy (PVR), diabetic retinopathy, age-rated macular degeneration, endophthalmitis and retinitis pigmentosa.

There are three main routes commonly used for administration of drugs to the eye: topical, intraocular and systemic.

The topical route is the most common method to administer a medication to the eye. Introducing the drug directly to the conjunctival sac localizes drug effects, facilitates drug entry that is otherwise hard to achieve with systemic delivery and avoids first-pass metabolism. The physiological factors affecting topical drug delivery and the approaches under development to optimize this type of delivery are described in detail below.

Intraocular drug delivery is more difficult to achieve practically. Research, as described below, is concentrating on the development of intravitreal injections and the use of intraocular implants to improve delivery to this region.

As regards the systemic route, several studies have shown that some drugs can distribute into ocular tissues following systemic administration. Oral administration of carbonic anhydrase inhibitors (CAIs; for the treatment of glaucoma), including acetazolamide, methazolamide and dichlorphenamide, demonstrates the capacity of a systemic drug to distribute into the ciliary process of the eye and to provide a concentration sufficient for inhibiting carbonic anhydrase isoenzyme II, resulting in an effective decrease in the secretion of aqueous humor. Systemic administration of CAIs has been used in the management of glaucoma.

It has also been demonstrated that steroids and antibiotics can penetrate into the aqueous humor following systemic administration. Systemic drug treatment is often considered as a first option for posterior eye diseases involving the optic nerve, retina and uveal tract. This is because drug distribution to posterior ocular tissues is difficult via the topical route due to the anatomical restriction posed by the eye. However, the systemic route has the significant disadvantage that all the organs of the body are subjected to the action of the drug, when only a very small volume of tissue in the eye may need the treatment.

12.2 STRUCTURE AND PHYSIOLOGY OF THE EYE

The function of the eye is to produce a clear image of the external world and to transmit this to the visual cortex of the brain. In order to do this the eye must have constant dimensions, an unclouded optical pathway and the ability to focus light on the retina. These requirements and the need for protection of the globe determine the special structure of the eye and its associated apparatus.

12.2.1 The cornea

The cornea is a five-layered structure, which comprises the epithelium (superficial layer), Bowman's membrane, stroma, Descemet's membrane and the endothelium, as shown in Figure 12.1.

The epithelium

Figure 12.1
Microscopic structure and characteristics of the corneal barrier

The epithelium is built up of several layers of cells and makes up about 10% of the total corneal thickness in man, and a similar proportion in

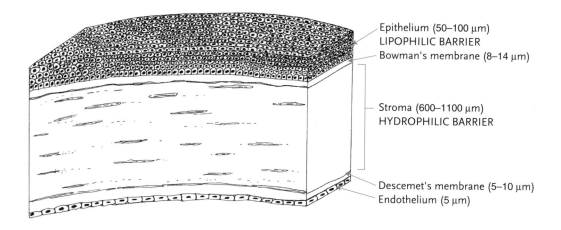

Epithelium (50–100 μm)
LIPOPHILIC BARRIER
Bowman's membrane (8–14 μm)

Stroma (600–1100 μm)
HYDROPHILIC BARRIER

Descemet's membrane (5–10 μm)
Endothelium (5 μm)

many other mammalian species. There are 5 layers in man with thickness 50–100 μm, which is similar to the rabbit, but the number of layers increases in thicker corneas to about 10, such as in the bovine cornea. This is a hydrophobic tissue and contributes 90% of the barrier to hydrophilic drugs and 10% to hydrophobic drugs.

The Bowman's membrane

This occurs in man as a thin homogenous sheet with a thickness of 8–14 μm. The rabbit eye does not possess this layer. It is not a true elastic membrane and does not regenerate when destroyed. This layer is not considered to be a barrier to drug absorption across the cornea.

The stroma

This represents about 90% of the thickness of the cornea in most mammals and is composed of a modified connective tissue; 70–80% of the wet weight is water, and 20–25% of the dry weight is collagen, other proteins and mucopolysaccharides. The stroma is the main barrier to extremely lipophilic drugs.

Descemet's membrane

This is a strong, homogenous and very resistant membrane. It is approximately 6 μm thick and is sharply defined from the stroma. This membrane is normally in a state of tension and regenerates when damaged.

The endothelium

This is a single layer of flattened epithelial-like cells interlocked by alternating, twisting surfaces, which completely covers the posterior surface of the cornea. Gap junctions exist between adjacent cells allowing the permeation of various substances. The endothelium is not rate-determining as its permeability is 200 or more times greater than that of the epithelium. This layer houses a Na^+/K^+-ATPase pump which is bicarbonate-dependent, and operates at a constant level to control a balance between the passive movement of water into the stroma and the active movement of fluid out of it, responsible for maintaining corneal transparency and a constant corneal thickness. If the active pump breaks down or the bicarbonate efflux is attenuated by carbonic anhydrase inhibitors, the stroma will absorb water, swell and become opaque, resulting in the thickening and clouding of the cornea. The change in corneal thickness affects the absorption of a drug by increase in path length.

12.2.2 The tear film

Proteins dissolved in the lacrimal fluid influence the viscosity of human tears, which ranges from 1.3 to 5.9 cps with a mean value of 2.92 cps. The tears have a pseudoplastic character with a yield value of about 32 cps at 33 °C. During a blink the lid moves at a high velocity and the film is submitted to a high rate of shear of about 10,000–40,000 sec^{-1}.

12.3 TOPICAL DRUG DELIVERY

There are three main routes commonly used for administration of drugs to the eye: topical, systemic and intra-ocular. These are summarized in Figure 12.2.

The topical route is the most common method to administer a medication to the eye. Introducing the drug directly to the conjunctival sac localizes drug effects, facilitates drug entry that is otherwise hard to achieve with systemic delivery and avoids first-pass metabolism. In practice, topical application frequently fails to establish a therapeutic drug level for a desired length of time within the target ocular tissues and fluids. The major problem of this inefficient ocular treatment results from many factors, including the precorneal clearance mechanism, the highly selective corneal barrier, the unproductive drug loss by the conjunctival route and the difficulty that old people have in dosing eyedrops to the eye. Typically, less than 5% of the instilled dose reaches the aqueous humor.

12.3.1 Physiological factors affecting topical drug delivery

The main factors affecting the topical absorption of drugs across the cornea cavity are physiological in origin. In addition to the hydrophilic and lipophilic barriers presented by the tear film and cornea described above, various other factors affect topical drug absorption.

Figure 12.2
Anatomical features of the eye in cross-section, illustrating major routes of administration

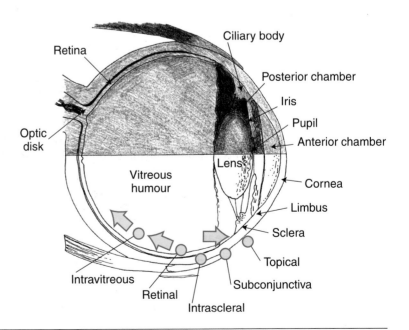

12.3.1.1 Nasolacrimal drainage

Nasolacrimal drainage is the major factor contributing to precorneal drug loss and associated poor ocular bioavailbility. Under normal conditions the human tear volume is about 7–9 μl and it is relatively constant. The maximum amount of fluid that can be held in the lower eyelid sack is 25–30 μl, but only 3 μl of a solution can be incorporated in the precorneal film without causing it to destabilize. When eyedrops are administered, the tear volume is suddenly increased which can cause rapid reflex blinking. Most of the eyedrop is pumped through the lacrimal drainage system into the nasolacrimal duct, and some is spilled on the cheeks and splashed on the eyelashes. The drainage rate of the solution is related to the instilled volume; the smaller the volume the slower the drainage rate. The instilled drop has been suggested to have an optimum volume of 8–15 μl. However, the typical volumes delivered by commercial eyedroppers are in the range of 35–56 μl. Only a small proportion of the eyedrop can therefore be retained by the eye. Formulations often disappear from the cul-de-sac within 5 to 10 minutes following instillation in rabbits and 1 to 2 minutes in humans. Severe systemic side-effects may be result from absorption of some drugs through the mucous membrane of the nasolacrimal duct.

12.3.1.2 pH

The pH of the normal tears has been determined by many investigators to have a mean value of 7.4, but there are wide variations. It is lowest on awakening as a result of acid by-products associated with relatively anaerobic conditions in prolonged lid closure and increases because of loss of carbon dioxide as the eyes open. The tears are more acid in contact-lens wearers due to the impediment of the efflux of carbon dioxide, and more alkaline in the case of diseases such as dry eye, severe ocular rosacea and lacrimal stenosis.

When an ophthalmic solution is instilled onto the eye surface, it is mixed with the tears present in the conjunctival sac and with the precorneal tear film. Tears have a weak buffering capacity and therefore the pH of the mixture is mainly determined by the pH of the instilled solution. The exposure of the eye surface to an acid fluid may cause damage to the ocular tissues resulting from a reaction with cellular proteins, forming insoluble complexes. Alkalinization of the tear film tends to produce an interaction of the hydroxyl ions with the cell membranes. At a high pH the lipids in the cell membranes will be saponified causing disruption of the structural integrity of the cells. The damage is dependent on the concentration of hydrogen and hydroxyl ions and on the exposure time. Reflex tears and drainage remove the irritant solution.

To avoid reflex lachrimation and to prolong the retention of a drug at the eye surface, it is desirable that the ophthalmic solution has a pH between 7.0 and 7.7. Some drugs are unstable in this pH range, and therefore need to be formulated at other pH values, but it is preferred that little or no buffering is employed.

12.3.1.3 Surface tension

The surface tension of tear fluid at the eye temperature has been measured as 43.6 to 46.6 mNm^{-1} for normal eyes and 49.6 mNm^{-1} for patients with dry eye. The instillation of a solution containing drugs or adjuvants that lower the surface tension may disrupt the outmost lipid of the tear film into numerous oily droplets, which become solubilized. The protective effect of the oily film against evaporation of the tear film aqueous layer disappears and dry spots will be formed. The dry spots are painful and irritant and elicit reflex blinks to eliminate the material. This irritation does not always occur immediately after the instillation. In many cases it appears 30 minutes to 1 hour following the application and is dependent on the substance and on its concentration. The tear film is destabilized when the surface tension of the instilled solution is much lower than the surface tension of the lacrimal fluid.

12.3.1.4 Osmolality

The osmolality of tears is of prime importance, since optical integrity of the cornea is significantly influenced by the tonicity of the tears. The normal osmolality of tears varies from 290 to 310 $mOsmkg^{-1}$, which is almost equivalent to that of normal saline solution. Variations in osmotic pressure between 100–640 $mOsmkg^{-1}$ appear to be well tolerated by the eye; beyond these values irritation takes place, eliciting reflex tears and reflex blinking.

When the eye surface is covered with a hypotonic solution the permeability of the epithelium is increased considerably and water flows into the cornea. The corneal tissues swell, increasing the pressure on the nerves and causing an anesthetizing action on the cornea. In the case where the eye surface is covered with hypertonic solution, water flows from the aqueous layer through the cornea to the eye surface. A desquamation of superficial cells is also observed after instillation of hypertonic solution in rabbits. Although the instillation of a non-isotonic solution will cause a change in tear osmolality, it will regain the original value within 1 to 2 minutes following dosing. This is mainly due to a rapid flow of water across the cornea.

In general, however, hypotonic solutions are well tolerated in the eye and can lead to better corneal absorption of the drug due to a concentration effect on the formulation and increased permeability of the cornea (both by virtue of uptake of water from the formulation by the corneal tissue).

12.3.2 The absorption of topically applied drugs

There are two pathways for ocular absorption, the corneal route and the conjunctiva/scleral route as shown in Figure 12.3. Conjunctival absorption is nonproductive and constitutes an additional loss following instillation of a topical dose.

12.3.2.1 Corneal route

The corneal route is often considered to be the main pathway for ocular absorption. Most drugs cross this membrane into the intraocu-

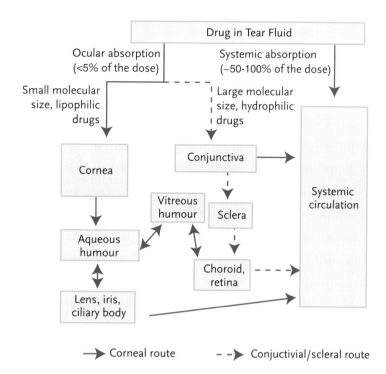

Figure 12.3 Pathways for entry of drugs into the eye

Drug in Tear Fluid

Ocular absorption (<5% of the dose)
Systemic absorption (~50-100% of the dose)

Small molecular size, lipophilic drugs
Large molecular size, hydrophilic drugs

Cornea

Conjunctiva

Vitreous humour

Sclera

Systemic circulation

Aqueous humour

Choroid, retina

Lens, iris, ciliary body

→ Corneal route   - -▶ Conjuctivial/scleral route

lar tissues by either intercellular or transcellular diffusion. Lipophilic drugs are transported via the transcellular route, and hydrophilic drugs penetrate mainly through the intercellular pathway. There is little evidence that ophthalmic drugs penetrate into ocular compartments by active transport. In general, corneal penetration is mainly governed by the lipophilicity of the drug but it is also affected by other factors, including solubility, molecular size and shape, charge and degree of ionization. These pathways and the factors affecting the absorption by these mechanisms are discussed in detail in Section 1.3.

12.3.2.2 *Noncorneal route*

The noncorneal route of absorption involves penetration across the conjunctiva and sclera into the intraocular tissues. There are three pathways for drug penetration across the sclera:

- through the perivascular spaces;
- through the aqueous media of gel-like mucopolysaccharides;
- through the empty spaces within the collagen network.

The noncorneal route is usually not productive, as drug penetrating the surface of the eye beyond the corneal-scleral limbus is picked up by local capillary beds and removed to the general circulation. This route in general precludes drug entry into the aqueous humor, which would have an impact on ocular drug delivery.

It is interesting that the noncorneal route of absorption may be important for hydrophilic compounds with large molecular weights such as timolol maleate and gentamicin. This route may also be attractive in potentially facilitating the transport of peptides and proteins, either as drugs or drug carriers, to their target sites within the eye.

12.3.3 Approaches to optimize topical ocular drug delivery

12.3.3.1 *Proper placement of the eyedrops*

Accurate and proper placement of an eye drop may considerably improve the efficacy in drug delivery as the capacity of the conjunctival sac is dependent on the position of the patient's head and technique of instillation. A drop is placed in the inferior cul-de-sac by gently pulling the lower lid away from the globe and creating a pouch to receive the drop. After gently lifting the lid to touch the globe, a small amount of liquid is entrapped in the inferior conjunctival sac, where it may be retained up to twice as long as when it is simply dropped over the superior sclera. Drainage from the cul-de-sac may further be reduced by punctual occlusion or simple eyelid closure, which not only maximizes the contact of drug with the periocular tissues but also slows the rate of the systemic absorption.

Following dosing, the normal manoeuvre results in a gradient across he eye as illustrated in Figure 12.4. This suggests that dosing under the upper lid would improve delivery: however, this method of dosing would be difficult for the patient.

Figure 12.4 Practical difficulties in treating the upper hemisphere of the eye with topical formulations. Flow from the lacrimal gland dilutes the concentration of drug in the tear film pulled up from the lower marginal strip

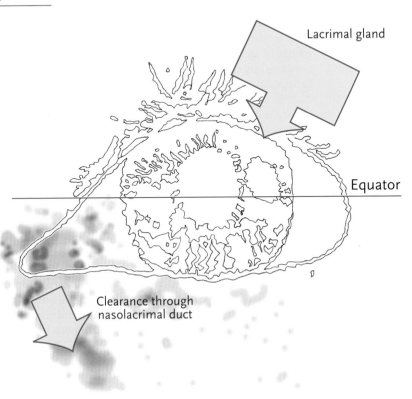

12.3.3.2 Reducing the instilled volume of an eyedrop

As indicated in Section 12.3.1.1, nasolacrimal drainage is the major factor contributing to precorneal drug loss and systemic side-effects. The local/systemic effect balance can be improved by reducing the size of the eyedrop and tips capable of delivering a drop of 8–10 μl have been designed by varying the relationship between the inner and outer diameters of the end of the tip. The use of smaller eye droppers results in a reduced systemic drug absorption, but their use in commercial containers has not been popular. Although a smaller drop may be retained longer in the conjunctival sac, the instilled volume less than 8 μl is not recommended due to the difficulty in making up a suitable concentration for the eyedrop.

12.3.3.3 Formulation factors affecting ocular bioavailability on topical application

For most membranes, passive diffusion is the main mechanism by which drug traverses membrane barriers. The process of passive diffusion initially involves partition of a drug between the aqueous fluid at the site of the application and the lipoidal cell membrane. The drug in solution in the membrane then diffuses across the membrane followed by a second partition of drug between the membrane and the aqueous fluids within the site of absorption.

Two approaches can be used to enhance corneal drug permeability:

- modify integrity of the corneal epithelium transiently;
- modify the chemical structure of the drug.

The first approach can be accomplished by exposing the eye to compounds such as chelating agents and surfactants, but it has hardly been explored due to the sensitivity of this particular tissue.

The second approach commonly focuses on changing the physicochemical properties of the drug, such as lipophilicity, solubility and pKa.

Physicochemical factors associated with the drug moiety

The physicochemical properties of a molecule which affect its absorption across the cornea are broadly the same as those affecting transepithelial absorption at any site and have been discussed extensively in Chapter 1 (Section 1.3.4). These factors influence the mechanism and rate of drug absorption through the cornea.

This is well illustrated by efforts in developing topically effective carbonic anhydrase inhibitors such as dorzolamide through significant alternations in chemical structure. Other efforts have been based on simple chemical modifications, i.e. a prodrug approach.

Prodrug approach

In ophthalmic research, a prodrug is designed to be inactive with some degree of biphasic solubility as the cornea is a biphasic tissue in structure. It will be transformed into the active drug by either an enzymatic or a chemical processes in the eye. Dipivefrin is an epinephrine prodrug. Due to its increased lipophilicity, dipivefrin penetrates the corneal epithelium 10 times more readily than epinephrine. The higher penetration of the drug results in a smaller dose being required, thus reducing systemic side-effects. For potent drugs such as timolol, which has the potential to cause serious systemic side-effects, such a corresponding reduction would be clinically valuable.

12.3.3.4 *Formulation approaches to improve precorneal retention*

In ophthalmic delivery the area of contact is necessarily restricted to approximately 3 cm^2 and thus the concentration gradient is the major determinant of absorption of a particular drug. By other routes, this can be achieved by adhering a reservoir of drug as a membrane-controlled patch or osmotic pump on the epithelium (see Chapters 4 and 8). However, the function of the eye as a visual apparatus limits the possibility of such an attachment of these dosage forms to the cornea.

To optimize ocular drug bioavailability by increasing concentration gradient of the drug, considerable efforts have been devoted to minimize solution drainage. This would improve drug residence time on the sclera and cornea, thereby modifying the drug pulse entry characteristics. The simplest excipients, such as hydroxyethylcellulose or poly(vinyl alcohol) (PVA), provide a thickened solution, which increases residence at the target site. Other techniques include the use of novel formulations allowing drugs to be delivered in a controlled manner over a long period. A suitable placement of an eyedrop and a reduced instilled volume also contribute to the improved ocular bioavailability.

Viscous systems

A popular approach to improve ocular drug bioavailability is to incorporate soluble polymers into an aqueous solution to extend the drug residence time in the cul-de-sac. It is reasoned that the solution viscosity would be increased and hence solution drainage would be reduced. The more commonly used viscolyzing agents include PVA and derivatives of cellulose. Cellulosic polymers, such as methylcellulose, hydroxyethylcellulose (HEC), hydroxypropyl-methylcellulose (HPMC) and hydroxypropylcellulose (HPC), are widely used as viscolyzers showing Newtonian properties. They have common properties:

- a wide range of viscosity (400 to 15,000 cps);
- compatibility with many topically applied drugs;
- increased stability of the lacrimal film.

PVA can lower the surface tension of water, reduce interfacial tension at an oil/water interface and enhance tear film stability. These together with ease of sterilization, compatibility with a range of ophthalmic drugs and an apparent lack of epithelial toxicity have led to the widespread use of PVA as a drug delivery vehicle and a component of artificial tear preparations.

Bioadhesives

Bioadhesion is an interfacial phenomenon in which a synthetic or natural polymer becomes attached to a biological substrate by means of interfacial forces. If it involves mucin or mucous-covered membrane, the narrow term *mucoadhesion* is employed. Bioadhesion has been used to enhance bioavailability of drugs via various other routes including oral (Section 6.7.1), transmucosal (Section 7.7.2.3) and vaginal (Section 11.7.6). Bioadhesion may offer several unique features:

- localizing a dosage form within a particular region, increasing drug bioavailability;
- promoting contact with the absorbing surface, permitting modification of tissue permeability in a restricted region;
- prolonging residence time and reducing dosing frequency.

Given the considerable challenge of ocular drug delivery, i.e. short contact time and low drug bioavailability, mucoadhesives are attractive excipients in ophthalmic drug formulations. The presence of mucin in the eye allows bioadhesive polymers to thicken the tear film in the front of eye.

The hydrophilic groups on mucoadhesive polymers and the large amount of water associated with mucin present two possible adhesion mechanisms: (i) hydrogen bonding and (ii) interpenetration of a swollen gel network with hydrated mucin. Many methods have been used for the assessment of bioadhesive properties, including fluorescent techniques and tensile tests. By using these methods, a number of natural and synthetic polymers have been discovered possessing mucoadhesive properties.

Natural polymers

Sodium hyaluronate is a high molecular weight polymer extracted by a patented process from sources including chicken coxcombs. It consists of a linear, unbranched, non-sulphated, polyanionic glycosaminoglycan, composed of one repeating disaccharide unit of D-sodium glucuronate and N-acetyl-D-glucosamine. Products based on hyaluronates are widely used in intraocular surgery as a substitute for vitreous humor and as an adjuvant to promote tissue repair. Hyaluronates show a topical protective effect for the corneal endothelium and other delicate tissues from mechanical damage through providing a stabilized hydrogel. Sodium hyaluronate with its unusual rheological quality, producing a rapid transformation from a liquid to a solid character with increasing stress frequency, appears to be beneficial for topical vehicles. The pseudoplastic behavior of hyaluronate solutions, where viscosity is higher at the resting phase, provides a thickened tear film, slow drainage and an improved distribution on the cornea during blinking. Furthermore, the carboxyl groups of hyaluronate form hydrogen bonds with sugar hydroxyl groups of mucin when sodium hyaluronate is applied in the eye, producing an intimate contact with the cornea. These unique properties give hyaluronates great potential in ocular drug delivery.

Chondroitin sulphate is another polysaccharide derivative (glycosaminoglycan) with a repeat unit containing β-D-glucoronic acid and D-N-acetyl galactosamine, very similar to hyaluronic acid except for modification of the position of a hydroxyl group and the addition of sulphate groups to the galactosamine residue. Chondroitin sulphate has a good affinity to the corneal surface, preventing premature breakup of the tear film between blinks. Formulations containing chondroitin have been used for the treatment of dry eye and showed superiority to hyaluronic acid in treating severe cases of *keratoconjunctivitis sicca*.

Synthetic polymers

Carbomers are poly(acrylic acid) polymers widely used in the pharmaceutical and cosmetic industries. They have several advantages, including high viscosities at low concentrations, strong adhesion to mucosa without irritation, thickening properties, compatibility with many active ingredients, good patient acceptability and low toxicity profiles. These properties have made carbomers very valuable in the field of ophthalmic formulations. Artificial tear products and novel drug delivery systems based on carbomers have been extensively formulated. Leogel containing 0.5% carbomer increases the ocular bioavailability of prednisolone acetate following repeated topical application and allows reduction in the frequency of administration. A recent scintigraphic study on Geltears (a Carbopol 940 based product) showed that the precorneal residence is significantly prolonged by carbomer gel when compared to the saline control. 40% of administered dose was retained in the eye at 8 minutes after topical application of Geltears while clearance of the label delivered in the saline vehicle was complete well before this time period.

Phase transition systems

The introduction in the early 1980s of the concept of *in situ* gel systems demonstrated that a considerable prolongation in duration of action could be obtained. *In situ* gelling systems have unique properties, which can make a liquid change phase to a gel or solid phase in the cul-de-sac upon its instillation into the eye. Three methods have been employed to induce phase transition on the eye surface: change in pH and temperature as well as activation by ions.

Cellulose acetate phthalate forms a pH-triggered phase transition system, which shows a very low viscosity up to pH 5. This system will coacervate in contact with the tear fluid (pH 7.4), forming a gel in few seconds and releasing the active ingredients over a prolonged period of time. The half-life of residence on the rabbit corneal surface was approximately 400 seconds compared to 40 seconds for saline. However, such systems are characterized by a high polymer concentration, and the low pH of the instilled solution may cause discomfort to the patient.

An alternative approach utilizes temperature-sensitive systems. Poloxamer F127 undergoes phase transition induced by changes in temperature. At room temperature the poloxamer remains a solution. When the solution is instilled onto the eye surface (34 °C) the elevated temperature causes the solution to become a gel, thereby prolonging its contact with the ocular surface. One of the disadvantages of such a system is that it is characterized by a high polymer concentration (25% poloxamer), and the surfactant properties of poloxamer may be detrimental to ocular tolerability.

An alternative approach is to utilize the effects of changes in ionic strength. Gellan gum is an anionic polysaccharide formulated in aqueous solution, which forms clear gels under the influence of an increase in ionic strength. The gellation increases proportionally to the amount of either monovalent or divalent cations. It has been reported that the concentration of sodium in human tears (~2.6 μg μL^{-1}) is particularly suitable to induce gelation of the gellan gum following topical instillation into the conjunctival sac. The reflex tearing, which often leads to a dilution of ophthalmic solutions, further enhances the viscosity of the gellan gum by increasing the tear volume and thus the increased cation concentration. Several studies have shown that Gelrite (0.6% w/v) significantly prolongs the ocular retention in man. The mean precorneal residence half-times were around 1,089 s, 891 s and 22 s for Gelrite, HEC (0.5% w/v) and saline respectively.

It is also possible to develop systems which undergo both temperature and pH dependent changes in structure. Carbomers form acidic, low viscosity, aqueous dispersions that transform into stiff gels when the pH is raised. Although these aqueous materials can form gels *in situ* in the conjunctival sac upon instillation, they often cause irritation to the eye due to their high acidity and sometimes the dispersions are not easily neutralized by the buffering action of the tear fluid. Other *in situ* gels are most characterized by a high polymer concentration, such as 25% poloxomer and 30% CAP (cellulose acetophthalate) which may cause discomfort. Various polymer combinations have been investigated in attempts to improve the gelling properties and reduce the total polymer content of formulations, thereby improving their tolerability.

Dispersed systems

These can be grouped into suspensions, particulates, liposomes and emulsions.

Suspensions

Suspensions are commonly formulated by dispersing micronized drug powder (< 10 μm in diameter) in a suitable aqueous vehicle. Ophthalmic suspensions, particularly for the steroids, are thought to be acceptable as delivery systems since it is assumed that drug particles persist in the conjunctival sac giving rise to a sustained release effect. However, suspensions have a disadvantage that the concentration of dissolved drugs cannot be manipulated due to their relative insolubility in the vehicle.

Several investigators have shown the importance of particle size of the suspension in ocular drug delivery. An increase in drug particle size enhances the ocular bioavailability. Unfortunately, a particle size above 10 μm in diameter may result in a foreign body sensation in the eye following ocular application causing reflex tearing. A reduction in particle size generally improves the patient comfort and acceptability of suspension formulations.

Particulates

Although the suspension technique may be useful in extending drug release under certain conditions, it is only applicable to drugs that are practically insoluble in water, such as corticosteroids. For drugs that are somewhat water-soluble, the particulate approach may be considered.

Particulates are commonly classified into micro- and nanoparticles based on the size of the particles. Nanoparticles are colloidal particles ranging from 10 to 1,000 nm, in which drug may be entrapped, encapsulated, and/or absorbed. Microparticulates are drug-containing small polymeric particles (erodible, non-erodible or ion-exchange resins) within the size of 1–10 μm, which are suspended in a liquid carrier medium.

Several distinct approaches have been used to formulate drugs in a microparticulate dosage form suitable for topical application. These include erodible microparticulates, swelling mucoadhesive particulates, pH responsive microparticulates, latex systems, ion-exchange resins, etc. Upon administration of particle suspension to the eye, the particles reside at the delivery site (cul-de-sac, sub conjunctiva or vitreous humor) and the drug is released from the particles through diffusion, chemical reaction, polymer degradation, or ion-exchange mechanism, resulting in increased ocular absorption.

Piloplex was one of the first commercial exploration of nanoparticle formulations in ocular drug delivery. The formulation consists of pilocarpine-loaded nanospheres of poly(methylmethacrylate-acrylic acid) copolymer. Following this introduction, many nanoparticle systems have been investigated for the prolongation of contact time in order to increase the ocular absorption. A significant reduction in intra-ocular pressure was noted following administration of betaxolol-poly- ϵ caprolactone nanoparticles, compared to the commercial eyedrops. The enhancement was ascribed to two factors: one because the nanoparticles increased the precorneal retention of the drug by agglomeration; and secondly because the entrapped drug was in the non-ionized form in the oily core of the carrier and could diffuse at a great rate into the cornea. Similar improvements were obtained with carteolol (β-blocker) which induced a better penetration of the drug from the nanosphere formulation.

Liposomes

Liposomes can be defined as microscopic vesicles, composed of membrane-like lipid bilayers surrounding aqueous compartments (see Section 5.3.1). Phospholipids commonly used in the preparation of liposomes are phosphatidylcholine, phosphatidylethanolamine, phosphatidylserine, phosphatidic acid, sphingomyelin, cardiolipins and cerebrosides. The versatility in manufacturing and use of liposomes is attributed to their amphiphilic nature. Both hydrophilic and lipophilic drugs can be encapsulated within the lipid vesicles. It has been shown that drugs with very low or very high logP values exhibit prolonged liposomal retention. The first application of liposomes in ocular drug delivery involved the application of a liposomal suspension of idoxuridine to rabbits for the treatment of herpes simplex keratitis. The liposmal formulation was found to be more efficient results compared to the aqueous solution.

Liposomes can be easily prepared from non-toxic materials, which are non-irritant and do not obscure vision. Unfortunately, routine use of liposomes in topical ocular drug delivery is presently limited by short shelf life of the formulation, limited drug loading capacity and obstacles in sterilizing the preparation.

Emulsions

Emulsions have been used for centuries for the oral administration of medical oils and vitamins and as dermatological vehicles. Recently, their application has been extended as drug carriers in the delivery and targeting of ophthalmic drugs. An indomethacin emulsion has been reported to increase ocular bioavailability and efficacy compared to commercially available formulation in rabbits. 0.4% indomethacin emulsion showed 2.2 fold increase in the area under the anterior aqueous drug concentration/time curve compared to a 1% indomethacin suspension. The emulsion formulation also reduced ocular surface irritation caused by indomethacin. Similar advantages have been shown for a pilocarpine emulsion which produced a prolonged therapeutic effect in comparison with pilocarpine hydrochloride eyedrops in man. It can be administered only twice a day, rather than four times daily for conventional formulation.

Other ophthalmic emulsions have been used to formulate prednisolone, piroxicam and amphotericin B emulsion. Although emulsions can produce sustained therapeutic effects and reduced irritancy of drug, their application in ophthalmology have been limited due to problems of stability.

Soft contact lenses and ocular inserts

The rationale for corneal contact devices has not been fully explored in therapy. In conventional dosing, there is a gradient across the eye caused by lacrimal flow, opposing drag of material above the equatorial axis by the upper lid as illustrated in Figure 12.4. Thus it is difficult to sustain high drug concentrations in the upper hemisphere unless the eye is bathed or the patient is supine. A corneal device such as a collagen shield or contact lens overcomes this problem by providing a slowly equilibrating reservoir.

It is generally accepted that soft contact lenses can act as a reservoir for drugs, providing improved release of the therapeutic agent. The therapeutic value of contact lenses was first demonstrated in a study which showed a significant increase in aqueous humor levels produced by drug-soaked lenses when compared with the conventional eyedrop. The use of Bionite contact lenses for delivery of idoxuridine, polymyxin B and Pilocarpine also showed that instillation of a drug solution onto an unmedicated contact lens was significantly more effective than instillation of a more concentrated drug solution directly to the cornea.

Presoaked lenses are considered a more efficient and reliable delivery system. However, the soaking of lenses in ophthalmic formulations to incorporate the drug into the lens may cause toxicity to corneal epithelium because preservatives, such as benzalkonium chloride, have a great affinity for the hydrophilic contact lens material and are concentrated in the contact lens. Contact lens for sensitive wearers may also cause foreign-body sensation, blurring and decreased oxygen tension on the corneal surface resulting from occlusion by contact lens.

An alternative system, manufactured as a wafer-like insoluble implant, has been developed (Ocusert). The system is preprogrammed to release pilocarpine at a constant rate of 20 or 40 μg/hr for a week to treat chronic glaucoma; however, release from inserts may be incomplete and approximately 20% of all patients treated with the Ocusert lose the device without being aware of the loss. The device also presents problems including foreign-body sensation, expulsion from the eye, and difficulty in handling and insertion. An alternative to the advanced non-erodible systems is an erodible insert for placement in the cul-de-sac.

Erodible implants

Collagen and fibrin are the common polymers used in the erodible implants. Three erodible devices have been marketed to date.

- Lacrisert is a rod-shaped device made of hydroxypropyl cellulose without any preservatives which is used for treatment of dry eye syndromes.
- SODI (Soluble Ocular Drug Insert) is a small oval wafer of polyacrylamide impregnated with drug.
- Porcine collagen shields, which are designed to promote corneal healing and provide lubricity to the eye.

An erodible implant system based on PVA has also been investigated. The bioavailability of pilocarpine was shown to be increased sixteen-fold using this system. The system showed considerable promise for prolonged drug delivery since vision is minimally affected by the presence of an insert positioned on the sclera. When the device is placed in the lower fornix, the contact area for the released drug is the sclera and little material is in contact with the cornea.

12.4 Intraocular drug delivery

The poor intravitreal penetration of systemically, topically or periocularly administered drugs limits the effectiveness of treatment of the posterior segment disorders. Furthermore, topical application of drugs for the treatment of posterior segment disorders is severely limited by the highly efficient clearance mechanisms and attempts to improve precorneal residence time of the drugs by addition of viscosity enhancing agents, gelling agents, mucoadhesive polymers etc., have failed to provide sufficient concentrations in the vitreous. This has prompted the development of alternative routes of drug administration. Moreover, most diseases affecting the posterior segment are chronic in nature and require prolonged drug administration.

12.4.1 Intravitreal delivery

Intravitreal injections remain the main route of delivery in order to avoid concomitant side-effects seen with systemic administration. An intravitreal injection provides therapeutic concentrations of the drug adjacent to the intended site of activity and a much smaller dose is required. However, retinal toxicity of the injected dose must be considered. Usually an intravitreal injection is restricted to a volume of 0.1/0.2 ml administered following both anterior chamber and vitreal taps. Following injection, the drug diffuses through the vitreous gel with little restriction to diffusion. For most drugs the diffusion coefficient through the vitreous humor is close to that through water. Once distributed throughout the vitreous humor, rapid elimination of the drug is observed. Drug loss from the vitreous takes place via two routes:

- anteriorly – by simple diffusion to the posterior chamber and followed by removal to the systemic circulation along with the aqueous humor drainage;
- posteriorly – across the retina where it is removed by active secretion.

Drugs lost primarily by anterior chamber diffusion have a long half-life in the vitreous, usually in the order of 20–30 hours. In contrast, drugs lost via the trans-retinal route, such as the penicillins, have typically much shorter half-lives of 5–10 hours. Ocular inflammation results in the breakdown of blood retinal barrier and increases the elimination of non-transported drugs from the vitreous. In contrast to the elimination of non-transported drugs, drugs that are removed by the active transport systems reside longer in the vitreous following ocular inflammation due to the failure in the transport system. Systemic probenecid is known to inhibit these active transport mechanisms. Rate of drug loss is also enhanced in vitrectomized and lensectomized eyes.

As the majority of the posterior segment disorders are chronic in nature, sustained delivery of medications is highly desirable. Liposomes and microparticulates are such systems designed to release the encapsulated drug gradually and over an extended period of time.

For reviews on intra-ocular drug delivery systems see Gregoriadis and Florence (1993), Metrikin and Anand (1994), and Peyman and Ganiban (1995) detailed at the end of this chapter.

12.4.1.1 Liposomes

Liposomal encapsulation has the potential not only to increase the activity and prolong the residence of the drug in the eye, but also to reduce the intraocular toxicity of certain potent drugs such as antimetabolites, antivirals and antibiotics to the retina. For example, liposome-encapsulated amphotericin B produced less toxicity than the commercial amphotericin B solution when injected intravitreally. Liposomes have also been used to study the release and distribution of dyes, which in turn reflect the integrity of the retinal vascular constitution. Direct intravitreal injection of liposomal-encapsulated drugs has shown enhanced vitreal levels for extended periods of time in the vitreous of rabbit models. Liposomal encapsulation of the antiviral, HPMPC, reduces the toxic effects to the retina and provides therapeutic levels against CMV retinitis for up to 8 months.

Biodistribution of dexamethasone sodium phosphate has been evaluated following intraocular delivery in rabbits. The liposomes were found to bind to various ocular tissues including the retina, iris, sclera and cornea. Using gold-colloid loaded liposomes, it was demonstrated that retinal bound liposomes were attached to the inner limiting membrane and did not penetrate the inner cells of the retina. This suggests that liposomes are suitable for targeted delivery to these areas. Heat-sensitive liposomes containing carboxyfluorescein have also been used to examine the potential of liposomes for targeted drug delivery to selected areas of the retina.

Liposomes to deliver cyclosporin A (CsA) have been incorporated into collagen shields. This delivery system provided the highest levels of CsA in both the cornea and sclera with higher levels in the aqueous humor compared to unencapsulated and capsulated CsA but not loaded into collagen shields.

The main drawbacks associated with liposomes are their short shelf life and difficulty in storage, limited drug-loading capacity and instability on sterilization and finally, transient blurring of vision after an intravitreal injection. Despite these disadvantages, they have a potential as drug delivery systems as they are composed of substances that are non-toxic and totally biodegradable.

12.4.1.2 Microparticulates and nanoparticles

Intraocular disposition of microencapsulated and nanoencapsulated antivirals have been of interest to several groups. Except for transient interference with vision, they seem to be attractive as drug delivery systems, especially because of their binding abilities to certain intraocular tissues.

Both microspheres and nanoparticles are retained within the eye for extended periods and provide slow, sustained release of the drugs. Microparticulates for intraocular drug delivery have been formulated as:

- erodible microparticulates;
- mucoadhesive particulates;
- pH responsive particulates;

- latex systems;
- ion-exchange resins.

Ganciclovir released from biodegradable polymer microspheres placed intravitreally into the rabbits inoculated with HCMV is efficacious with a decrease in vitritis, retinitis and optic neuritis. Microspheres have also been used to provide sustained delivery of retinoic acid in proliferative vitreoretinopathy. The use of microspheres for selective drug targeting to the retinal pigment epithelium has also been investigated. Surface modified PLA microspheres were loaded with a fluorescent dye, 1,4-bis(2-(5-phenyloxazolyl)-benzene. The cellular uptake by the retinal pigment epithelium was monitored at 4 °C and 37 °C. Phagocytosis was observed only at 37 °C when the cell fluorescence was found to increase for up to 24 hours. Gelatin-precoated microspheres showed enhanced uptake by the retinal pigment epithelium and the authors suggested that this technique could be used as the basis for selective delivery.

A rabbit model has been used to investigate the intracameral, intravitreal and retinal delivery of adenovirus-mediated heme oxygenase-1 (HO-1) gene. The results of these studies suggest that this technique may be promising means for delivering HO-1 gene *in vivo*. HO-1 provides a protective mechanism against oxidative stress that contributes to the pathogenesis of ocular diseases such as cataract, age-related macular degeneration and diabetic retinopathy

Intravitreal injection provides the potential to deliver large quantities of drug into the eye and effectively treats or prevents posterior segment diseases. Intravitreal injections are preferred in certain disease states and are used in combination with systemic administration to enhance the effectiveness of the treatment. However, this is an unsuitable method for treating chronic ocular diseases: repeated intravitreal administration carries significant risks, such as clouding of the vitreous humor, retinal detachment and endophthalmitis. Moreover, it is a potentially painful route of administration. Novel approaches, such as depot devices, have been developed to treat proliferative vitreoretinopathy and retinitis associated with cytomegalovirus. Various implantable devices, such as a gentamicin osmotic minipump, a polyvinyl alcohol/ethylene vinyl acetate cup containing ganciclovir, a polysulfone capillary fiber with daunomycin in tristearin and ganciclovir intraocular implant have also been suggested.

Although liposomes and microparticulates have been extensively investigated these systems have failed to be accepted as a drug delivery system in the clinical setting as the preparations can cause clouding of the vitreous and moreover can prolong the release of the drug for only up to a month.

12.4.2 Intraocular devices

Sustained delivery of ophthalmic medications is a novel approach in treating chronic intraocular infections in conditions where systemic administration is accompanied by undesirable side-effects and repeated intravitreal injections carry the risk of infection. The administration of medications by implants or depot devices is a very rapidly developing technology in ocular therapeutics. The various types of implant and mechanisms of drug release have been discussed in general in Chapter 4.

Implantable ocular devices have been developed that serve two major purposes:

- release of the drug at zero-order rates, improving the selectivity of drug action;
- release of the drug over several months, thus reducing dramatically the frequency of administration.

The first osmotically driven minipump was investigated using a rabbit model of endophthalmitis in 1979. The osmotic minipump was implanted subcutaneously in the ear region. This device had tubing connected that was directed to the vitreous cavity through a pars plana incision. The device was tested for delivery of gentamicin and the authors succeeded in maintaining a calculated dose of 0.01 mg/hr for 4.5 days. Similar designs have been investigated in animals but success has been variable and none have reached clinical acceptance.

Vitrasert is a commercially available sustained release intraocular device approved for use in patients suffering from cytomegalovirus retinitis. The device consists of a 6 mg pellet of ganciclovir coated with EVA and PVA to give the sustained release effect. The current device is designed to release ganciclovir at a rate of 2 μg/hr. Apart from the anticipated problems of endophthalmitis and retinal detachment, dislocation of implant and poor intravitreal drug levels due to its placement into the suprachoroidal space have been observed. Further details of this system are given in Chapter 4 (Section 4.4.1.3 and Figure 4.5).

Sustained release intravitreal dexamethasone implants have a potential use in reducing ocular inflammation and treating PVR. The device consists of a 5 mg pellet of dexamethasone coated with 10% PVA and EVA giving a mean release rate of 1.2 ± 0.1 μg/hr over a period of 5 months. A slow release daunomycin implant was fabricated by loading the polysulfone capillary fibre with 1% w/w of daunomycin in tristearin. The controlled release is attributed to the diffusion-retardant properties of the fat. An experimental evaluation of the kinetics and efficacy of this device in a rabbit model at 15 μg and 30 μg/device resulted in a therapeutically sustained level of daunomycin for up to 21 days after device implantation. Exhausted devices have to be removed surgically, which is an important limitation.

One way of overcoming this problem is the use of a biodegradable polymer in the fabrication of the intravitreal implant. Polycaprolactone polymer matrices containing 5-FU and ganciclovir were studied for their release characteristics. The porous reservoir type devices were manufactured and the porosity imparting agents included. Suitable pore-forming agents include NaCl, KCl, potassium acetate and low molecular weight polyvinyl alcohol. A tubular reservoir having a diameter of 2 mm and length of 8 mm was filled with the drug and heat sealed. The results show that using the matrix-type device, ganciclovir was released at a rate of 1.5 μg/day over a period of 160 days. In the porous reservoir-type devices, using 20% wt of pore-forming agent, ganciclovir was released for 160 days at a rate of 8.0 μg/day. Devices containing 50% wt of the pore-forming agents released ganciclovir at a rate of 20 μg/day. Similar results were obtained with foscarnet loaded, 5-FU loaded and carboxyfluorescein loaded devices, all showing zero-order kinetics. The advantages of the use of a 20%, 5-FU device in the prevention of PVR and tractional retinal detachment seem to be slow release of the drug, reducing toxicity and providing a constant concentration of the drug, and ease of surgical implantation into the eyes with no significant complications.

More recently, cylindrical solid biodegradable implants have been evaluated for the delivery of 5-FU in the treatment of proliferative vitreoretinopathy. The poly(lactic-co-glycolic) acid implant was evaluated in a rabbit. Intravitreal concentrations of 5-FU were approximately 2.6 μg mL^{-1} for at least 14 days after implantation. No toxic effects due to either the implant or the drug itself were observed. Other groups have undertaken developmental studies with a scleral plug made of poly(lactic-co-glycolic) acid containing 1% doxorubicin. The device was placed at a sclerectomy site in the pars plana after vitrectomy of the rabbit eye; 26% of doxorubicin was released gradually over a 4-week period.

Other studies have investigated the feasibility of preparing and utilizing a PLGA device for delivering drugs to the vitreous. The release kinetics of sodium fluorescein, as a water-soluble marker, in rabbit eyes has been studied using fluorospectrophotometry. Two types of devices have been prepared using different molecular weight polymers. Both devices released sodium fluorescein for over 20 days *in vitro*. In the *in vivo* studies, detectable concentrations sodium fluorescein were seen in the vitreous for up to 17 days with one device and up to 28 days with the other.

Another group have recently evaluated the release kinetics of ganciclovir from PLGA scleral implants in rabbit eyes. Using a 25% ganciclovir loaded PLGA implant, they found that the vitreal concentration of ganciclovir was maintained above the ED90 value for 3 months and in the retina/choroid for 5 months.

In summary, deficiencies in the current intraocular therapy using implants include:

- risk of endophthalmitis or retinal detachment;
- short and/or variable duration of therapy;
- requirement for surgical removal of the implant in the case of a non-degradable polymeric implants;
- evaluation of tissue toxicity and safety of the polymers.

12.4.3 Iontophoresis

Iontophoresis is a novel drug delivery system that involves the use of electric current to drive charged ions across membranes (see Section 8.6.2). The technique generates an electrical potential gradient that facilitates the movement of solute ions. Iontophoresis has a long history and the earliest documented use dates back to 1740.

The versatility of the technique has made it a useful investigative tool for local drug delivery in several areas of medicine, including dermatology, dentistry, ophthalmology, otolaryngology and for systemic delivery of proteins and peptides. The attractiveness of the method lies in the non-invasive nature and the suitability for transferring high molecular weight, charged ions. The advantage in local drug delivery lies in reducing the risk of side-effects and provides an important alternative to parenteral administration.

In ophthalmology, both trans-scleral and transcorneal drug delivery has been studied. Drugs investigated include fluorescein, tobramycin, gentamicin, ticarcillin, cefazolin, dexamethasone and ketoconazole. Iontophoresis has been found to be both safe and effective in delivering the required doses locally, at the intended site of action. Excepting for lidocaine, which has been tested in human volunteers, all the other drugs have been tested in rabbits.

Retinotoxic effects associated with iontophoresis have been evaluated by slit lamp microscopy, indirect ophthalmoscopy, light and electron microscopy. Commonly reported toxic effects include slight retinal and choroidal burns and retinal pigment epithelial and choroidal necrosis, corneal epithelial edema, persistent corneal opacities and polymorphonuclear cell infiltration. Disadvantages of iontophoresis include side-effects such as itching, erythema and general irritation. Although the technique is found to be suitable for a range of compounds like NSAIDS, antivirals, antibiotics, anaesthetics and glucocorticoids, its acceptability as a routine drug delivery system is limited by the little information available on its side-effects from repeated or multiple applications on the same or different sites.

12.5 CONCLUSIONS

In conclusion, the eye continues to present significant challenges in the sustained delivery of drugs. Although many systems have been developed, very few have really tackled the overwhelming difficulty of delivering the medication to the eye.

At the front of the eye, the efficient clearance mechanism and the nature of the precorneal and scleral barriers oppose retention of drug in periocular tissue. The penalty for prolonged delivery may be blurring of vision or the need to use an implant. Drug delivery to the back of the eye is fraught with difficulties and the poor penetration severely limits the treatment of sight-threatening diseases. Developments in the next century will have to focus on the need to provide prolonged release of disease modulators with less risk and easier access than the present generation of devices.

12.6 FURTHER READING

Davies, N.M., Greaves, J.L., Kellaway I.W. and Wilson C.G. (1993) Advanced corneal delivery systems: liposomes. In *Ophthalmic Drug*

Delivery Systems (A.K. Mitra, ed.), Drugs and the Pharmaceutical Sciences. Dekker, New York, 58, pp. 289–306.

Greaves J.L., Olejnic O. and Wilson C.G. (1992) Polymers and the precorneal tear film. *STP Pharma. Sci.*, 2:13–33.

Gregoriadis, G. and Florence, AT. (1993) Liposomes in drug delivery. Clinical, diagnostic and ophthalmic potential. *Drugs*, 45:15–28.

Gurny, R., Boye, T. and Ibrahim, H. (1985) Ocular therapy with nanoparticulate systems for controlled drug delivery. *J. Contr. Rel.*, 2:353–360.

Hashizoe, M., Ogura, Y., Kimura, H. *et al.* (1994) Scleral plug of bideogradable polymers for controlled drug release in the vitreous. *Archives of Ophthalmology*, 112:1380–1384.

Kimura H.-O.Y., Hashizoe, M., Nishiwaki, H., Honda, Y. and Ikada, Y. (1994) A new vitreal drug delivery system using an implantable biodegradable polymeric device. *Investigative Ophthalmology and Visual Science*, 35:2815–2819.

Kunou N.-O.Y., Hashizoe, M., Honda, Y., Hyon, S.H. and Ikada, Y. (1995) Controlled intraocular delivery of ganciclovir with use of biodegradable scleral implant in rabbits. *Journal of Controlled Release*, 37:143–150.

Metrikin, D.C. and Anand R. (1994) Intravitreal drug administration with depot devices. *Current Opinion in Ophthalmology*, 5:21–29.

Mitra, A.K. (ed.) (1993) *Ophthalmic Drug Delivery Systems*. Marcel Dekker, New York.

Moritera, T.-O., Y., Yoshimura, N., Kuriyama, S., Honda, Y., Tabata, Y. and Ikada, Y. (1994) Feasibility of drug targeting to the retinal pigment epithelium with biodegradable microspheres. *Current Eye Research*, 13:171–176.

Peyman, G.A. and Ganiban, G.J. (1995) Delivery systems for intraocular routes. *Advanced Drug Delivery Reviews*, 16:107–123.

Singh, P. and Maibach, H.I. (1994) Iontophoresis in drug delivery: Basic principles and applications. *Critical Reviews in Therapeutic Drug Carrier Systems*, 11:161–213.

12.7 SELF-ASSESSMENT QUESTIONS

1. Outline the structure and physiology of the cornea relevant to drug delivery and adsorption.

2. List the physiological factors that affect topical drug delivery to the eye.

3. Describe the two pathways for ocular adsorption of topically applied drugs.

4. Describe the formulation approaches used to enhance corneal permeability.

5. List the various disperse systems which have been employed to enhance topical ocular drug delivery.

6. Describe the use of liposomes, microparticulates and nanoparticulates in intraocular drug delivery.

7. Outline the use of implantable devices in intraocular drug delivery.

8. Outline the advantages and disadvantages of iontophoresis in ophthalmic drug delivery.

Drug Delivery to the Central Nervous System

William M. Pardridge and Pamela L. Golden

OBJECTIVES

On completion of this chapter the reader should be able to:

- Describe the structure and function of the blood-brain barrier
- Outline the physiological factors affecting drug delivery to the CNS
- Describe the physicochemical factors affecting drug delivery to the CNS
- Describe the current approaches to CNS drug delivery
- Discuss the latest developments in CNS drug delivery

13.1 INTRODUCTION

Drugs that act on the CNS include those used for the treatment of psychosis, affective (mood) disorders, such as depression and mania, anxieties and related disorders, seizure disorders (epilepsies), Parkinson's disease, Alzheimer's disease, pain (opioid analgesics) and brain tumors. Furthermore, the AIDS virus has a special affinity for the brain, where it attacks neurons and their structural supports (glial cells) causing memory loss, palsy, dementia and, finally, paralysis.

Ideally, drugs used in the treatment of diseases affecting the CNS would be delivered directly to the site of action. However, drugs generally do not readily enter the brain from the circulating blood. Access to the brain is particularly difficult for the "new biotherapeutics" such as peptide, protein and nucleic-acid based biopharmaceuticals.

Entry of molecules to the brain is regulated by a selective barrier that exists between the brain and the blood, known as the blood-brain barrier (BBB). This chapter reviews the structure and physiology of this barrier and the new and emerging technologies to overcome this barrier and achieve drug delivery to the CNS.

13.2 STRUCTURE AND FUNCTION OF THE BLOOD-BRAIN BARRIER

Figure 13.1 Sagittal section film autoradiogram of a mouse killed 5 minutes after intravenous injection of [^{14}C] histamine, a small molecule that readily crosses the porous capillary beds in peripheral tissues, but does not cross the blood-brain barrier (BBB) in brain or spinal cord

Blood capillaries in the brain are structurally different from the blood capillaries in other tissues; these structural differences result in a permeability barrier between the blood within brain capillaries and the extracellular fluid in brain tissue. This permeability barrier, comprising the brain capillary endothelium, is known as the Blood-Brain Barrier (BBB).

The BBB phenomenon is demonstrated in Figure 13.1, which shows a film autoradiogram of a mouse following intravenous injection of radiolabeled histamine, a small molecule that readily crosses the porous capillaries in peripheral tissues, but cannot cross the BBB in brain or spinal cord.

The brain capillary endothelium comprises the lumenal and ablumenal membranes of capillaries, which are separated by approximately 300 nm of endothelial cytoplasm (Figure 13.2). The structural

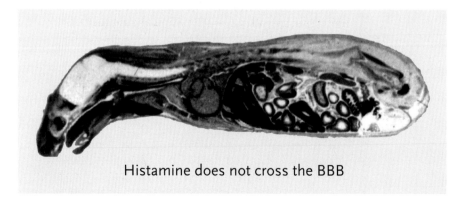

Histamine does not cross the BBB

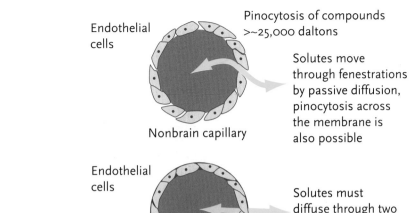

Endothelial cells

Pinocytosis of compounds >~25,000 daltons

Solutes move through fenestrations by passive diffusion, pinocytosis across the membrane is also possible

Nonbrain capillary

Endothelial cells

Solutes must diffuse through two membranes, the lumenal and ablumenal membranes of the capillary endothelium. There is minimal pinocytosis across the membrane

Ion pumps (Na⁺, K⁺, ATPase)

Brain capillary

Figure 13.2 Structural differences between non-brain (a) and brain (b) capillaries, that account for the existence of the BBB

differences between brain capillary endothelium and non-brain capillary endothelium are associated with the endothelial tight junctions. The non-brain capillaries have fenestrations (openings) between the endothelial cells through which solutes can move readily via passive diffusion. In brain capillaries, the endothelium has epithelial-like tight junctions which preclude movement via paracellular diffusion pathways. There is also minimal pinocytosis across brain capillary endothelim, which further limits transport of moieties from blood to brain.

In addition to the endothelial cells, the cerebral micro-vasculature (Figure 13.3) also contains pericytes (phagocytic cells) located on the brain side of the endothelium, which share a common basement membrane with the endothelial cell. There are about 3 endothelial cells for every pericyte. They probably play an important role in drug passage across the BBB, but have not been studied very extensively. In the brain, neurons are supported by a scaffold of glial cells called astrocytes. Extending from the sides of these cells are foot processes; or limbs, that spread out, and abutting one another, encapsulate the capillaries. There is a very close relationship between the endothelial cells and the astrocyte foot processes, they are separated by a distance of only 20 nm, or approximately the thickness of the basement membrane. Although the astrocyte invests >99% of the brain surface of the capillary, the astrocyte foot process does not constitute part of the permeability barrier of the BBB. Neuronal endings also occasionally innervate endothelial cells directly.

In addition to the permeability barrier of the capillary endothelium, highly active enzymes present in the brain endothelial cells, pericytes and astrocytes, represent a further metabolic component of the BBB that also restricts the entry of substances to the brain. This is further

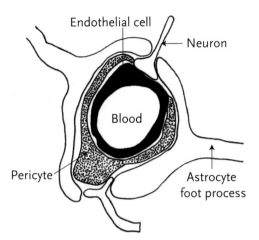

Figure 13.3 The four cell types comprising the cerebral micro-vasculature (endothelial cells, pericytes, astrocytes, neurons)

compounded by the presence of the p-glycoprotein active efflux system in the astrocyte membranes (see below); these various components work in parallel with the permeability barrier of the capillary endothelium, to form a multicomponent BBB.

The BBB is found throughout the brain and spinal cord except for a small number of isolated regions of brain that line the ventricles, the large cavities in the middle of the brain. These circumventricular organs (CVOs) include the choroid plexus (a patch of tissue that lines the floors of the ventricles and manufactures cerebrospinal fluid), the median eminence of the hypothalamus, the subfornical organ at the roof of the third ventricle and the area postrema at the base of the fourth ventricle.

The BBB acts as a safety shield, limiting the entry of circulating substances and thus protecting the CNS from the potentially deleterious effects of many compounds. However, the presence of the BBB also poses a considerable problem for drug delivery to the CNS, as the entry of potential drug candidates is also restricted.

13.3 PHYSIOLOGICAL FACTORS AFFECTING DRUG DELIVERY TO THE CNS

Various transport mechanisms exist in the brain endothelium for the uptake of nutrients into the CNS. These transport mechanisms may also potentially take up drugs. The types of transport mechanisms available include:

13.3.1 Passive diffusion

In the majority of cases, drug absorption into the CNS occurs by passive diffusion. The existence of the endothelial tight junctions means that passive diffusion between the cells is prohibited (paracellular route), so that passive diffusion is limited to the transcellular route. Lipid soluble drugs move across the lipid-rich plasma membranes of the endothelial cells, down a concentration gradient according to Fick's Law (see Section 1.3.3.2).

13.3.2 Specialized transport systems

Passive diffusion readily allows the transport of such lipid-soluble substances as oxygen and carbon dioxide, nicotine and heroin across the BBB, whereas none of the water-soluble nutrients and messenger molecules used by the brain can gain access via this route. Their access to the CNS is achieved by specialist transport systems, which selectively carry substances across the barrier.

13.3.2.1 Carrier-mediated transport

Several carrier systems have been shown to be present in the brain endothelium, allowing for the selective transport of a group of common substrates (Table 13.1). The most common system is the one that mediates the transport of glucose, which provides the brain with virtually all its energy. Carrier-mediated mechanisms are also responsible for the absorption of two other energy sources: ketone bodies, which are derived from lipids, and lactic acid, a by-product of sugar metabolism. Carrier-mediated transport systems are also involved in the uptake of amino acids by the brain. The brain can manufacture its own small neutral and acidic amino acids; however, large neutral and basic amino acids are obtained from the bloodstream.

The ionization state of the substrate can affect BBB transport of carrier-mediated substrates. For example, histidine is an imidazole amino acid that is highly charged under acidic conditions and crosses the BBB via the basic amino acid carrier. However, under neutral conditions, histidine is 90% neutral and traverses the BBB via the neutral amino acid carrier.

The ionization state of a drug may be affected by factors other than pH. When citrate, a tricarboxylic acid, chelates metals such as aluminum, the tetravalent citrate–aluminum complex leaves a free non-complexed monocarboxylic acid which is a substrate for the monocarboxylic acid or lactate carrier in the brain endothelium. When citrate is not chelated, it has no affinity for these carriers and, as there is no di- or tri-carboxylic acid carrier within the BBB, citrate is not significantly transported through the BBB via carrier-mediated transport.

Table 13.1 Carrier-mediated transport systems within the BBB

Transport System	Substrate
Hexose carrier	D-glucose (but not L-glucose), mannose, galactose
Neutral amino acid carrier	phenylalanine (and 13 other neutral amino acids)
Monocarboxylic acid (MCA) carrier	lactate, pyruvate, and the ketone bodies β-hydroxybutyrate and acetoacetate
Adenosine carrier	adenosine

Adenosine, which crosses the BBB via the adenosine carrier, is converted to inosine via adenosine deaminase. This enzyme is localized in the astrocyte foot processes of the brain, with minimal localization in capillary endothelial cells. This astrocytic enzymatic barrier to adenosine movement into brain interstitial fluid is an example of how the permeability barrier of the endothelium can work in tandem with the enzymatic barrier in astrocyte foot processes, to provide a multicomponent blood-brain barrier.

13.3.2.2 *Receptor-mediated transcytosis*

Receptor-mediated transcytosis has been described in Chapter 1 (Section 1.3.3.2). In brief, a macromolecular drug combines with a membrane-bound receptor and is internalized into endocytic vesicles. Transcytosis is achieved if the endocytic vesicles containing the drug-receptor complexes can reach the basal membrane without fusion with lysosomes. The macromolecule is then exocytosed and released into the brain.

Polypeptides are substrates for receptor-mediated transcytosis. Cerebral insulin reaches the brain from the circulation via receptor-mediated transcytosis through the BBB on the brain endothelial insulin receptor. This receptor is upregulated in development and downregulated in streptozotocin-induced diabetes mellitus. Similarly a BBB transferrin receptor mediates the transcytosis of transferrin across the BBB and this explains how the brain is able to extract iron from the circulation. Other RMT pathways consituting portals of entry to the brain for circulating peptides include receptors for insulin-like growth factors, cationic proteins, lectins, acetyl-low density lipoprotein and leptin.

13.4 PHYSICOCHEMICAL FACTORS AFFECTING DRUG DELIVERY TO THE CNS

13.4.1 Physicochemical factors affecting passive diffusion

As described above, the majority of drugs gaining access to the CNS do so via passive diffusion across the capillary endothelial membranes. Physicochemical factors associated with the drug which facilitate this process have been discussed extensively in Chapter 1 (Section 1.3.4). The more important physicochemical factors with respect to CNS drug delivery are discussed below:

13.4.1.1 *Lipid solubility and molecular weight*

Increasing the lipid solubility of a drug increases its permeability across the BBB. This linear relationship is clearly demonstrated by plotting log (BBB permeability) versus the log partition coefficient$_{(octanol-saline)}$ for various drugs, as demonstrated in Figure 13.4.

However, this linear relationship is only applicable if the molecular weight of the molecule is under a threshold of 400–600 Da (Figure 13.4). If the molecular weight of the drug exceeds this threshold, the BBB

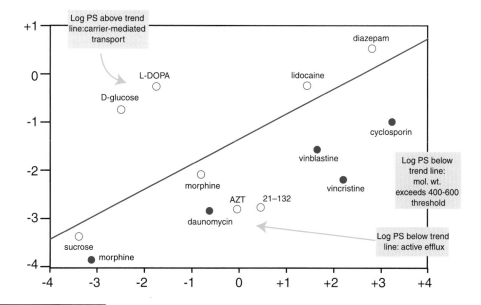

Figure 13.4 The log (blood-brain barrier permeability-surface area (PS) product) is plotted versus the log (partition coefficient) 1-octanol/saline for different molecules of varying molecular weight. The line in bold font denotes the lipid solubility trend line.

permeability is decreased by one to three log orders of magnitude from the value predicted on the basis of the lipid solubility of the compound. Examples of decreased permeability due to high molecular weight include morphine-6-glucuronide (molecular weight = 461 Da), somatostatin analog 201–995 (1,019 Da), vinblastine (814 Da), vincristine (825 Da), or cyclosporin (1,203 Da).

There are occasional exceptions to the molecular weight threshold rule. For example, although molecules 36–733 and BCECF-AM have molecular weights above the threshold (590 and 809 Da respectively), they nevertheless lie on the lipid solubility trend line. This is thought to be due to their compact molecular volume. Size exclusion is associated primarily with the molecular volume of the molecule and not strictly with the molecular weight (see Section 1.3.4.3). Apparently these molecules assume a more compact conformation that facilitates movement through the BBB in spite of their high molecular weight.

Small molecules with molecular weights of approximately 200 Da, such as AZT or 21–132, have permeability values below the lipid solubility trend line, and are presumed to be actively effluxed from the BBB (see below). Molecules such as D-glucose and L-DOPA have permeability values 3–4 log orders of magnitude *above* the lipid solubility trend line, owing to carrier-mediated transport through the BBB *in vivo* which results in enhanced transport.

13.4.1.1 *p-Glycoprotein*

An alternative explanation to that of the molecular weight threshold of BBB transport is thought to be due to the action of an active efflux system at the BBB. It is proposed that such an active efflux system is p-glycoprotein based (see Sections 1.3.2 and 6.3.4). For example, vinblastine, vincristine, and cyclosporin are all potential substrates for p-glycoprotein.

Recent studies have shown that p-glycoprotein is located in the astrocyte membranes (and not in the brain capillary endothelium as previously accepted) and that it functions by reducing the volume of distribution of the drug in the brain. Thus this efflux system, by restricting the transcellular flux of some molecules, may serve as a further barrier to drug delivery to the CNS.

13.4.1.2 *Ionization of the drug*

The passive diffusion of a drug that is a weak electrolyte across a membrane is generally a function of the pKa of the drug and the pH of the two compartments (Section 1.3.4.2). The unionized form of the drug is the lipophilic form which can cross membranes, whereas negligible transport occurs for the ionized form. Thus lipophilic amine drugs are transported through the BBB at reduced rates under conditions of acidosis, when such moieties will become positively charged. Conversely, monocarboxylic acid drugs are transported through the BBB at increased rates under acidotic conditions, as such moieties will become less negatively charged.

13.4.1.3 *Plasma protein binding*

Plasma proteins, *per se*, do not undergo significant exodus from the plasma compartment into the brain. Thus conventional theory holds that drugs that bind strongly to plasma proteins are also excluded from permeating the BBB. However, a drug which is plasma protein bound may still be operationally available for transport through the BBB via an "enhanced dissociation" mechanism. In this process, the plasma protein collides with the endothelial glycocalyx and this microcirculatory event triggers conformational changes in the plasma protein. These conformational changes may involve the drug binding site on the plasma protein, so that the drug undergoes enhanced dissociation from that binding site within the brain capillary. Thus the drug becomes available for transport through the BBB without significant egress of the plasma protein, *per se*, from the plasma compartment. The enhanced dissociation of a drug from its binding site on plasma proteins *in vivo* in the brain capillaries has been demonstrated for a number of different drugs and ligands (Table 13.2).

Table 13.2 Examples of drugs demonstrating increased dissociation from plasma proteins in the brain microvasculature	Protein	Drug
	Bovine albumin	testosterone, dihydrotestosterone, tryptophan, corticosterone, estradiol
	Human a_1 acid glycoprotein	Propanolol
	Human albumin	Diazepam
	Human very low density lipoprotein	Cyclosporin

13.4.2 Physicochemical factors affecting other transport mechanisms

Drugs which have structures similar to that of endogenous nutrients may be taken up by a specialized transport system (carrier-mediated transport, receptor-mediated transcytosis) existing in the brain endothelium for nutrients. For example, drugs having a molecular structure similar to a large neutral amino acid may cross the BBB via the neutral amino acid carrier; such drugs include melphalan (phenylalanine mustard), L-dopa, α-methyldopa, and p-chlorophenylalanine.

Strategies such as modifying the physciochemical properties of a drug to enhance uptake by specialized transport systems are described below.

13.5 CURRENT TECHNOLOGIES IN CNS DRUG DELIVERY

Various strategies have been developed to overcome the BBB and deliver drugs to the CNS, which can be divided into:

- invasive strategies;
- pharmacologically based strategies;
- physiologically based strategies.

13.5.1 Invasive strategies

13.5.1.1 Intracerebroventricular drug infusion

Intracerebroventricular (icv) drug infusion involves direct injection of the drug into the ventricles, the large cavities in the middle of the brain. This is a highly invasive procedure requiring the intervention of a neurosurgeon. Following icv infusion, drug diffusion in the brain is limited by such factors as:

- physical barriers such as synaptic regions protected by ensheathing glial processes;
- catabolic enzymes;
- high- and low-affinity uptake sites;
- low diffusion coefficients of macromolecules.

The situation is further complicated by the cerebrospinal fluid (CSF), which is manufactured in the choroid plexus and stored in the ventricles. CSF moves through CSF flow tracks in the brain, and is ultimately cleared into the peripheral bloodstream via absorption at the arachnoid villi. Bulk CSF flow moves rapidly in comparison to the relatively slow rate of solute diffusion within brain. Due to the rapid rate of bulk CSF flow, a drug infused into the ventricles is rapidly distributed to the peripheral venous system. For example, within 30 minutes of administering cholecystokinin to the brain via icv infusion, the neuropeptide has reached the plasma and inhibits feeding via a peripheral rather than a central mechanism of action. The distribution of drug rapidly to the peripheral bloodstream following icv infusion has been demonstrated repeatedly for both large molecules, such as cytokines, and small molecules. A further limitation is that CSF flow through the flow tracts of the brain is unidirectional, thus following icv, drug distribution is limited to unilateral brain surfaces.

These factors combine to limit drug delivery via icv to the surface of the brain, with minimal distribution of drug into brain parenchyma. This may be beneficial when target receptors are found on the surface, or for diseases confined to areas near the ventricle wall. Also, opioid peptides exert profound analgesia following icv infusion in rodents. However, this analgesia is caused by distribution of opioid peptides to neurons which are immediately contiguous with the CSF flow tracks. Therefore in most cases, icv infusion represents a poor mode of delivery for drugs to the CNS.

13.5.1.2 *Implants*

An alternative invasive drug delivery strategy is implantation within the brain of either genetically engineered cells secreting a drug or polymeric matrix or reservoir containing the drug.

The use of genetically engineered cells to secrete a drug is currently at a very preliminary stage of development. However, the use of polymeric implants for CNS delivery is well established and commercial products (for example, Gliadel) are available. A wide variety of polymeric implants are available, with different rate-controlling mechanisms, degrees of biodegradability, shapes, sizes etc. They are discussed in detail in Chapter 4 and will not be discussed further here.

As for icv infusion, this is a highly invasive approach. The distribution of drug into the brain following the intracerebral implantation of a polymeric implant is also limited by diffusion, with a maximal penetration of drug into brain parenchyma of < 1 mm.

13.5.1.3 *Reversible BBB disruption*

Transient opening or disruption of the BBB may be achieved by the intracarotid infusion of hyperosmolar (2 M) solutions of mannitol, or vasoactive substances, such as leukotrienes or bradykinin.

Both methods are transitory and the barrier closes within 10–20 minutes of the initiation of BBB disruption. Hyperosmolar BBB disruption selectively opens the BBB in normal brain, as compared to the barrier in brain tumors. Conversely, biochemical BBB disruption selectively increases barrier permeability in brain tumors, with minimal disruption of barrier permeability in normal brain.

BBB disruption is associated with significant side-effects including seizures in experimental animals and neuropathologic changes. The mechanism of the neurotoxicity of BBB disruption is not clear, but may be related to the influx of albumin into brain interstitium from the circulation. Albumin is neurotoxic for astrocytes and normally exists at concentrations in brain interstitial fluid that are approximately 1,000-fold lower than the concentrations of albumin in the circulation. This approach is not therefore recommended as an effective strategy for drug delivery to the CNS.

13.5.2 Pharmacologically based strategies

The objective of pharmacologically based strategies is to turn water-soluble (and thus poorly penetrable) compounds into lipid-soluble ones, thereby increasing their passive transport across the BBB. A number of approaches have been investigated:

13.5.2.1 Drug delivery systems

Liposomes (see Section 5.3.1), even small unilamellar vesicles, are usually too large to cross the BBB. Multivesicular liposomes of the order of 0.3–2 μm in diameter are retained by brain following systemic administration; however, this is due to embolization of these large structures within the brain microvasculature. Since 40–80 nm liposomes do not undergo significant transport through the BBB, it is expected that nanoparticles, which typically have diameters of 140–300 nm, would also have insignificant transport properties at the BBB. Newer strategies involving the use of drug delivery systems include the use of immunoliposomes to target vesicles to the brain, as discussed below (Section 13.6.1).

13.5.2.2 Lipidization

The lipophilicity of a drug may be increased by blocking hydrogen bond-forming functional groups on the drug structure or covalently binding the drug to lipidic moieties, such as long chain fatty acids.

BBB permeability may be increased by a log order of magnitude by blocking a pair of hydrogen bonds on the drug structure. For example, blocking one hydroxyl group on morphine via O-methylation to form codeine increases the BBB permeability to morphine by a log order of magnitude; blocking two hydroxyl groups via acetylation to form diacetylmorphine (heroin) increases the BBB permeability by 2 log orders of magnitude. Peptide lipidization strategies such as forming cyclic derivatives or diketopiperazines have also been applied to small peptides such as the C-terminal dipeptide of TRH.

One of the simplest methods of improving the uptake of a drug to the brain involves the conversion of the drug to a more lipophilic prodrug (see Section 1.3.4.1). Using this approach, moderate increases in transport across the BBB have been achieved for enkephalin analogs and TRH.

The problems with the various lipidization strategies described include the limitations posed by the 400–600 Dalton molecular weight threshold of the BBB. Increased lipidization will also cause enhanced drug distribution into peripheral tissues, thereby offsetting the enhanced BBB permeability effects, and active concentrations in the CNS can only be maintained if the blood concentrations are maintained at adequately high levels.

13.5.3 Physiologically based strategies

13.5.3.1 Exploitation of carrier-mediated transport systems

As discussed above, certain nutrients are taken up into the brain by carrier-mediated systems. If a drug possesses a molecular structure similar to that of a nutrient which is a substrate for carrier-mediated transport (Table 13.1), the "pseudo-nutrient" drug may be transported across the BBB by the appropriate carrier-mediated system. For example, the drug L-dopa crosses the BBB via the neutral amino acid carrier system. Other neutral amino acid drugs that are transported through the BBB on this transport system are α-methyldopa, α-methyl-paratyrosine, and phenylalanine mustard.

Due to the high structural specificity of the carriers, it is more advantageous to convert the drug into a structure similar to that of an endogenous nutrient, rather than conjugating the drug to the nutrient. For example, the BBB transport of morphine is 20-fold greater than that of morphine-6-glucuronide, which correlates with the much greater lipid solubility of morphine as compared to morphine-6-glucuronide. The glucose carrier forms a highly stereospecific pore that only tolerates minimal molecular substitutions on the parent hexose; glucuronidation of morphine therefore does not increase its BBB transport.

13.5.3.2 *Exploitation of receptor-mediated transcytosis systems*

The process of receptor-mediated transcytosis may be exploited to facilitate drug transport across the BBB. This strategy (essentially a prodrug strategy) involves coupling the drug to a peptide or protein "vector" which normally undergoes receptor-mediated transcytosis, to form a so-called "chimeric peptide" (Figure 13.5). The chimeric peptide is endocytosed at the luminal side of the BBB, carried through the membrane and then exocytosed into the brain interstitial fluid. The chemical linker joining the therapeutic agent to the transport vector is cleaved, freeing the therapeutic agent to bind to the appropriate target receptor.

Design considerations in the development of effective chimeric peptides include vector specificity for the brain, vector pharmacokinetics, coupling between vector and drug, and intrinsic receptor affinity for the released drug.

Figure 13.5
Exploitation of receptor-mediated transcytosis for drug delivery to the CNS. A: transport vector; B: non-transportable drug; A-R: receptor for transport vector; B-R: Receptor for peptide

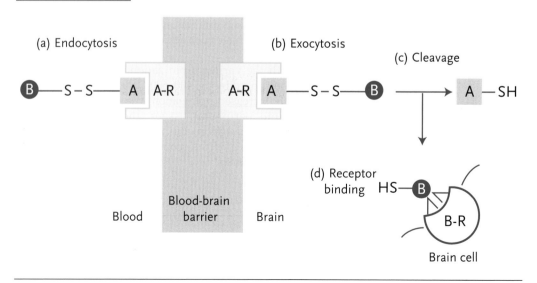

The use of a native peptide or protein such as insulin, insulin-like growth factor or transferrin as transport vectors is associated with a number of disadvantages, including rapid clearance of the peptide from the bloodstream. The use of insulin *per se* triggers insulin receptors in peripheral tissues and causes hypoglycemia. If transferrin is used as a vector, the exogenous transferrin competes for uptake with endogenous transferrin. As the endogenous concentration of transferrin in the plasma is very high (25 μM), only limited uptake is therefore possible.

Alternatively, monoclonal antibodies (Mabs) to the relevant receptors can be used as transport vectors. Anti-insulin (Mab83-7 and Mab83-14) and anti-transferrin (OX26) receptor antibodies have been proposed as efficient and selective BBB transport vectors. The anti-transferrin receptor antibody binds to a site removed from the transferrin binding site and therefore does not compete with endogenous transferrin for transport across the BBB. Studies using radiolabeled peptides have shown that significant uptake of a peptide conjugated with the anti-insulin Mab83-7 antibody is possible, even though the free peptide is unable to cross the BBB.

A number of constraints may be associated with exploiting receptor-mediated transcytosis systems for drug delivery to the CNS. These include poor stoichiometry of the drug to the transport vector which thus limits the mass transport of the drug. However, this problem is circumvented with the use of pegylated immunoliposomes, which increases by several log orders the drug-carrying capacity of the vector. Alternatively, many "large molecule" drugs are active in brain in nM concentrations, and such concentrations are easily achieved with the a 1:1 stoichiometry of drug and transport vector. Furthermore receptor-mediated transcytosis is a saturable process (see Section 1.3.3.2) which might prevent pharmacologically significant amounts of drug from reaching the CNS. However, this problem is obviated by the use of peptidomimetic monoclonal antibodies as BBB drug targeting vectors, and the antibodies bind to BBB receptor sites that are removed from the binding site of the endogenous ligand, and thus, are not saturated *in vivo*. The method also requires that the linker will be cleaved *in vivo* and that the drug will retain biological activity after release, if a disulfide linker is utilized to conjugate the vector and the drug. However, this problem is solved simply by conjugating the drug and vector with non-cleavable (amide) linkers, and in this approach, the drug binds to its cognate receptor in brain while still conjugated to the BBB transport vector.

13.6 NEW TECHNOLOGIES IN CNS DRUG DELIVERY

13.6.1 Immunoliposomes

Liposomes can be targeted to the brain by exploiting receptor-mediated transcytosis systems. For example, a bi-functional PEG-linker has been used to couple anti-transferrin (OX26) receptor antibodies to one end of the PEG strands and liposomes at the other end of the PEG

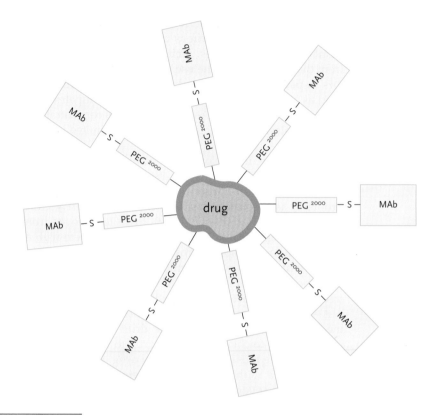

Figure 13.6
PEG-ylated
immunoliposomes for
CNS drug delivery. The
drug is entrapped
within a liposome
vector to which is
attached antibodies on
poly(ethylene glycol)
linkers

strands (Figure 13.6). Classically, immunoliposomes are prepared by attaching the MAb to the surface of the liposomes (see Section 5.3.1.3). However, this can lead to steric hindrance by the PEG strands with respect to antibody binding to the appropriate receptor. The use of the bifunctional PEG linker overcomes this problem.

This study showed that the brain volume of distribution (V_D) of the drug (tritiated daunomycin) increased with time following a single intravenous injection, indicating that the liposomes were sequestered by the brain. The receptor-mediated endocytosis of the OX26 pegy-lated immunoliposomes (loaded with the fluorescent marker, rho-damine) into rat glioma cells bearing transferrin receptors was demonstrated by confocal microscopy. When pegylated immunolipo-somes were prepared with a mouse IgG_{2a} isotype control instead of the OX26 MAb, there was no specific uptake of the immunoliposomes by rat brain capillaries.

13.6.2 Antisense drug delivery to the brain

Peptide nucleic acids (PNA) are novel antisense oligonucleotides (see Section 1.6.2) which contain a polypeptide backbone. Receptor-mediated transcytosis can be exploited to promote their delivery to the CNS. For example, the attachment of PNAs to the anti-transferrin (OX26) receptor antibodies has been shown to increase the brain uptake of the PNAs, without loss of the ability of the PNAs to hybridize to target mRNA. However, antisense agents will not exert pharmacologic effects *in vivo* following delivery to cells via receptor-mediated endocytosis systems unless there is endosomal release of the antisense agent into the cytosol. Therefore, present-day antisense drug delivery systems need to be designed and optimized to facilitate endosomal release.

13.7 CONCLUSIONS

More than 99% of the worldwide CNS drug development effort is devoted to CNS drug discovery and less than 1% is devoted to CNS drug delivery. This imbalance is the major impediment to future progress in the overall CNS drug development mission. The vast majority of new drugs that emerge from CNS drug discovery programs will not be effective pharmaceuticals because they do not cross the BBB *in vivo*. Even though the drug does not undergo significant transport through the BBB, the decision is frequently made to take a CNS pharmaceutical into clinical trials. For example, >$100,000,000 has been spent on clinical trials of neurotrophins for CNS disorders. These molecules do not undergo transport through the BBB and have (unsurprisingly) failed in clinical trials. If only a fraction of the funds for clinical trials had been devoted to CNS drug delivery strategies, then the fate of the overall CNS drug development mission could be much different.

However, in spite of the lack of funding and resources dedicated to CNS drug delivery, some new approaches are emerging with considerable potential, particularly those based on the exploitaton of natural transport mechanisms.

13.8 FURTHER READING

Aird, R.B. (1984) A study of intrathecal, cerebrospinal fluid-to-brain exchange. *Exp. Neurol.*, 86:342–358.

Carter, D.C. and Ho, J.X. (1994) Structure of serum albumin. *Adv. Protein Chem.*, 45:153–203.

Diamond, J.M. and Wright, E.M. (1969) Molecular forces governing non-electrolyte permeation through cell membranes. *Proc. Roy. Soc. B.*, 172:273–316.

Levin, V.A. (1980) Relationship of octanol/water partition coefficient and molecular weight to rat brain capillary permeability. *J. Med. Chem.*, 23:682–684.

Oldendorf, W.H. (1974) Blood-brain barrier permeability to drugs. *Ann. Rev. Pharmacol.*, 14:239–248.

Pardridge, W.M. (1991) *Peptide Drug Delivery to the Brain*. Raven Press, New York, pp. 1–357.

Pardridge, W.M. (1997) Drug delivery to the brain. *J. Cereb. Blood Flow Metab.*, 17:713–731.

Pardridge, W.M. (1993) *The Blood-Brain Barrier: Cellular and Molecular Biology.* Raven Press, N.Y., pp. 1–496.

Pardridge, W.M. (1998) *Introduction to the Blood-Brain Barrier: Methodology and Biology*, Cambridge University Press, Cambridge, UK, pp. 1–500.

Pardridge, W.M. (1998) Targeted delivery of hormones to tissues by plasma proteins. In: *Handbook of Physiology: Section 7, Endocrinology*, Volume I (P.M. Conn, ed.). Oxford University Press, NY.

Pardridge, W.M. (1998) CNS drug design based on principles of blood-brain barrier transport. *J. Neurochem.*, 70:1781–1792.

Träuble, H. (1971) The movement of molecules across lipid membranes: a molecular theory. *J. Membrane Biol.*, 4:193–208.

13.9 SELF-ASSESSMENT QUESTIONS

1. Describe the function of the blood-brain barrier.
2. Explain the differences between the brain capillary endothelium and the non-brain capillary endothelium.
3. Outline the physiological factors affecting drug delivery to the brain.
4. Explain how the physicochemical properties of a drug molecule affect CNS drug delivery.
5. Describe the current invasive strategies employed in CNS drug delivery.
6. Describe the different pharmacological-based strategies employed in CNS drug delivery.
7. Explain how carrier-mediated transport systems may be exploited in CNS drug delivery.
8. Give examples of where receptor-mediated transcytosis systems have been exploited in CNS drug delivery.
9. Outline the new technologies which are presently under evaluation for use in CNS drug delivery.

| | |
| 14 | **Plasmid-based Gene Therapy** |

Ram I. Mahato and Eric Tomlinson

OBJECTIVES

On completion of this chapter the reader should be able to:

- Describe the use of plasmid-based approaches for gene therapy
- Discuss the components of gene expression systems
- Describe the various gene delivery systems
- Explain how formulations may be modulated to improve biodistribution, pharmacokinetics, cellular uptake and intracellular trafficking
- Describe the clinical applications of gene therapy

14.1 Introduction

Genes are segments of deoxyribonucleic acid (DNA) and provide information needed by the cells for protein production. The absence or overproduction of a specific protein in the body can lead to a variety of clinical manifestations depending on the structural or functional role that the protein normally plays in the body. Many severe and debilitating diseases (e.g. diabetes, hemophilia, cystic fibrosis) and several chronic diseases (hypertension, ischemic heart disease, asthma, Parkinson's disease, motor neuron disease, multiple sclerosis) remain inadequately treated by conventional pharmaceutical approaches.

Recombinant DNA technology has allowed the large-scale production and biological characterization of several therapeutic proteins, including granulocyte-macrophage colony stimulating factor (GM-CSF), erythropoietin (EPO), interleukins, insulin-like growth factor-I (IGF-I), human factor VIII and IX and tissue plasminogen activator (t-PA). However, the clinical use of many protein drugs is limited by their inappropriate concentration in blood, poor oral bioavailability, high manufacturing cost, chemical and biological instability and/or rapid hepatic metabolism and renal excretion. In addition, few protein drugs can efficiently enter target cells unless administered at very high doses, which can lead to toxic side-effects. These limitations lead to their frequent administration with an increased treatment cost and reduced patient compliance (also see Section 1.6.1).

Gene therapy is a method for the treatment or prevention of disease that uses genes to provide the patient's somatic cells with the genetic information necessary to produce specific therapeutic proteins needed to correct or to modulate a disease. The promise of somatic gene therapy is to overcome limitations associated with the administration of therapeutic proteins, including low bioavailability, inadequate pharmacokinetic profiles and high cost of manufacture. Providing a therapeutic gene as a "pre-drug" to a patient to allow either the production of therapeutic proteins that may be difficult to administer exogenously or the inhibition of abnormal protein production may circumvent some limitations associated with the use of recombinant therapeutic proteins.

Plasmid-based gene medicine contains three components:

- a therapeutic gene that encodes a specific therapeutic protein in the form of a plasmid;
- a plasmid-based gene expression system that controls the functioning of a gene within a target cell;
- a gene delivery system that controls the delivery of the plasmid expression system to specific locations within the body.

The gene and the gene expression system are the components of the plasmid. The gene delivery system distributes the plasmid to the desired target cell, after which the plasmid is internalized into the cell. Once inside the cytoplasm, the plasmid can then translocate to the nucleus, where gene expression begins, leading to the production of a therapeutic protein through the steps of transcription and translation.

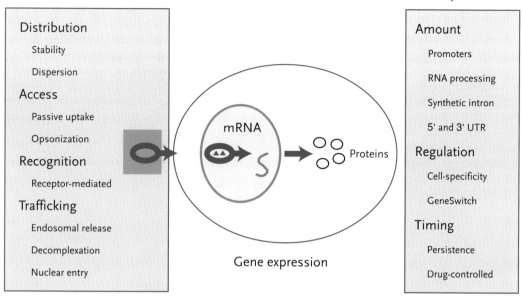

Gene delivery systems

Gene expression systems

Distribution
Stability
Dispersion

Access
Passive uptake
Opsonization

Recognition
Receptor-mediated

Trafficking
Endosomal release
Decomplexation
Nuclear entry

mRNA

Proteins

Gene expression

Amount
Promoters
RNA processing
Synthetic intron
5' and 3' UTR

Regulation
Cell-specificity
GeneSwitch

Timing
Persistence
Drug-controlled

Figure 14.1
Modulation of gene expression. A) Gene delivery systems are designed to control the location of a gene within the body by affecting distribution, and access of a gene expression system to the target cell receptor followed by intracellular and nuclear translocation. B) Plasmid-based gene expression systems are designed to control the level and duration of *in vivo* production of a therapeutic gene product

The gene expression system can be engineered to control whether the resulting protein will remain within the cell for an intracellular effect or will be secreted out of the cell for either a local or systemic action. The gene expression system can also be adjusted to control the level of protein production, as well as the fidelity and duration of gene expression (Figure 14.1).

A viral vector consists of genetic material encapsulated in a particle that can be taken up by the target cell, leading to transgene expression of virally encoded genes. Several different viral vectors have been developed for gene therapy including those derived from retrovirus, adenovirus, adeno-associated virus (AAV) and herpes simplex virus-1. Retroviruses are RNA viruses that have the ability to insert their genes permanently into host cell chromosomes after infection. For gene expression, retrovirus must reverse transcribe its positive-strand RNA genome into double-stranded DNA, which is then integrated into the host cell DNA. "Defective" retroviral vectors are devoid of the genes encoding viral proteins, but retain the ability to infect cells and insert their genes into the chromosomes of the target cell. Retroviruses infect only dividing cells and thus are often used to introduce genes into cells *ex vivo* where cell division can be stimulated with growth-promoting media. Retroviral vectors can also be directly administered to patients, though the applicability of this approach is limited by the rapid inactivation of retroviruses by human complement. However, retroviral vectors are not safe to use because of its random insertion into the host cell chromosome, which may lead to insertional mutagenesis and oncogenesis.

Adenoviral vectors infect both dividing and non-dividing cells in many different tissues including airway epithelial cells, endothelial cells, hepatocytes and various tumors. The adenovirus genome is much larger (about 35 kb) and its organization is much more complex than retroviruses. Adenoviral vectors do not integrate into the host cell chromosomes. Genes introduced into cells using adenoviral vectors are maintained in the nucleus episomally and provide transsient expression of transgenes. AAV is a small virus containing linear single-stranded DNA. AAV vectors are capable of permanently inserting their genomes into the host cell chromosomes. AAV vectors preferentially infect cells in S phase during the replicative cycle. However, it is often difficult to develop packaging cell lines that will produce sufficient titers of AAV for clinical use without the presence of helper virus. Table 14.1 summarizes the important characteristics and limitations of these viral vectors.

Compared to viral vectors, gene medicines present several potential advantages, including:

- low cost;
- non-infectivity;
- absence of immunogenicity;
- good compliance;
- well-defined characteristics;
- possibility of repeated clinical administration.

In spite of their lower transfection efficiencies, the advantage of these systems over viral vectors with respect to safety has been highlighted following the recent deaths in clinical trials of viral vector-based gene products in the US.

14.2 GENE EXPRESSION SYSTEMS

Gene expression plasmids contain a cDNA sequence coding for either a full gene or a minigene and several other genetic elements, including introns, polyadenylation sequences and transcript stabilizers to control transcription, translation, protein stability and secretion from the host cell. Basic components of a gene expression plasmid are illustrated in Figure 14.2. Plasmids encode bacterial origin of replication, usually derived from a high copy plasmid and a selectable marker, usually a gene that confers resistance to an antibiotic, such as kanamycin or neomycin.

These "prokaryotic" plasmid segments permit the production of large quantities of a given plasmid in bacteria. The prokaryotic origin of replication is a specific DNA sequence that binds to factors that regulate replication of plasmid and, in turn, control the number of copies of plasmid per bacterium. The minimal transcription unit required for the expression of a therapeutic protein consists of 5′ enhancer/promoter upstream of the gene encoding for the therapeutic protein and a poly(A) signal downstream of the gene. A heterologous intron is often inserted into the 5′ or 3′ untranslated region (UTR) of the transcription unit. This kind of "insertion" leads to elevation in mRNA levels. A single intron inserted into the 5′ UTR of the transcription unit is the most common arrangement

Viral Vectors	Characteristics	Limitations
Retrovirus	• has RNA genome • integrate into host chromosomes • sustained gene expression • incorporate up to 8kb of DNA	• do not infect post-mitotic cells • random integration • problematic large-scale production • possible insertional mutagenesis
Adenovirus	• contains linear double stranded DNA • infect dividing and non-dividing cells • high titer (10^{11}–10^{12} virus particle/ml) • large DNA (» 35 kb) insertion capacity	• transient gene expression • antigenic against viral proteins • possible toxicity at high doses
Adeno-associated virus	• contains linear single-stranded DNA • genome comprising only rep and cap genes • non-immunogenic • replication requies co-infection with	• lack of suitable packaging cell lines • low titers (10^5–10^6) virus particles/ml) • small DNA insertion capacity (» 4.7kb) adenovirus or other viruses

Table 14.1
Characteristics of viral
vectors commonly used
for gene transfer

14.2.1 Promotor

A promoter is defined as a DNA region, usually at the 5′ end of a gene, that binds to transcription factors and RNA polymerase during the initiation of transcription of a gene at the correct nucleotide site. Several promoters originating from eukaryotic viruses, such as cytomegalovirus (CMV), simian virus 40 (SV40), Moloney murine leukemia virus (MoMLV), and Rous Sarcoma virus (RSV) are widely used. Tissue-specific promoters are designed to interact with transcription factors or other nuclear proteins present in the desired target cells. The chicken skeletal α-actin promoter contains positive *cis*-acting elements required for efficient transcriptional activity in myogenic cells. Therefore, an α-actin promoter could direct high expression of recombinant protein in skeletal muscle. Muscle-specific expression of insulin-like growth factor-I (IGF-I), human growth hormone (hGH) and human factor-IX (hFIX) has been demonstrated after intramuscular administration of plasmids that encode these genes and contain skeletal α-actin promoter/enhancer.

14.2.2 Cap structure

The 5′ untranslated region (5′ UTR) is the region of the mRNA transcript that is located between the cap site and initiation codon. The linkage between methylated G residue and a 5′ to 5′ triphosphate bridge is known as the cap structure, which is essential for efficient initiation of protein synthesis. The 5′ UTR is known to influence mRNA translation efficiency. In eukaryotic cells, initiation factors first interact with the 5′ cap structure and prepare the mRNA by unwinding its secondary structure. An efficient 5′ UTR is usually moderate in length,

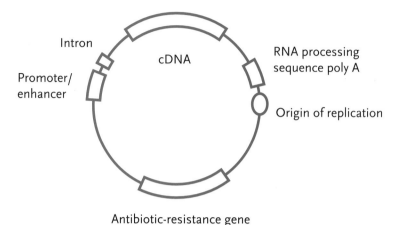

Coding sequence for therapeutic gene

Intron

Promoter/
enhancer

cDNA

RNA processing
sequence poly A

Origin of replication

Antibiotic-resistance gene

Figure 14.2 Basic components of a gene expression plasmid

devoid of strong secondary structure, devoid of upstream initiation codons, and has AUG within an optimal context.

14.2.3 3'-UTR

The 3' UTR is defined as the mRNA sequences following the termination codon. The 3' UTR is thought to play a potential role in mRNA stability. AU-rich motifs are commonly found in the 3' UTR of mRNA of cytokines, growth factors and oncogenes. These motifs are mRNA instability elements and should be eliminated for maximal levels of expression. This is usually accomplished by using standard 3' UTR sequences in place of the one found in the cDNA. The most commonly utilized 3' UTR sequences are from the bovine growth hormone and rabbit β-globin genes. Another approach is to minimize the length of the 3' UTR by placing the hexanucleotide of the poly(A) signal immediately downstream of the stop codon. Inclusion of 5' and 3' UTR introns may provide tissue specificity and long-term gene expression.

14.2.4 poly(A) tail

The poly(A) tail is a homopolymeric stretch of A residues added to the primary transcript by polyadenylation. A poly(A) signal is required for the formation of the 3' end of most eukaryotic mRNA. The signal directs two RNA processing reactions: site-specific endonucleolytic cleavage of RNA transcript, and stepwise addition of adenylates to the newly generated 3' end to form the poly(A) tail. The efficiency of polyadenylation is important for gene expression, as transcripts that fail to be cleaved and polyadenylated are rapidly degraded in the nuclear compartment. The poly(A) signals utilized in gene expression plasmids are chosen from a set of mammalian poly(A) signals, such as bovine growth hormone, rabbit β-globin and SV40.

14.2.5 Gene switches

Many endogenous proteins are produced according to circadian rhythms. Therefore, *in vivo* pulsatile production of certain therapeutic proteins may be beneficial for their clinical applications. This can be achieved by including gene switches in a gene expression system to turn on or off the transcription of an administered gene. A gene switch is designed to be part of a gene expression system that contains both the gene switch and a therapeutic gene. In the positive system, the target gene will be inactive until the administration of an exogenous compound or ligand. Such inducing agents or drugs include progesterone antagonists, tetracycline, ecdysone and rapamycin.

14.3 GENE DELIVERY SYSTEMS

Gene delivery systems are designed to control the location of a gene within the body by affecting the distribution and access of a gene expression system to the target cell, and/or recognition by a cell-surface receptor followed by intracellular trafficking and nuclear translocation. This section describes the development of several lipid, peptide and polymer-based gene delivery systems.

14.3.1 Lipid-based gene delivery

Plasmids may be incorporated into anionic or neutral liposomes (for further details on liposomes see Section 5.3.1) to ensure protection against *in vivo* degradation, to control disposition profiles and to enhance intracellular delivery. However, the encapsulation efficiency of plasmids is very low, because of the large dimension of plasmids compared to the internal diameter of the vesicles.

14.3.1.1 *pH-sensitive liposomes*

pH-sensitive liposomes are fusogenic at acidic pH and thus can be used to facilitate the endosomal disruption and subsequent release of plasmids in the cytoplasm. pH-sensitive liposomes usually consist of dioleoylphosphatidylethanolamine (DOPE) and a lipophilic anionic component containing a titratable head group. The pH-sensitive immunoliposomes have been shown to mediate 6~8 times higher levels of transgene expression into mouse lymphoma cells, compared to non-pH-sensitive immunoliposomes.

14.3.1.2 *Proteoliposomes*

Proteoliposomes, also known as virosomes or chimerasomes, incorporate viral proteins, fusogenic peptides, nuclear proteins or nuclear localization peptides, which induce fusion of liposomes with the cell membranes and facilitate DNA release and transport through the cytoplasm.

14.3.1.3 *Cochleates*

Cochleates can also be used for plasmid delivery. A negatively charged phospholipid such as phosphatidylserine, phosphatidic acid or phosphatidyl glycerol, in the absence or presence of cholesterol, are utilized to produce a suspension of multilamellar vesicles containing plasmids, which are then converted to small unilamellar vesicles by sonication. These vesicles are dialyzed against buffered divalent cations (e.g. calcium chloride) to produce an insoluble precipitate referred to as cochleates. Cochleates have been shown to encapsulate plasmid and enhance plasmid stability and transfection efficiency.

14.3.1.4 *Cationic liposomes*

Since the introduction of the transfection reagent Lipofectin, a cationic liposome composed of 1:1 (w/w) mixture of the cationic lipid N[1-(2,3-dioleyloxy)propyl]-N,N,N-trimethylammonium chloride) (DOTMA) and the colipid DOPE, many cationic lipid formulations have been tested for gene transfer. Cationic lipids interact electrostatically with the negatively charged phosphate backbone of DNA, neutralizing the charges and promoting the condensation of DNA into a more compact structure. Usually, cationic lipids are mixed with a zwitterionic or neutral colipid such as DOPE or cholesterol, respectively to form liposomes or micelles. Inclusion of a colipid is not always essential. For instance, the cationic lipid DOTAP is active in the absence of a colipid in a variety of cells *in vitro*.

A cationic lipid consists of:

- a hydrophobic lipid anchor group
- a linker group
- a positively charged headgroup.

The hydrophobic lipid anchors can be either fatty chains (e.g. derived from oleic or myristic acid) or a cholesterol group. Lipid anchors help in forming liposomes (or micellar structures) and determine the physical properties of a lipid bilayer, such as membrane rigidity and rate of lipid exchange between lipid membranes. The linker group is an important component, which determines the chemical stability and biodegradability of a cationic lipid. The head groups of cationic lipid appear to be critical for transfection and cytotoxicity of corresponding liposome formulations. The cationic amphiphiles differ markedly in structure and may be single or multiple charged as primary, secondary, tertiary and/or quaternary amines. Examples are lipospermine, cationic cholesterol, cationic detergent or lipopolysine.

The relative proportions of each component and the structure of the head group influence the physicochemical properties of plasmid/lipid complexes. Many effective cationic lipids contain protonatable polyamines linked to dialkyl or cholesterol anchors. In case of DOTMA, the hydrophobic domain is an oleoyl alcohol group that is connected to a glycerol-like, three-carbon backbone via an ether bond. A trimethyl quaternary amine is linked directly to the three-carbon backbone. To increase the biodegradability of cationic lipids, a series of cationic lipids have been synthesized in which the ether bonds were replaced with ester bonds. The structure of 1,2-bis(oleoyloxy)-3-(trimethylammonio)propane (DOTAP) is similar to DOTMA except that DOTAP contains ester bonds. $3\beta(N', N'$-dimethylaminoethane)-

carbamoyl] cholesterol (DC-Chol) contains a cholesterol linked via carbamoyl bond and ethyl group to a trimethyl, quaternary amine. Several cationic lipids, including 2,3-dioleyloxy-N-[2(sperminecarboxyamido)ethyl]-N,N-dimethyl-1-propanaminium trifuoroacetate (DOSPA), contain a spermine group for binding to DNA. Chemical structures of commonly used cationic lipids as well as that of colipid DOPE are shown in Figure 14.3.

Cationic lipid-based gene delivery systems lack target specificity, which results in low transfection efficiency in certain tissues due to the interference from cationic lipid-binding macromolecules either in the circulation or in the extracellular matrix. To circumvent this problem, neutral plasmid/lipospermine complexes containing a trigalactolipid have been prepared and shown to efficiently transfect hepatoma HepG2 cells bearing asialoglycoprotein receptor. Addition of 25% (mol mol^{-1}) of the triantennary galactolipid increased the transfection efficiency by a thousand fold, compared to the lipid-based system with no targeting ligand. An efficient transfection of β-galactosidase into HeLa cells has been shown with the combination of transferrin and cationic liposome Lipofectin, whereas Lipofectin alone had low transfection efficiency.

Asialofetuin is an asialoglycoprotein containing terminal galactosyl residues that have been used to target liposomes to the liver. There

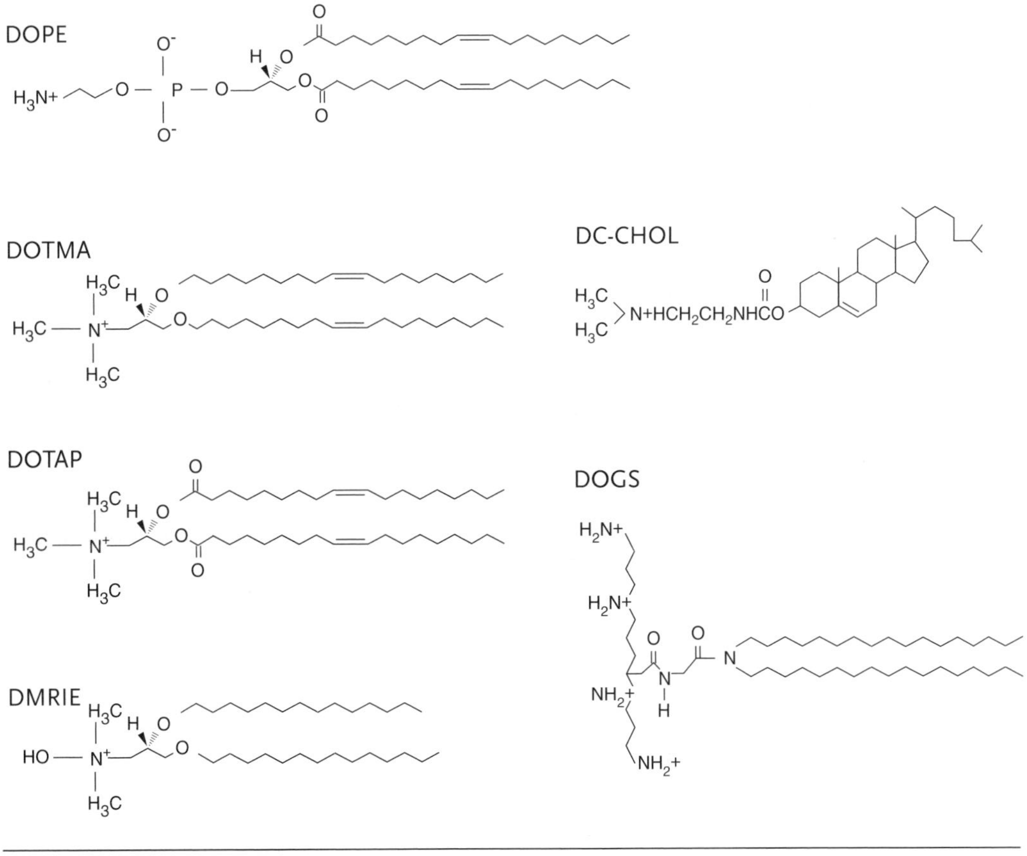

Figure 14.3 Chemical structures of colipid DOPE and some cationic lipids commonly used for gene transfer

was seven-fold enhancement in CAT expression in the liver when succinylated asialofetuin was added to preformed plasmid/ DOTAP:Chol complexes to provide a ligand for hepatic asialoglyco-protein receptor.

14.3.2 Peptide-based gene delivery

For site-specific gene delivery, positively charged macromolecules such as poly(L-lysine) (PLL), histones, protamine, or poly(L-ornithine) may be linked to a cell-specific ligand, and then bound to plasmids via electrostatic interaction. The resulting complexes retain their ability to interact specifically with target cell receptors, leading to receptor-mediated internalization of the complex into the cells. Receptor ligands currently being investigated include glycoproteins, transferrin, polymeric immunoglobulin, insulin, epidermal growth factor (EGF), lectins, folate, malaria circumsporozoite protein, α_2-macroglobulin, CD3-T cell, sugars, integrins, thrombomodulin, surfactant protein A and B, mucin and the c-kit receptor.

Site-specific gene delivery and expression are influenced by the extent of DNA condensation, the method of complexation, the molecular weights of both polycations and plasmid, and the number of ligand residues bound per polycation molecule.

To avoid high cytotoxicity and molecular heterogeneity of poly(L-lysine), molecularly homogenous lysine-rich synthetic peptides have been used for gene transfer. It is known that the active sites of enzymes, receptor ligands and antibodies usually involve about 5 to 20 amino acids. Thus, it should be possible to design small synthetic peptides to mimic the active sites of viral proteins and formulate synthetic peptide/DNA complexes that are as efficient as viruses, but do not have their limitations. The major components of a peptide-based delivery systems are:

- a DNA binding peptide to condense the plasmid;
- a targeting peptide to confer cell and/or tissue specificity;
- a lytic peptide to induce endosomal release of the plasmid;
- an NLS peptide to enhance nuclear entry of the plasmid.

Synthetic peptide-based gene delivery systems consisting of a lysine-rich DNA binding motif and endosomolytic motif have been developed for *in vivo* gene delivery. One example of such a gene delivery system comprises:

- a galactosylated peptide that both condenses the plasmid into monodisperse nanoparticles of about 100 nm in diameter and enables specific recognition and binding to asialoglycoprotein receptors;
- an amphipathic, pH-selective peptide that enables the plasmid to leave the endosomes prior to their fusion with lysosomes and entry into the cytoplasm.

Chapter Fourteen

The improved DNA binding and condensation provided by amino acids such as tryptophan suggests that the inclusion of hydrophobic interactions within DNA complexes may be beneficial. Peptides with moities that provide cooperative hydrophobic behavior of alkyl chains of cationic lipids would improve the stability of the peptide-based DNA delivery systems. Two general classes of lipopeptide analogs of Tyr-Lys-Ala-Lys_n-Trp-Lys peptides have been prepared by including a hydrophobic anchor. The general structures are N, N-dialkyl-Gly-Tyr-Lys-Ala-Lys_n-Trp-Lys and N^α,N^ϵ-diacyl-Lys-Lys_n-Trp-Lys. These peptides differ from the parent structures in that they self-associate to form micelles in aqueous solutions. The inclusion of dialkyl or diacyl chains in the cationic peptides improves the peptide ability to bind DNA and reduces aggregation of the complexes in ionic media.

Recent research has suggested that short synthetic peptides containing different analogs of the first 19–23 amino acid residues of influenza hemaglutinin protein (HA) terminus may be attractive because of their pH-dependent lytic properties, with little activity at pH 7 but $\geq$ 100-fold increase in transfection efficiency at pH 5. The lytic characteristics are revealed as the carboxyl groups of the aspartyl and glutamyl side chains are protonated, which allows the peptides to assume a α-helical conformation that can be inserted into the membrane bilayer.

Similarly an amphipathic membrane associating peptide, JTS-1, Gly-Leu-Phe-Glu-Ala-Leu-Leu-Glu-Leu-Leu-Glu-Ser-Leu-Trp-Glu-Leu-Leu-Leu-Glu-Ala has also been recently developed. The hydrophobic face contains only strongly apolar amino acids, while negatively charged glutamic acid residues dominate the hydrophilic face at physiological pH. The hydrophobic face of JTS-1 appears to cause self-association and leads to the formation of pores in one side of the endosomal membrane, thereby destabilizing the membrane, which leads to its rupture. The cationic DNA complex formed with the condensing peptide Tyr-Lys-Ala-Lys_8-Trp-Lys is rapidly mixed with negatively charged JTS-1, which spontaneously incorporates through electrostatic interactions to form the ternary complex. At a given charge ratio of condensing peptide to plasmid, the transfection efficiency has been shown to be proportional to the concentration of the endosomolytic peptide added to the complex. *In vitro* transfection efficiency up to 10,000-fold higher than that of DNA/Tyr-Lys-Ala-Lys_8-Trp-Lys complex alone has been reported.

14.3.3 Polymer-based gene delivery

14.3.3.1 *Polyvinyl pyrrolidone (PVP)-based formulations*

Polyvinyl pyrrolidone (PVP)-based formulations are hyperosmotic and result in an improved dispersion of plasmids through the extracellular matrix of solid tissues (e.g. muscle), possibly by:

- protecting plasmids from nuclease degradation;

- dispersing plasmids in the muscle;
- facilitating their uptake by muscle cells.

By increasing the hydrophobicity of plasmids and reducing their net negative surface charge, PVP may facilitate the uptake of plasmids by muscle cells. Intramuscular injection of PVP-based plasmid formulations in rats significantly increased the number and distribution of expressing cells, as compared to unformulated plasmid. The formation of condensed interpolyelectrolyte complexes between PVP and DNA has been proposed to both protect DNA from nuclease degradation and facilitate its cellular uptake by hydrophobic interaction with cell membranes. The increased hydrophobicity of the complex may enhance interaction with cell membranes and facilitate cell uptake.

14.3.3.2 *Cationic polymers*

Cationic polymers such as polybrene and diethylaminoethyldextran (DEAE-dextran) have been used for transfection of genes into cultured cell. However, these polymers cannot be used for *in vivo* application due to their poor transfection efficiency and high cytotoxicity.

Dendrimers

Starburst polyamidoamine (PAMAM) dendrimers are a class of highly branched spherical polymers whose surface charge and diameter are determined by the number of synthetic steps. For example, five polymerization cycles produce the 5th generation dendrimers. The major structural differences in PAMAM dendrimers relate to the core molecules, either ammonia or ethylenediamine, with which the stepwise polymerization process begin and which dictates the overall shape, density and surface charge of the molecule. Dendrimers can condense plasmids through electrostatic interactions of their terminal primary amines with the DNA phosphate groups. The effect of colloidal and surface characteristics of plasmid/dendrimer complexes on gene transfer has been examined. These complexes were monodisperse, with a mean hydrodynamic diameter of about 200 nm. The particle size, surface charge and gene transfer efficiency of plasmid/dendrimer complexes prepared with the 5th generation of dendrimers has been shown to be influenced by dendrimer concentration in the complexes.

Polyethyleneimine(PEI)

PEI is a branched cationic polymer and has been shown to condense plasmids into colloidal particles that effectively transfect genes into a variety of cells *in vitro*. In addition to enhancing cellular uptake of plasmids, PEI may also enhance the intracellular trafficking of plasmids by buffering the endosomal compartments, thus protecting plasmids against degradation and enabling endosomal release of plasmid via lysosomal osmotic swelling and disruption. Conjugation of targeting ligands, such as transferrin or anti-CD3 antibody, to PEI has recently been shown to enhance transfection efficiency by 30~1,000 fold compared to ligand-free PEI in various tumor cell lines.

Chitosan

Chitosan is a biodegradable polysaccharide and has been shown to interact with the phosphate groups of DNA, condensing plasmids into spherical and toroidal particles. The colloidal and surface properties of plasmid/chitosan complexes have been shown to depend on the molecular weight of chitosan, the ratio of plasmid to chitosan and the preparation medium. Smaller nanoparticles have been observed with low molecular weight chitosan (2 kDa) as compared to high molecular weight chitosan (540 kDa). A number of cell lines have been transfected with plasmid/chitosan complexes.

Poly(2-dimethylamino)ethyl methacrylate (PDMAEMA)

PDMAEMA has also been evaluated for transfecting plasmids encoding β-galactosidase gene in COS-7 cell lines *in vitro*. The optimal transfection efficiency was found at a PDMAEMA/plasmid ratio of 3:1 (w/w), the ratio at which homogeneous complexes of about 150 nm in diameter could be formed. Interestingly, the transfection efficiency of the complexes was not affected by the presence of serum proteins, even though the presence of serum is known to adversely affect the transfection efficiency. Poly(ethylene glycol)-poly(L-lysine) block copolymers have been shown to form complexes with DNA that can transfect human embryonal kidney cells *in vitro*.

14.4 BIODISTRIBUTION AND PHARMACOKINETICS

Biodistribution of plasmid to either extracellular or intracellular targets is dependent on the structure of capillary walls, (patho)physiological conditions, the rate of blood and lymph supply, the physicochemical properties of plasmid and its carrier molecules. The fate of plasmid after *in vivo* administration is illustrated in Figure 14.4. The blood capillary walls are comprised of four layers, namely plasma–endothelial interface, endothelium, basal lamina, and adventia. Macromolecules can cross the endothelial barrier:

- through the cytoplasm of endothelial cells themselves;
- across the endothelial cell membrane vesicles;
- through inter-endothelial cell junctions;
- through endothelial cell fenestrae.

Based on the morphology and continuity of the endothelial layer, capillary endothelium can be divided into three categories: continuous, fenestrated, and discontinuous endothelium (see Section 5.1.3).

The continuous capillaries are found in skeletal, cardiac, and smooth muscles, as well as in lung, skin, subcutaneous and mucous membranes. The endothelial layer of brain microvasculature is the tightest endothelium, with no fenestrations. Capillaries with fenestrated

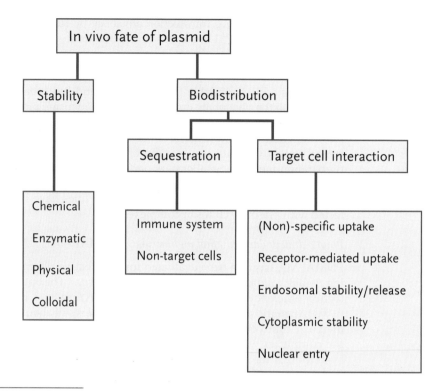

```
In vivo fate of plasmid
├── Stability
│   └── Chemical
│       Enzymatic
│       Physical
│       Colloidal
└── Biodistribution
    ├── Sequestration
    │   └── Immune system
    │       Non-target cells
    └── Target cell interaction
        └── (Non)-specific uptake
            Receptor-mediated uptake
            Endosomal stability/release
            Cytoplasmic stability
            Nuclear entry
```

Figure 14.4 Fate of plasmid DNA after *in vivo* administration (modified with permission from: Site-specific gene therapy: design and use of plasmid-based gene medicines to control *in vivo* production, delivery and effect of therapeutic proteins, Eric Tomlinson (1998). In *Peptide and Protein Drug Delivery, Alfred Benzon Symposium 43."* Eds. Sven Frøkjaer, Lona Christrup and Povl Krogsgaard-Larsen; Munksgaard, Copenhagen, 1998, pp. 462–477

endothelia and a continuous basement membrane are generally found in the kidney, small intestine and salivary glands. Most of these capillaries have diaphragmed fenestrae, which are circular openings of 40–60 nm in diameter. The discontinuous capillaries, also known as sinusoidal capillaries, are common in the liver, spleen, and bone marrow. These capillaries show large interendothelial junctions (fenestrations up to 150 nm). Highly phagocytic Kupffer cells line the sinusoids of the liver, and those of the bone marrow by flattened, phagocytic reticuloendothelial cells. In the spleen, the endothelial cells contain a large number of pinocytic vesicles (up to 100 nm in diameter).

Due to their large molecular weight (> 1,000 kDa) and hydrodynamic diameter in aqueous suspension of 100 nm, plasmids extravasate poorly via continuous capillaries because of tight junctions between the cells. However, plasmids can easily extravasate to sinusoidal capillaries of liver and spleen. Formulating plasmids into unimeric particles of 20–40 nm in diameter may enhance extravasation of plasmids across continuous and fenestrated capillaries.

The (patho)physiology and microanatomy of tumors is significantly different from normal tissues (see Section 5.1.3). A tumor contains vessels recruited from the pre-existing network and vessels resulting from angiogenic response induced by cancer cells. There is a considerable variation in the cellular composition, basement membranes and in the size of the interendothelial cell fenestrations. Tumor interstitium is characterized by large interstitial volume and high diffusion rate. High interstitial pressure of the tumor retards the extravasation of plasmids,

Figure 14.5
Biodistribution of
plasmid/cationic
liposome complexes
after systemic
administration. PCMV-
CAT/DOTMA:DOPE
[2:1 mol/mol, 1:3
(−/+)] complexes were
injected into the tail
vein of mice at a dose
of 60 mg DNA. Fifteen
minutes, 2 hr and 24 hr
after injection, tissues
were collected and
processed for PCR
analysis. The percent of
recovered dose was
calculated from the
sum of the total
amount of DNA
recovered from all the
organs examined. The
data are presented as
the group mean value
+/− S.D. (n= 4–6).
Reproduced with
permission from:
Biodistribution and
gene expression of
plasmid/lipid
complexes after
systemic
administeration,
Mahato R.I. et al. (1998)
Human Gene Therapy, 9:
2083–2099

whereas large vascular permeability facilitates their migration to tumor tissues. Tumor accumulation of plasmid could result from the enhanced permeability of the tumor vasculature, combined with their reduced clearance from the tumor due to the absence of the lymphatic system.

The biodistribution of plasmid can be determined by measuring the rate of disappearance of radiolabeled DNA from the bloodstream and its accumulation in tissues or by the use of fluorescence microscopy to trace the leakage of dye-labeled plasmids from the vasculature. Pharmacokinetic analysis of *in vivo* disposition profiles of radiolabeled plasmid provides useful information on the overall distribution characteristics of systemically administered plasmids, with one critical limitation. The radiolabel represents both intact plasmid and its metabolites. The plasma half-life of plasmid is less than 10 min, and hence tissue distribution and pharmacokinetic parameters of plasmid calculated on the basis of total radioactivity are not valid at longer time points. Thus, polymerase chain reaction and Southern-blot analysis are required to establish the time at which the radiolabel is no longer an index of plasmid distribution.

The deposition of plasmids after systemic administration is restricted to the intravascular space due to its low microvascular permeability in most organs with continuous capillary bed. Some organs with fenestrated capillaries, such as liver, spleen, and bone marrow, provide some opportunities for extravasation of plasmids. Intravenously injected plasmids initially perfuse the pulmonary vascular beds, maximizing the potential uptake of plasmid DNA in the lung endothelial cells soon after administration. Plasmid DNA was rapidly cleared from the circulation due to the extensive uptake by the lung and liver, while it was not susceptible to glomerular filtration because of the presence of the basement membrane. Liver accumulation increased with time, while there was rapid decrease in the DNA accumulation in the lung (Figure 14.5). In addition, plasmid DNA was

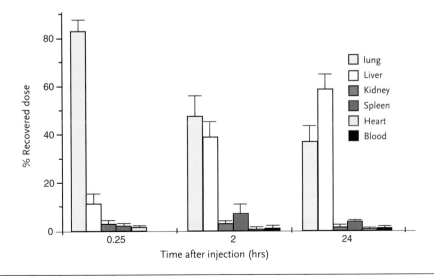

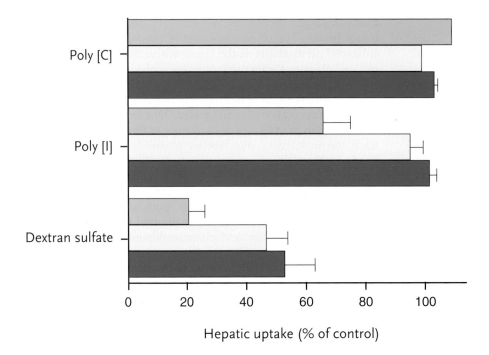

Poly [C]

Poly [I]

Dextran sulfate

0   20   40   60   80   100

Hepatic uptake (% of control)

Figure 14.6 Inhibitory effects of polyanions on the hepatic uptake of ^{32}P-labeled plasmid/cationic liposome complexes administered intravenously into mice at 1 minute after DNA iv injection of excess polyanions. Hepatic accumulation was determined at 10 minute post-injection. Key: (orange) free plasmid, (pale orange) 1:5 w/w plasmid/LipofectACE, (blue) 1:5 w/w plasmid/LipofectACE. Reproduced with permission from: Physicochemical and pharmacokinetic characteristics of DNA/cationic liposome complexes, Mahato R.I. et al. (1995) *J. Pharm. Sci.*, 84: 1267–1271

preferentially taken up by the liver nonparenchymal cells as huge anionic molecules via the scaveger receptor-mediated process in a specific manner for polyanions (Figure 14.6).

Autoradiography of mouse whole body after intravenous injection of [^{33}P]plasmid/lipid complexes has shown DNA localization predominantly in the lung, with notable uptake in the liver and other tissues containing RES cells. In contrast, the autoradiograph of mouse whole body after intravenous injection of free [^{33}P]plasmid showed the highest levels of radioactivity in the liver, followed by other tissues containing RES cells. Southern-blot analysis of blood showed the rapid degradation of plasmid, with a half-life of less than 5 min for intact plasmid, and was no longer detectable at 1 hr postinjection. By Southern-blot analysis, there was no detectable plasmid in the brain, large intestine, small intestine, or gonads at the 1-hr timepoint. Southern blot analysis also demonstrated that plasmid remained in the liver, spleen, lung, marrow, and muscle, although at diminished levels, up to 24 hr postinjection. After 7 days, no intact plasmid was detectable by Southern-blot analysis. However, the plasmid was detectable by PCR analysis in all tissues examined at 7 and 28 days postinjection. PCR analysis at the 6-month timepoint revealed that only muscle had any significant levels of plasmid above background.

14.4.1 Cellular uptake and intracellular trafficking

Interaction of formulated plasmids with biofluids and penetration of the extracellular matrix, if present, are the major extracellular barriers. The plasma membrane is the next obstacle to be overcome in delivering genes into a cell. Gene delivery systems rely on binding to cell surface molecules, either specific, non-specific or both, prior to cellular internalization. The surface bound material usually gains entry into the cell either by endocytosis or membrane fusion. Successful intracellular trafficking of plasmids must surmount several barriers, including release from endosomes, DNA uncoating, movement through the cytoplasm, association with the nuclear membrane, and transport to the nucleus probably through the nuclear pore before transcription factors become limiting. The schematic representation of the process of gene delivery and expression is shown in Figure 14.7.

Gene delivery systems can distribute plasmids to the desired target cells, after which the plasmid is internalized into the cell by a number of mechanisms, such as adsorptive endocytosis, receptor-mediated endocytosis, micropinocytosis, caveolae-mediated endocytosis and phagocytosis (see Section 1.3.3.2). The intracellular fate of plasmids depends on the means by which they are internalized and translocated to the cytoplasms and then to the nucleus. In coated-pit endocytosis, DNA complexes first bind to the cell surface, then migrate to clathrin-coated pits about 150 nm in diameter and are internalized from the plasma membrane to form coated vesicles.

Figure 14.7 Schematic representation of the process of gene delivery and expression. Extacellular environment → tissue targetability → cellular uptake → intracellular trafficking → nuclear entry → gene expression

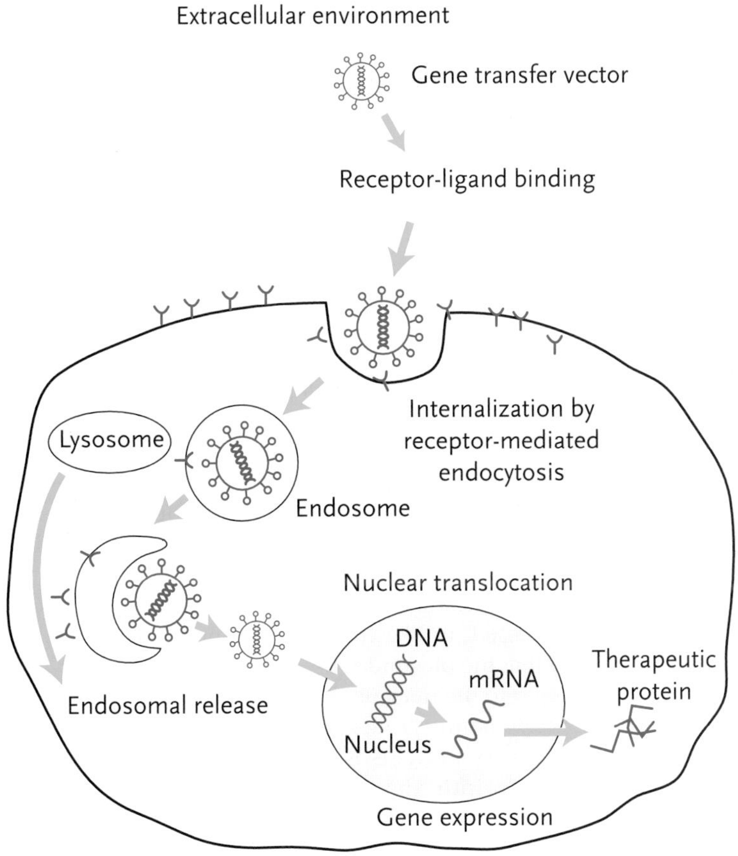

Extracellular environment

Gene transfer vector

Receptor-ligand binding

Internalization by receptor-mediated endocytosis

Lysosome

Endosome

Endosomal release

Nuclear translocation

DNA

mRNA

Therapeutic protein

Nucleus

Gene expression

The transition from coated vesicle to early endosome is accompanied by acidification of the vesicular lumen that continues into the late endosomal and lysosomal compartments, reaching a final pH in the perinuclear lysosome of approximately 4.5. Such acidification associated with endosome maturation provides the means by which certain viruses gain access to the cytosol. Acid-induced conformational changes in the viral proteins trigger translocation across the endosomal membrane via a fusion process. By taking advantage of the endosomal acidification, pH-sensitive liposomes, adenovirus and endosomolytic peptides have been used to facilitate the release of plasmids into the cytoplasm prior to lysosomal degradation.

Non-clathrin-coated pit internalization can occur through smooth invagination of 150–300 nm vesicles or via potocytosis. This pathway has been shown to be involved in the transport of folate and other small molecules into the cytoplasm. Plasmids are taken up by muscles through the T-tubules system and caveolae via potocytosis. Muscle cells appear to take up plasmids through the T-tubule system and caveolae via potocytosis. Apart from coated or uncoated pit pathways, cells may also take up plasmid/cationic carrier complexes via plasma membrane destabilization. Particles greater than 200 nm in diameter are not efficiently taken up by endocytosis, but cells may also take up some larger plasmid/cationic carrier complexes via phagocytosis.

Plasmid/cationic carrier complexes have been proposed to internalize into the endosome and initiate the destabilization of endosomal membranes. This destabilization would induce diffusion of anionic lipids from the external layer of the endosomal membrane into the complexes and form charge neutralized ion pairs with the cationic lipids. Destabilization and/or fusion of the complex with the plasma membrane would permit the same anionic lipids to diffuse to the surface, as would fusion with the endosomal membrane. Release of the condensed DNA from the cationic lipid in the endosome is likely to generate a mechanical or osmotic stress that ruptures the endosomal bilayer and releases DNA into the cytoplasm. In contrast, DNA release from complexes on the cell surface might be unable to stress the membrane to a degree sufficient to rupture.

Transfection efficiency is dependent on mitotic activity, as cells prevented from going into mitosis after transfection express transgenes much less efficiently than proliferating cells. In search for an explanation, the transport of plasmids across the nuclear membranes has been studied. Plasmids injected into the cytoplasm of quiescent human fibroblasts are not expressed, in contrast to plasmid injected into the nucleus. This has been found to be true for the cationic lipid-based systems; as plasmid injected into the cytoplasm of Xenopus oocytes is not expressed, unlike that injected into the nucleus, it must be concluded that the plasmid must dissociate from the cationic lipids before entering into the nucleus.

A fundamental limitation to gene expression using most of the gene delivery systems is the inability of plasmid in the cytoplasm to migrate into the nucleus. To design strategies to enhance intracellular and nuclear trafficking of plasmid, a thorough understanding of cytoskeletal components, nuclear envelope, nuclear pore complex, nuclear localization of plasmids as well as nuclear localization signal sequences (NLSs) will be needed. Microtubules and actin filaments have been proposed to be involved in intracellular trafficking of macromolecules, including plasmids. These cytoskeletal components maintain intracellular distribution of organelles and facilitate trafficking between organelles. Motor proteins, motor protein receptors, or the relevant peptide sequences may be conjugated to or complexed with plasmid. This may result in association of plasmids with myotubules or actin filaments for more efficient transport through the cytoplasm to regions bordering the nucleus.

The nucleus is a dynamic structure, which disassembles at the onset of mitosis and reassembles during telophase. The major barrier between the cytosolic and nucleoplasmic compartments is the hydrophobic double-bilayered barrier of the nuclear envelope. Access of macromolecules into the nucleus is restricted and regulated by the nuclear envelope and the nuclear pore complex (NPC). The NPC accommodates both passive diffusion and active transport. Macromolecules of $<\sim$ 70 kDa passively diffuse through the NPC in and out of the nucleus, although passive diffusion becomes rate-limiting at approximately 20 kDa. Larger macromolecules require active transport for nuclear entry. Plasmids may gain access into the nucleus through the NPC during telophase, when the nuclear envelope reassembles after cell division.

NLS sequences are short mono- or bipartite sequences that induce nuclear import when transferred genetically or chemically to a carrier protein. These sequences generally contain a high proportion of the basic amino acids lysine and arginine. There is often a proline residue to break α-helix formation upstream of the basic residues. NLS sequences are frequently present within viral proteins, or, as in the case of adenovirus, the nuclear localizing proteins are covalently linked to the 5' end of the DNA at the terminal dCMP. A variety of viral nucleic acids (HIV-2, influenza virus, SV40, and adenovirus) are guided through the nuclear pore complex with assistance from at least one NLS-containing viral protein. The first characterized signal shown to be necessary and sufficient to direct nuclear import was the NLS exemplified by the 92-kDa SV40 large T-antigen NLS (Pro[126]-Lys-Lys-Arg-Lys-Val[132]) and the bipartite nucleoplasmin NLS (Lys-Arg-Pro-Ala-Ala-Ile-Lys-Lys-Ala-Gly-Glu-Ala-Lys-Lys-Lys-Lys). The NLS of SV40 large T-antigen has been shown to increase the nuclear accumulation of different nonkaryophilic proteins, such as bovine serum albumin and immunoglobulin into the nucleus of frog oocytes or mammalian cells following their microinjection into the cytoplasm. Mutations of any lysine residue of SV40 large T-antigen are reported to abolish nuclear accumulation.

14.5 CLINICAL APPLICATIONS OF GENE THERAPY

Gene therapy is being investigated for monogenic diseases such as adenosine deaminase, cystic fibrosis, familial hypercholesterolemia,

Gaucher's disease, Duchenne muscular dystrophy as well as for more complex disease processes such as cancer and infectious diseases, such as AIDS (see also Section 1.6.2.1.1). This section discusses biological opportunities for systemic, cancer and pulmonary gene therapy, as well as genetic vaccines.

14.5.1 Systemic gene therapy

Both systemic and local administration of gene medicines offers several biological opportunities for gene therapy. The systemic route allows non-invasive access to many target cells that are not accessible otherwise by direct administration. Systemic gene delivery can broadly be categorized as passive and active targeting. Passive targeting refers to the exploitation of natural disposition profiles of gene medicines, which depends on the physicochemical properties of formulated plasmid DNA and the anatomical and physiological characteristics of the body. Active targeting refers to an alteration in the natural disposition pattern of plasmids by means of target-specific ligands, which can bind specifically to receptors on the surface of target cells.

Passive targeting is an attractive approach for delivery and expression of therapeutic genes to normal endothelia of lung and liver, various phagocytic cells, and potentially disseminated tumors and metastases. Following intravenous injection of plasmid/lipid complexes, gene expression was detected in various organs, with high expression in the lung. Numerous genes, including human growth hormone, α-antitrypsin, prostaglandin G/H synthase and cystic fibrosis transmembrane conductance regulator (CFTR) genes, have been shown to be expressed in the lungs after intravenous administration. Intravenous injection of prostaglandin G/H synthase expression plasmid complexed with DOTMA:DOPE liposomes has also been shown to protect rabbits and pigs against endotoxin-induced pulmonary hypertension.

The liver is the site of many essential metabolic and secretory functions and thus also constitutes an important target for gene therapy. Potential therapies include the treatment of inherited hepatic metabolic and infectious disorders, such as hyperlipidemia, phenylketonuria, familial hypercholesterolemia, organic acidemia, urea cycle disorders, hepatitis, cirrhosis and hemophilia. The liver may also be used as a bioreactor for the sustained production and secretion of therapeutic proteins, such as blood clotting factors (factor VIII or factor IX), erythropoietin, growth factors and α-1 antitrypsin. Gene expression in the liver after intravenous injection of plasmid/lipid complexes often remains low, as Kupffer cells largely take up these complexes via phagocytosis, which presumably leads to the degradation of the DNA and inefficient gene expression. Gene expression in the mouse liver has been shown to be significantly increased after intravenous injection of plasmid/lipid complexes prepared using 1-[2-(9(Z)-octadecenoyloxy ethyl]-2(8-(Z)heptadecenyl-3-hydroxyethylimidazolium chloride (DOTIM):Chol (1:1 mol mol^{-1}) multilamellar vesicles, as compared to DOTIM:Cholesterol (1:1 mol/mol) small lamellar vesicles.

Prolonged retention of gene medicines in the blood circulation might be beneficial for passive distribution of genes to both the intravascular spaces and the highly vascularized tissues, such as tumors. Cationic liposomes containing amino-polyethylene glycol (PEG)-phosphatidylcholine may be used to minimize the non-specific interaction of cationic-lipid based gene medicines with the blood components and their uptake by the reticuloendothelial cells. Even without the use of sterically stabilized liposomes, passive targeting may still be possible for gene delivery to certain tumors. For example, repeated tail vein injection of the tumor suppressor gene p53 complexed with DOTMA:DOPE liposomes into breast tumor-bearing nude mice has been shown to significantly decrease the tumor size as well as the number of metastatic cells in the lung.

Endothelial cells, hepatocytes, tumor and blood cells may be able to process both soluble macromolecules and particulate materials via receptor-mediated endocytosis. Hepatocytes represent an attractive target for the treatment of many hepatic disorders; and the potential of utilizing normal hepatocytes for the secretion of therapeutic proteins. Effective hepatocyte gene therapy requires particulate systems with the appropriate size (<100 nm in diameter) and colloidal properties, for extravasation through the sinusoidal hepatic endothelium and access to the Space of Disse, while avoiding non-specific uptake into numerous non-target sites. The receptor-binding ligand on the surface of the formulated plasmid must also compete with endogenous ligands for cell binding and internalization, and must avoid masking by adsorbed serum proteins. Hepatocytes are quiescent cells that normally do not undergo mitosis. Incorporation of hepatocyte-specific promoter that contains binding sites for hepatocyte transcription factors within plasmid constructs may allow long duration and high levels of tissue-specific gene expression.

Plasmid/asialo-orosomucoid-poly(L-lysine) complexes have been used to obtain expression of genes in hepatocytes of normal animals, as well as expression of low-density lipoprotein (LDL) receptor in LDL-deficient rabbits, albumin in analbuminemic rats and methylated CoA mutase in mice. Evidence of hepatocyte cell-specific gene expression *in vivo* has been obtained with the use of hepatocyte-specific promoters. However, prolonged gene expression required partial (66%) hepatectomy 15 minutes before intravenous injection of the complex into rats, probably due to stimulation of liver cell regeneration. Hepatocyte-specific gene expression has been shown using synthetic peptide-based gene delivery.

14.5.2 Cancer gene therapy

Gene therapy provides a significant opportunity to devise novel strategies for the control or cure of cancer. Several approaches of cancer gene therapy are currently being investigated:

- enhancing cellular and humoral immune responses to tumors;
- inserting genes into tumor cells to evoke "cell suicide";

- modifying tumor suppressor genes or anti-oncogenes.

Such therapeutic genes include the ones that convert prodrugs into toxic metabolites, such as the herpes simplex thymidine kinase (HSV_{tk}) gene driven by T7 promoter, followed by ganciclovir treatment, cytokine genes, which stimulate the immune system to eliminate cancer cells (e.g. IL-2); costimulatory molecules (e.g. gene B7–1) that augment antigen-presentation of tumor-specific antigens by the tumor to the T cells; foreign histocompatibility genes that stimulate a poly-clonal alloreactive immune response; genetic vaccines that generate tumor-specific immunity; replacement of wild-type tumor suppressor genes, such as p53, and antisense genes targeted at oncogenes (e.g. *ras* oncogenes).

Cytokine genes

Several cytokine genes have been found to reduce tumors by stimulat-ing localized inflammatory and/or immune responses. These include interleukin-1 (IL-1), IL-2, IL-4, IL-6, IL-7, IL-12, interferon gamma (IFN-γ), tumor necrosis factor-α (TNF-α), and granulocyte-macrophage colony-stimulating factor (GM-CSF).

Activation and differentiation of cytotoxic T lymphocytes (CD8+ T cells) (CTLs) require interplay of various cytokines and cells. During the presentation of tumor-specific antigens by antigen-presenting cells (APCs) to helper T cells (CD4+ T cells), cytokines present in the micro-environment control the helper immune response to develop into either a cellular or a humoral response. CD4+ T cells have been classified into Th1 and Th2 subsets according to the pattern of cytokines they produce. Th1 clones secrete IL-12 and IFN-γ, whereas Th2 clones secrete IL-4, IL-5, IL-6 and IL-10. Th1 immune response is beneficial for the develop-ment of the cellular cytotoxic (CD8) immune response, whereas Th2 immune response is inhibitory to cytotoxic response. IFN-γ is a type 1 interferon that also promotes Th1-type anti-tumor immunity, reduces tumor cell growth, and inhibits angiogenesis.

Upregulation of the immune system

The immune system has the ability to react very strongly to foreign histocompatability antigens, even ones that have not been seen before. This property of the immune system has been utilized to generate immune responses against tumors. A Phase I/II clinical trial is under way using intratumoral injection of plasmid/lipid complex that results in the expression of HLA-B7, a class I major histocompatibility antigen (MHC class-I), on the tumor cell surfaces. The plasmid used in this study encodes a biscistronic mRNA that produces HLA-B7 (heavy chain) and β-microglobulin (light chain) in equimolar amounts. The expression of the HLA-B7 protein by cancer cells is expected to stimu-late the patient's immune system to recognize these transfected cells as "foreign" and to selectively destroy the tumor. This may also facilitate the presentation of tumor-specific antigens to the immune system, and help the development of tumor-specific immunity. Preclinical results obtained after intratumoral injection of plasmid encoding a murine allogeneic MHC antigen and complexed with cationic liposomes also suggest that the immune response generated against the primary tumor may be effective in eliminating secondary tumors or metastases.

Tumor suppressor genes

Tumor suppressor genes actively repress cell growth and their loss leads to tumor development. The p53 gene has been shown to be involved in the control of the cell cycle, transcriptional regulation, DNA replication and induction of apoptosis. The p53 gene can suppress cell transformation and malignant cell growth. Introduction of the wild-type p53 gene in a colon cancer xenograft model has been shown to induce tumor regression due to apoptosis. Lung cancer cells are frequently deficient in p53 and are susceptible to the induction of apoptosis by overexpressed p53, making this tumor particularly suitable for gene therapy by p53. Systemic administration of the tumor suppressor gene p53 complexed with cationic liposomes significantly reduced tumor growth and metastases of nude mice injected with cancer cells.

14.5.3 Pulmonary gene therapy

Pulmonary gene therapy is attractive for the treatmment of chronic bronchitis, cystic fibrosis, α-1 antitrypsin deficiency, familial emphysema, asthma, pulmonary infections, surfactant deficiency, pulmonary hypertension, lung cancer, and malignant mesothelioma. The pulmonary endothelium may act as a bioreactor for the production and secretion of therapeutic proteins, such as clotting factors and erythropoietin into the blood circulation. There is a potential benefit for acquired lung diseases, as well as cancers, to be controlled and possibly treated by expression of cytokines, surfactant, antioxidant enzymes, or mucoproteins within lung cells.

Plasmid can be delivered to the lung by intravenous injection, intratracheal by instillation or inhalation. Gene delivery to the submucosal glands of the upper airway is of particular interest, though challenging for treatment of cystic fibrosis, where correction of the genetic defects in the glands may improve the alterations in the patients' secretions. Aerosolization requires monodisperse particles, since the deposition of inhaled particles in the airway depends on particle size (see Section 10.3.1). As has been detailed in Chapter 10, larger particles (>5 μm mass median diameter) tend to deposit mainly in the larynx and upper airways. With droplets < 5 μm , there is an increase in airway and alveoli deposition, but alveolar deposition is far greater. The inhaled dose is dependent on the minute volume and entrainment efficiency of the subject and therefore has considerable intersubject variability. Such variability will only be accentuated in many diseases in which the airways are obstructed by mucus. Still, aerosolization of plasmid/lipid complexes has been successfully used for gene delivery into the airways of mice and rabbits with a pump spray device and is under clinical trials for gene delivery to the nasal epithelium.

Intratracheal instillation bypasses the barrier of the endothelial cell layer that is associated with systemic gene delivery. Almost 80–90% of

---

the starting material is wasted in aerosol gene delivery irrespective of the inhalation device employed. Therefore, intratracheal instillation of plasmid/lipid complexes is being investigated as an alternative to deliver transgenes to the lung. Plasmid/lipid complexes, not plasmid alone, are effective in aerosolization, whereas plasmids alone can efficiently be transfected to rat and mouse airway epithelial tissues when given by the intratracheal route. Altering the physicochemical characteristics of the formulated plasmids can vary the distribution of plasmid to the bronchial tree. Immunohistochemical studies of lung tissues after intratracheal administration of plasmid/lipid complexes have shown gene expression mainly within the epithelial cell layer lining the bronchus.

14.5.4 Genetic vaccines

Genetic vaccination can be carried out by injecting plasmids encoding antigens directly into muscle or skin, resulting in host immunity against this antigen. Depending on the site of expression and the nature of antigen, *in vivo* expression of plasmids encoding antigen can provide superior cellular, humoral and mucosal immunity. The efficacy of genetic vaccines could be enhanced or modulated through the use of formulations that increase nucleic acid stability or distribution in the tissue, the coexpression of immune molecules that affect the processing of antigens, or through the use of adjuvants that affect the immune response. Genetic vaccines have been applied to several systems, including immune responses against cancer antigens, mycoplasma, tuberculosis, malaria, parasites, and viral infections.

Two types of immunity may be induced in response to an antigen, namely humoral immunity mediated by antigen-specific antibodies produced by B lymphocytes, and cell-mediated immunity produced by activated macrophages and cytotoxic T lymphocytes. Antibodies may neutralize pathogens, whereas cytotoxic T lymphocytes can destroy infected cells or control infection by noncytolytic means. Antibody-mediated immunity effectively prevents infection by binding to the infectious organisms and then eliminating either directly or via phagocytic ingestion by neutrophils and/or monocytes. Antibodies also bind to the surface of infected cells expressing the specific antigen.

Cell-mediated immunity involves T cells, which recognize antigen presented by antigen-presenting cells (APCs) via molecules encoded by the major histocompatibility complex (MHC) genes. MHC class I molecules present peptides derived from antigens that are synthesized endogenously by the cells. CD8+ T cells differentiate into cytotoxic lymphocytes (CTLs) upon activation by such peptide-MHC class I complex expressing APCs. CD4+ T cells differentiate upon recognition of peptide-MHC class II complexes, which are generated from the processing of exogenous antigens, developing to T helper cells. The CD4+T helper cells can broadly be divided into two major sub-types: Th1 CD4+ cells are implicated in delayed type hypersensitivity reactions and the generation and maintenance of CTL responses, while Th2 cells are necessary for the generation and maintenance of adequate antibody responses.

Several routes, including intramuscular, subcutaneous, intravenous, intradermal, nasal, and oral administration, have been investigated for the administration of genetic vaccines. Of these routes, intramuscular injection of genetic vaccines generated the best response. Mature myotube has been shown to be the target for the uptake of plasmid after intramuscular administration. Plasmid can enter the bloodstream and lymphatic system after intramuscular administration and traffic to the spleen, liver, kidney, lymph nodes and bone marrow. It is not clear whether the production of antigens in muscle has unique properties with respect to the elicitation of a prolonged immune response or whether expression in any tissue in the periphery is sufficient for the induction of an antigen-specific immune response.

Subcutaneous injection leads to DNA uptake and expression in keratinocytes, macrophages, and Langerhans cells. Single injection provides for a full humoral and T cell response for 60–70 weeks, with the antibody titer being higher than that achieved by intramuscular injection. The antigen-producing epidermal keratinocytes and myocytes cannot properly present to the immune system without special APCs, dendritic cells and macrophages. The latter are more abundant in epidermis than in muscle. DNA can be introduced in the epidermal cells by the ballistic method. In this method, small metal particles of tungsten or gold that are coated with DNA are accelerated to very high speeds to force the coated particles to deliver the DNA to the cytoplasm and then to nucleus.

Skin is rich in dendritic cells, which are potent initiators of immune responses and possess the co-stimulatory and adhesion molecules required for T cell activation. In addition, dendritic cells possess a unique ability to process and present extracellular antigens in the context of both class I and class II molecules. Thus, transfection of plasmids into these cells is likely to elicit both cellular and humoral responses. Specific targeting of dendritic cells residing in the lymph nodes will likely represent an attractive strategy for providing a robust immune response with nucleic acid vaccines.

14.6 CONCLUSION

Plasmid-based gene therapy holds great promise for improving the delivery and therapeutic use of proteins that have poor pharmacokinetic profiles. Plasmid-based (or non-viral) gene therapy has generated considerable research interest because of many inherent advantages over the viral vectors in terms of safety, immunogenicity and ease of manufacture. Gene therapy offers unique opportunities in the development of novel products that produce intracellular proteins. Several plasmid-based approaches are already in clinical trials and offer the potential of safe and effective gene therapy. To enhance the therapeutic efficacy of proteins using plasmid-based expression systems, many fundamental questions related to their pharmaceutical formulation, biodistribution and intracellular trafficking still need to be addressed.

14.7 FURTHER READING

Berg, P. and Singer, M. (1992) *Dealing With Genes: The Language of Heredity*. University Science Books, Mill Valley, California.

Brown, T.A. (1990) *Gene Cloning: An Introduction*. Chapman & Hall, London.

Drlika, K. (1996) *Understanding DNA and Gene Cloning: A Guide for the Curious*, 3rd edn. John Wiley & Sons, Inc., New York.

Eck, S.L. and Wilson, J.M. (1996) Gene-based therapy. In: Goodman and Gilman's *The Pharmacological Basis of Therapeutics*, 9th edn. McGraw-Hill, New York.

Felgner, P.L., Heller, M.J., Lehr, P., Behr, J.P. and Szoka, F.C., Jr (1996) *Artificial Self-Assembling Systems for Gene Delivery*. ACS Books, Washington.

Friedmann, T. (1998) *Development of Human Gene Therapy*. Cold Spring.

Jain, K.K. (1998) *Textbook of Gene Therapy*. Hogrefe & Company.

Kabonov, A.V., Felgner, P.L. and Seymour, L.W. (1998) *Self-Assembling Complexes for Gene Therapy: From Laboratory to Clinical Trials*. John Wiley & Sons.

Lasic, D.D. and Templeton, N.S. (1996) Liposomes in gene therapy. *Adv. Drug Del. Rev.*, 20:221–266.

Lemoine, N.R. and Cooper, D.N. (1996) *Gene Therapy*. Bios Scientific Publishers, Oxford, UK.

Mahato, R.I., Takakura, Y. and Hashida, M. (1997) Nonviral vectors for *in vivo* gene therapy: Physicochemical and pharmacokinetic considerations. *Crit. Rev. Ther. Drug Carrier Syst.*, 14:133–172.

Rolland, A. (1999) *Advanced Gene Delivery: From Concepts to Pharmaceutical Products*. Harwood Press.

Smith, A.E. (1995) Viral vectors in gene therapy. *Annu. Rev. Microbiol.*, 49:807–838.

Tomlinson, E. (1992) Impact of the new biologies on the medical and pharmaceutical sciences. *J. Pharm. Pharmacol.*, 44(suppl. 1):147–159.

Vega, M.A. (1995) *Gene Targeting*. CRC Press, Boca Raton, FL.

Vile, R.G. (1998) *Understanding Gene Therapy*. Springer-Verlag, New York.

Zanthopoulos, K. (1998) *Gene Therapy*. Springer-Verlag, New York.

14.8 SELF-ASSESSMENT QUESTIONS

1. Describe the three parts of a plasmid-based gene medicine.
2. Outline the advantages and disadvantages of using viral vectors for gene therapy.

3. List the advantages of plasmid-based gene medicines over viral vectors.
4. Describe the essential features of a gene expression system.
5. Outline the various types of lipid-based gene delivery systems.
6. Outline the various types of polymer-based gene delivery systems.
7. Describe the pharmacodynamic and pharmacokinetic barriers to effective plasmid-based gene delivery.
8. Give examples of the clinical application of gene therapy.
9. Outline the various approaches to cancer gene therapy presently being investigated.
10. Describe the use of plasmid-based gene delivery for vaccination.

15

Integrating Drug Discovery and Delivery

David Bailey and Andrew W. Lloyd

OBJECTIVES

On completion of this chapter the reader should be able to:

- Describe the principles of combinatorial chemistry
- Outline the uses of high-throughput screening in drug discovery
- Describe the uses of proteomics and genomics in identifying therapeutic targets
- Understand the importance of informatics in drug discovery
- Understand the future role of combinatorial chemistry, proteomics and genomics on drug delivery and targeting

15.1 INTRODUCTION

The recent revolution in drug discovery technologies has important consequences for drug delivery and targeting. Traditionally new chemical entities have been identified by the screening of natural products and chemical libraries to identify potential lead compounds. These lead compounds have then been optimized through an iterative lead-optimization process involving the synthesis of analogs, the development of quantitative-structure-activity relationships and the use of molecular modeling to obtain new chemical entities with high specificity and affinity for the therapeutic target for pharmaceutical development. The development of combinatorial chemistry has led to the ability to produce vast libraries of compounds for initial screening. The evaluation of combinatorial libraries using high-throughput screening technologies allows the rapid screening of potential lead compounds with a wider molecular diversity against a broad range of therapeutic targets.

Until recently, therapeutic targets were identified through the application of basic pharmacology and biochemistry with both receptor and enzyme targets being identified and isolated from specific tissues. The identification of potential therapeutic targets has been further enhanced through the recent development of genomics and proteomics. These techniques provide mechanisms to identify upregulated gene and protein expression in diseased tissue providing pointers towards potential means of therapeutic intervention.

The advances in molecular biology have also led to the ability to clone receptors into various cell types to facilitate screening of potential ligands against such targets. The parallel development of cell biology has led to the ability to utilize cell-based assays rather than tissue-based assays for drug screening and the advances in robotics have led to the development of high-throughput screening technologies.

The development of genomics, proteomics, high-throughput screening and combinatorial chemistry has led to an information explosion within pharmaceutical companies requiring better mechanisms for the storage and manipulation of biological and chemical data. This has driven the development of the field of bioinformatics which serves to provide searchable databases allowing comparison of molecular and biological information to potentially identify other therapeutic targets and lead compounds.

This chapter aims to provide a brief overview of these different technologies to provide a basis for the reader to develop their understanding of this field in order to appreciate how these technologies will underpin the future of drug delivery and targeting.

15.2 COMBINATORIAL CHEMISTRY

Combinatorial chemistry provides a means of synthesizing a vast array (libraries) of compounds in clean single pot reactions. The majority of combinatorial approaches utilize polymeric solid supports as a base onto which the compounds are synthesized. However, there are also approaches which utilize solution-based chemistries to generate combinatorial libraries.

15.2.1 Peptide synthesis

Combinatorial chemistry evolved from the field of solid state peptide synthesis in which peptides are prepared on a polymeric solid phase support. Such supports are traditionally composed of polymeric resin beads on to which the synthesis of a peptide is undertaken in a step-wise fashion with each amino acid being added sequentially to the peptide chain (Figure 15.1). In order to avoid the formation of side products each amino acid is protected so that only one reaction, that with the amino acid already bound to the support, is possible. After coupling the amino acid to the peptide chain, the protecting group is removed from the terminal amino acid exposing a reactive site to which another amino acid may subsequently be coupled.

This technique relies on the clean coupling of amino acids in peptide synthesis, the ability to easily remove reactants and solvents and wash the products between each stage of the synthesis and the ability to protect and deprotect reactive groups on the solid support as necessary.

Figure 15.1 Peptide synthesis

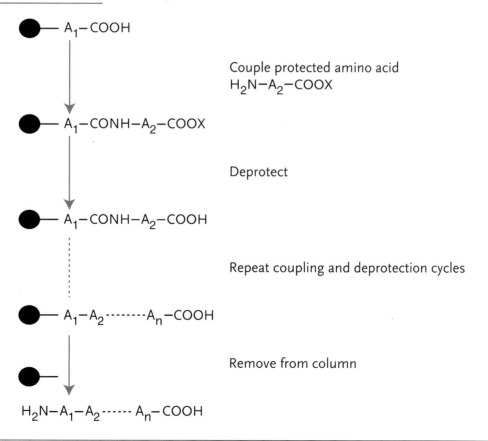

Integrating Drug Discovery and Delivery

15.2.2 Split and mix combinatorial synthesis

The split and mix approach forms the basis of all solid support-based combinatorial synthetic strategies.

An example of a $3 \times 3 \times 3$ combinatorial split and mix combinatorial synthesis is shown in Figure 15.2. The technique involves three initial batches of resin beads to which are initially coupled, for example, a different amino acid. These batches are then combined, mixed and split again into three batches; each batch now containing a mixture of beads containing different amino acids. A different amino acid is then coupled to each of these batches of beads, the beads mixed, split and the process repeated a third time. This simple $3 \times 3 \times 3$ combinatorial split and mix approach generates a library of beads containing 27 different compounds in only 6 coupling reactions. A $10 \times 10 \times 10 \times 10 \times 10$ split and mix reaction scheme will produce 10,000 compounds in only 50 reactions. It is therefore clear that these strategies can produce large libraries of compounds of wide molecular diversity.

As each resin bead contains only a single molecule the beads can be screened individually for bioactivity by either screening for activity of bound peptide in the biological assay or by cleaving the resultant peptide from the bead before undertaking the bioanalysis. The identity of any active compounds can then be determined by using mass spectrometry to sequence the active peptide.

15.2.3 Indexed libraries

Alternative approaches to the identification of active agents involve the synthesis of indexed or parallel array libraries. These involve the synthesis of a large number of combinatorial libraries making it possible to identify the sequence of the active agent from the identification of the libraries containing the active agent. For example, if we were interested in a 5 amino acid peptide we could use an indexed library approach. This approach involves the initial synthesis of 20 combinatorial libraries using 20 different amino acids as the first amino acid. By screening these libraries we would be able to identify a library containing the most active peptide against a therapeutic target – this library would indicate which amino acid is required in the first position of the peptide. If we then, keeping the first amino acid constant, synthesize a further 20 libraries using 20 different amino acids in the second position we will be able to identify the second amino acid required for optimal activity. This is then repeated until we have identified all five amino acids. Such a process allows the most active agent to be identified from a potential pool of 3.2 million possible peptide sequences using only 310 reactions.

Parallel array libraries use a similar strategy but the libraries are all synthesized in parallel. For example, if we were looking for a small molecule drug which could be synthesized from three basic building blocks A, B and C each of which had 12 different possible variants (e.g. 12 different carboxylic acids; 12 different aromatic amines and 12 different alkyl halides) we would synthesis 3 parallel sets of 12 libraries. The first set of libraries would each contain a known variant of A, the

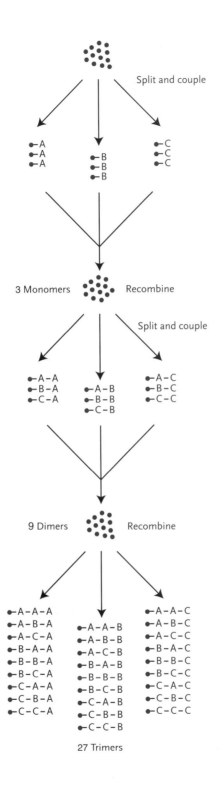

Figure 15.2 Split and mix combinatorial synthesis

Integrating Drug Discovery and Delivery

403

second set of libraries a known variant of B and the third set of libraries a known variant of C. By screening all the libraries and identifying the most active library from each set it is immediately possible to identify the structure of the most active compound, as only one compound will be common to the libraries (e.g. A3B5C13) containing the most active compounds from each set.

All these approaches assume that the only a single compound will be synthesized on each bead at each coupling stage, that there are no side-reactions and that other members of the libraries do not interfere with the binding of the most active compound to the ligand of interest during screening. Although these limitations may seem highly significant, these techniques have been successfully validated using combinatorial techniques to identify known endogenous receptor ligands. These techniques provide a wide range of molecularly diverse molecules with potential therapeutic applications.

In addition, the field of combinatorial chemistry has led to the development of (i) a vast range of clean chemical reactions which give rise to a single products, (ii) novel linker technologies allowing molecules to be readily linked to solid supports and subsequently cleaved on completion of the coupling reactions, (iii) novel protecting strategies and (iv) novel chemistries which allow the synthesis of a diverse range of molecules including benzodiazepines, saccharides and lactams, in addition to the more traditional peptides and oligonucleotides on solid supports.

The identification of peptidomimetics through combinatorial chemistry and high-throughput screening may negate the need to address the challenge of biopharmaceutical drug delivery.

15.3 High-throughput screening

The ability of combinatorial chemistry to produce large numbers of molecular entities led to the need to develop fast, efficient screening technologies for evaluating these entities as potential inhibitors and/or activators against therapeutic targets. The recent developments in molecular biology and robotics have provided the impetus for such technology. Initially bioassays were developed using 96-well microtitre plate technologies. However, more recently the industry has been considering 384 and even 1,536 microwell plates. The advances in robotics allow assays to be fully automated and run continually day and night with minimal operator intervention.

Molecular biology has provided the means to clone human receptors in a variety of cells and express different enzymes in model systems. These techniques also facilitate the monitoring of drug–receptor interactions by the use of biosystems which detect secondary processes mediated by receptor activation such as elevation in cAMP levels. This is achieved, for example, through the incorporation of luciferase reporter genes into cells systems which allow the rapid detection of changes in cAMP by bioluminscence monitoring.

Other detection systems use radioactive ligands, bioactivated fluorescent markers or fluorescent quenching approaches in which the interaction with the test compound causes a reduction in the fluorescence of a plate bound enzyme/receptor-conjugate. Novel, rapid methods of detecting both drug-ligand interations and receptor/enzyme activation are continually being developed in order to provide more rapid and sensitive detection systems. In many cases the amount of test compound is limited and HTS systems must be able to detect drug–ligand interactions at very low drug concentrations.

In this way HTS allows the rapid screening of combinatorial libraries for potential lead compounds. These lead compounds are then isolated and characterized, if necessary, before production and optimization on a larger scale.

Although HTS initially focused on assessing drug–ligand binding and activation, the development of cell-based assays has provided potential means for HTS toxicity and bioavailability screening at an early stage of drug development, allowing the industry to perhaps focus at an earlier stage on drugs with high ligand specificity, low toxicity and potentially good bioavailability. The integration of HTS with proteomics and genomics (see Section 15.6) may also allow the future early-stage screening of drug metabolism and interactions.

With the developments in high-throughput screening the issues of bioavailability and drug metabolism can be addressed at the earlier stages in the drug discovery/development program ultimately allowing the pharmaceutical industry to select compounds for development with acceptable bioavailability and metabolic profile, and reducing the development costs associated with developing a suitable means of delivering such agents.

15.4 GENOMICS

Genomics, the systematic study of the structure and function of mammalian genetic information, is radically expanding our understanding of the molecular basis of biology. Nowhere is the impact of this new science more dramatic than in medicine and pharmaceutical drug discovery.

Previously "invisible" traditional drug targets are today being examined in detail at the molecular level through the systematic analysis of the genes and proteins which encode them. Coupled with powerful approaches to determining protein structure, such as X-ray crystallography and Fourier-transform two-dimensional electron microscopy, their detailed molecular architecture and the molecular mechanisms by which they work are also being revealed.

As will be become apparent, genomics can define the molecular diversity of key receptors, ion channels, enzymes and transporters, and for the first time permits detailed structural comparison of pharmaceutically important gene "families" at the DNA and amino-acid level. This molecular information, when coupled with a detailed knowledge of the pharmacological behavior of the same receptors in specific tisssues, gives pharmacologists and medicinal chemists new starting points for drug discovery and optimization, leading to more selective and potentially safer medicines.

In the context of drug delivery, genomics allows an organism-wide appreciation of the molecular mechanisms which specific cells and tissues employ for drug absorption and metabolism, the traditional Absorption, Distribution, Metabolism and Excretion (ADME) arms of pharmaceutics (see Section 1.4). Importantly, defining the specific molecular components of target tissues not only raises our understanding of the molecular basis of ADME, but also provides the basis of exploiting these characteristics in designing new advanced drug delivery systems.

Currently, very few examples of the successful *ab initio* design of effective drugs exist, let alone their specific optimization for delivery. However, with the definition of robust molecular approaches for building specific delivery and activation characteristics into broad classes of drug, there is an increasing opportunity for converting already known drugs with limited selectivity into highly targeted agents. As the search for safer, more effective medicines continues, the availability of routine methods for optimizing delivery is one stage of the development process which offers considerable commercial potential.

15.4.1 Genomics: the technology

Progress in the field of molecular biology in recent years has been impressive. From the discovery of DNA in 1953, to the identification and mapping of the entire complement of human genes, published in spring 2001, has taken only 50 years. It has been a stimulating period for molecular biology, with a raft of innovative technologies providing the basis for profound advances in our appreciation of the inner workings of cells, tissues and, increasingly, whole organisms.

15.4.1.1 Obtaining the gene sequences

The story of the race to sequence the human genome and its component genes is enthralling. A heady mixture of scientific opportunism and commercial exploitation has led us to the point where virtually all the genes in the human genome are now known. However, as unfair as it may seem, this genetic heritage is not yet available to all scientists. A small number of companies still hold the keys to the majority of these genes, and, with recent developments, it looks as though the same may prove true for the framework sequence of the entire genome. Potentially more frustrating for the academic scientist, the patenting of such information may lock away the fruit of genomics for decades to come.

At the heart of the technologies underpinning genomics has been our ability to clone individual genes, as complementary DNA sequences, or cDNAs. Originating from pioneering work by Paul Berg at Stanford University in 1975, the ability to copy messenger RNA (mRNA) into the more stable complementary DNA (cDNA) and clone this into bacteria, thereby producing an endless source of target DNA simply by growing up the bacteria, has proved a robust technique and is still in use today.

Techniques for the production of individual cDNAs, "cloned" in bacteria at the rate of one cDNA per bacterium, were multiplexed to produce cDNA "libraries", large collections of cDNAs, simply by repeating the cloning procedure with complex cDNA mixtures. These complex cDNA mixtures, now in bacteria, can be surveyed by retrieving and sequencing each individual cDNA, giving a faithful representation of the abundance of each cDNA in the original mixture if sufficient cDNAs are sequenced.

The key to the utility of this technique in genomics is the observation that cDNA libraries, made from individual tissues and cell lines, preserve the relative levels of individual mRNAs found in the extracts as cDNAs within the library. From this it has proved possible to survey the majority of the genes expressed in a particular cell or tissue. The broad applicability of such techniques not only to tissues but also to established cell lines and model cell systems is illustrated in Figure 15.3.

Figure 15.3 Producing "expressed sequence tag" (EST) databases by random DNA sequencing of cDNA libraries

A subsequent technological advance, that of DNA sequencing, opened the way to the large-scale exploitation of the information in these libraries. The seminal invention was that of dideoxy terminator DNA sequencing by Fred Sanger in 1987, leading to his second Nobel

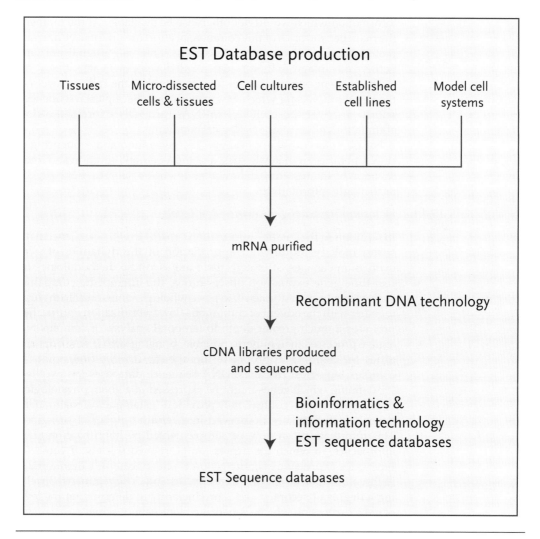

Prize and in 1989 to the commercial development of automated electrophoretic DNA sequencing systems.

In the space of only a few years, these technologies have allowed the determination of the complete DNA sequence of the first chromosome, the first bacterial genome, and the first entire eukaryotic genome, that of baker's yeast, *Saccharomyces cerevisiae*. The websites shown in Table 15.1 provide an overview of the current status of genome information. The MAGPIE website is particularly useful for obtaining a complete and current listing of genome sequencing projects.

Random genomic DNA sequencing and assembly, used so effectively for bacterial genomics, was originally devised to analyze the expressed human genome. The latter effort is still under way in companies as well as in public institutions. The economies of scale provided by industrial-scale sequencing have hastened progress to the point where at least two companies now have the majority of expressed human genes in their freezers. This has certainly had the effect of restricting access to key therapeutic genes, but on the other hand subscribers to these proprietary databases have early access to information which would not otherwise be available. At the moment, the main beneficiaries of this commercial effort are pharmaceutical and biotech companies who see such access as conferring a significant competitive advantage on their research and development activities.

The challenges now are two-fold: to complete the full sequences of the larger mRNAs for which we currently only have partial sequences, and to discover those elusive mRNAs, probably expressed at low abundance under unique biological conditions.

For pharmaceutical applications, the generation and sequencing of cDNA libraries from key tissues, and the assembly, curation and interrogation of the resulting enormous sequence databases, have proved particularly informative.

15.4.1.2 *Determining exact gene expression levels*

In addition to the "static" information present in DNA sequence databases, biology requires an appreciation of the dynamics of gene expression changes. Although there are as yet no methodologies for real-time gene expression observations, the attempt by companies such as Incyte and Affymetrix to place whole genomes on silicon chips, together with the advent of continuous flow hybridization approaches, promises a much greater depth to temporal analysis of complex biological processes than hitherto possible, bringing with it new opportunities for defining appropriate therapeutic intervention points in complex biological cascades. DNA sequence databases are excellent for defining which genes might be expressed in a given physiological or pharmacological context: they provide a "catalogue" of mammalian genes which have been observed in a certain number of situations. This information can now be complemented by hybridization array approaches, in which the expression of defined subsets of genes (or indeed the expression of entire genomes) can be carefully monitored at high volume across specific time courses and dose regimens, providing a degree of accuracy and reproducibility in determining the level of gene expression which sequencing alone cannot achieve.

It is interesting to note the technical synergies between these technologies. Together, sequencing and arraying techniques can be used to provide information on both the biology of disease and the behavior of compounds as they impact a biological system.

The scientific basis of hybridization arraying as a technique for the determination of gene expression levels is shown in Figures 15.4 and 15.5. The two currently available systems use either immobilized oligonucleotides or immobilized cDNAs as mRNA hybridization targets, but both require preparation and fluorescent-labeling of the mRNAs prior to quantitation. A full description of these hybridization arraying approaches has been published and is also available on the Web (see Table 15.1).

Access to comprehensive sequence databases and the bioinformatics tools to analyze them plays a central role in these gene expression monitoring approaches, illustrating their "reach-through" impact in genomics in general. Such databases provide the primary sequence information from which to design key oligonucleotides for chip immobilization, while the ability to compare and contrast individual cDNAs for immobilization from the large commercially available collections is equally vital for cDNA array design and production.

A further technique which holds considerable promise for evaluating individual gene expression at the histological or cellular level is *in situ* hybridization. This provides a cellular level of resolution to gene expression analysis which complements that of microarray analyses.

All the above techniques have major potential applications in drug delivery, from defining new members of key transporter and receptor gene families and their expression, to providing experimental systems for evaluating the efficacy of new delivery systems.

15.4.1.3 Assembling protein signaling networks

Key to the full exploitation of cell-based targeting is an intimate understanding of the protein networks present within each cell type. Careful biochemical analysis of both extracellular and intracellular signaling

Figure 15.4 Producing microarrays for gene expression analysis

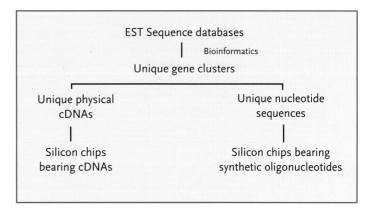

Expression microarray production

EST Sequence databases

| Bioinformatics

Unique gene clusters

Unique physical cDNAs

Unique nucleotide sequences

Silicon chips bearing cDNAs

Silicon chips bearing synthetic oligonucleotides

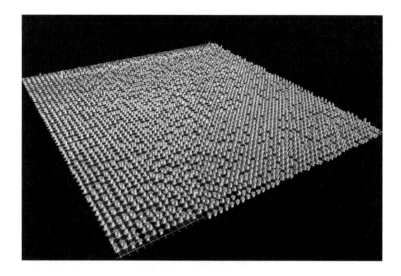

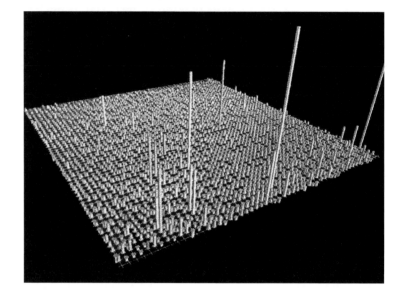

Figure 15.5 Gene expression changes amongst 3,000 selected human genes induced in human cells treated with the phorbol ester PMA, using a microarray.

pathways, such as those recently elucidated for TGF-β, provide exciting opportunities for multiple-target screening, while databases, such as the *E. coli* database EcoCyc, provide new ways of storing and enhancing such pathway information. Similar databases will undoubtedly emerge from mammalian systems as mammalian cell genome closure and proteomics advance.

An increasing emphasis on comparative genomics can be seen in the development of databases covering a broad spectrum of gene families, as well as specialist databases devoted to individual gene families (for example, the MEROPS protease database).

Table 15.1 Useful web-sites for genomic information	

Dictionary of Cell Biology	http://www.mblab.gla.ac.uk/~julian/Dict.html
JayDoc HistoWeb	http://www.kumc.edu/instruction/medicine/anatomy/histoweb/
MedWeb: Genetics and Molecular Biology	http://www.cc.emory.edu/WHSCL/medweb.gen.html
PathWeb, Virtual Pathology Museum	http://pathweb.uchc.edu/
Glaxo Virtual Anatomy Project	http://www.vis.colostate.edu/library/gva/gva.html
International Union of Pharmacology Home Page	http://iuphar.pharmacology.unimelb.edu.au/
MedWeb: Genetics and molecular biology	http://www.cc.emory.edu/WHSCL/medweb.gen.html
American Society of Human Genetics	http://www.faseb.org/genetics/gsa/gsamenu.htm
MicroArray Hompage	http://cmgm.stanford.edu/pbrown/
Caenorhabditis elegans WWW Server	http://elegans.swmed.edu/
The Catalog of Databases	http://www.infobiogen.fr/services/dbcat/
CBCG: Genome Databases	http://genome.cornell.edu/index.html
CGAP Home Page	http://www.ncbi.nlm.nih.gov/ncicgap/
Emotif: exploring the motif universe	http://dna.Stanford.EDU/emotif/
ESTablishing a Human Transcript Map, Boguski and Schuler	http://www.ncbi.nlm.nih.gov/Schuler/Papers/ESTtransmap/
EST Machine	http://office4.tigem.it/pages/ESTmachine.html
G-Protein Coupled Receptor Database	http://receptor.mgh.harvard.edu/GCRDBHOME.html/
GeneCards: integrating information about gene functions and biomedical applications	http://bioinfo.weizmann.ac.il/cards/
Gene Expression Information Resource Project	http://www.informatics.jax.org/doc/gxdgen.html
Gene Family Database	http://gdbdoc.gdb.org/~avoltz/home.html
GENETIC POLYMORPHISMS	http://ird04.pfizer.com/sptopic/poly/poly.html-ssi
The Genetics Society of America	http://www.faseb.org/genetics/acmg/acmgmenu.htm
The Genome Channel	http://compbio.ornl.gov/tools/channel/index.html
Genome database	http://gdbwww.gdb.org/
GenomeNet WWW server	http://www.genome.ad.jp/
Genome programs	http://megasun.bch.umontreal.ca/other/genomes.html
GenomeNet	http://www.genome.ad.jp/
GenWeb Home Page	http://www.genweb.com/
HGBASE (human SNPs site)	http://hgbase.interactiva.de/intro.html
Human Genome Program Home Page	http://www.er.doe.gov/production/oher/hug_top.html
Human Transcript Map	http://www.ncbi.nlm.nih.gov/SCIENCE96/
Human Genome Project Info	http://www.ornl.gov/TechResources/Human_Genome/home.html
KEGG - Kyoto Encyclopedia	http://www.genome.ad.jp/kegg/kegg.html
MEROPS Database. The	http://www.bi.bbsrc.ac.uk/Merops/

15.4.2 Genomics: relating cellular structure to biological function

The application of genomics to areas of biology such as drug delivery can be seen in two contexts:

- defining the system as a whole;
- defining specific molecular mechanisms which could be exploited for drug delivery.

Systematic approaches to biological function are encompassed within the broad area of "functional genomics".

For most of this century, our knowledge of cell biology has been primarily descriptive, reproducible *in vitro* work dating only from the 1960s. From the ability to induce neuronal cell differentiation to the observation of cellular apoptosis, cell culture is now offering radically new insights into the way in which genetic programs are executed at a functional level.

The advent of genomic biology places cell structure and structural biology in a new context. Processes fundamental to cell biology, such as protein translocation and apoptosis, can now be seen as variations on an evolutionarily conserved theme. The cysteine-containing aspartate-specific proteases, or caspases, which act in the apoptotic autocatalytic cascade, have largely been defined, often by homology searching of EST databases, while their characteristic tetrapeptide substrate sites have been used in motif searches to identify putative substrates. Interestingly, many of these important enzymes had already been identified by EST-based approaches, and patented, as early as 1994.

For drug discovery and delivery, this growing knowledge of cell biology is extremely useful. Not only has an intimate appreciation of cellular processes behind disease revealed new therapeutic targets, the inner workings of the cell have now become accessible to exploitation. The development of cell-based screening technologies, ranging from yeast-based screening to reporter gene assays, underlies the increasing trend towards directly harnessing cell biology to drug discovery.

Cell-based systems are biology's way of dividing the expressed genome into functional units. In drug discovery, a focus on specific cell systems, such as T-cells and fibroblasts for assembly of human immunodeficiency virus or herpes simplex virus particles and endothelial cells for demonstrating adhesion-dependent processes, often provides convenient primary drug screening systems.

Other single cell systems, such as yeast, and even entire organisms, such as *Caenorhabditis elegans*, have themselves been positioned as cell-based screening systems, capable of relatively high-throughput screening using appropriate reporters, or even visual analysis. The value of such systems for functional genomics and genetic engineering has been greatly enhanced by access to genome sequences of both organisms, and they may provide new and sensitive ways of examining the potential of new delivery mechanisms.

15.5 PROTEOMICS

Over recent years the realization that (i) most diseases are manifested at the protein level, (ii) therapeutic treatments primarily involve drug–protein interactions and (iii) there is often poor correlation between gene and protein expression has led to the development of the field of protein expression profiling – proteomics. The lack of correlation between gene and protein expression can be attributed to:

- differences in the location of gene expression and site of protein action within the cell;
- differences in the number of genes expressed and those which are ultimately translated into functional proteins;
- the differences in the relative stability and turnover of mRNA and the associated protein;
- post-transcriptional processing of mRNA yielding different protein products;
- post-transcriptional, such as glycosylation and phosphorylation of proteins which have important roles within cell biochemistry – for example in signal transduction pathways;
- formation of heterodimers and protein complexes which cannot be identified from the gene transcript alone.

Proteomics may therefore be more useful than genomics for identifying therapeutic targets within the cell. Until recently the development of proteomics was limited by the availability of technology to reproducibly separate protein components from the cellular pool and to specifically identify the protein sequence of small amounts of protein products. The development of 2 D polyacrylamide gels which separate proteins according to molecular weight in one dimension and charge in the other direction has provided a high-resolution quantitative method for separation of low levels of expressed proteins.

The generic proteomic processes is illustrated in Figure 15.6. Tissue extracts are pooled and initial protein purification undertaken using ion-exchange and affinity chromatography. The resultant protein fractions are further separated by reverse-phase high performance liquid chromatography. The fraction obtained from the HPLC separation are then further fractionated using 2 D polyacrylamide gel electrophoresis. This gives rise to a number of gels each containing individual protein bands. The bands are identified using standard techniques such as silver or fluorescent dyes and the expression profile may be used to compare expression of proteins in normal and diseased tissue or to examine changes in expression under stress conditions or following drug administration. In this way proteins associated with different diseased or stress conditions can be identified and the changes in protein expressions, for example, due to drug metabolism may be identified.

The specific proteins may be identified by *in situ* digestion and analysis by mass spectrometry. Recent developments in this technology have resulted in the technique being accepted as the primary tool for high-throughput, high-sensitivity protein analysis. The

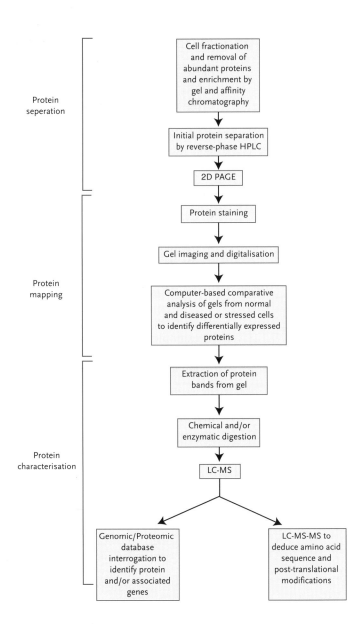

Figure 15.6 The generic approach to proteomic screening.

identification of the mass of individual peptide fragments allows the analyst to search genomic and protein sequence databases in order to find genes and/or proteins which would be expected to give the same fragmentation patterns. A highly matched database sequence will provide the full sequence and identify the protein.

Although reliable, this technique may lead to false positive results in some cases. To overcome this problem many proteomic companies are now adopting the technique of tandem mass spectrometry to unambiguously identify protein sequences. This technique subjects proteins to successive routines of fragmentation and mass analysis in order to provide the actual amino acid sequence.

15.6 Pharmacogenomics and pharmacoproteomics

In addition to screening for new therapeutic targets for lead candidate selection, pharmacogeneomics and pharmacoproteomics have a number of other preclinical and clinical applications.

Mode of drug action

By probing drug treated cells for expression of genes and proteins it may be possible to more precisely identify the specific mode of action of a drug of known therapeutic value, for example natural herbal remedies, thereby offering opportunities to develop new drugs for such therapeutic conditions.

Toxicology

The monitoring of expression of certain genes and proteins in, for example, hepatic cells offers a means of detecting upregulation of metabolic enzymes such as P450 isoenzymes. This may provide a means, in combination with HTS, of identifying potential drug interactions at an early stage in the drug development process. Similarly, such profiling may also provide opportunities to identify the mechanisms of drug toxicity of therapeutic agents in order to design new drugs to overcome these problems.

Clinical applications

These technologies will also allow the screening of patients for particular diseases or metabolic polymorphisms, which may dictate whether a patient is a rapid or slow metabolizer of certain drugs. Such response markers will allow more stringent selection criteria to be applied to clinical trials selection and could also be used to more specifically adjust a drug dosing regimen to a particular patient's metabolic profile. Such diagnostic screens allow more effective patient treatment and the development of therapeutic agents specifically designed for the treatment of specific patient subpopulations.

In the future these screening techniques will allow us to more readily identify upregulated enzymes in diseased tissues which will facilitate the development of prodrug-based technologies for the site-specific chemical delivery of drugs to these diseased cells. The identification of surface-expressed disease-specific ligands will allow targeting of polymeric and microparticulate drug delivery systems to these particular diseased cells through the use of molecular entities specifically targeted against these ligands.

It is clear that genomics and proteomics are complementary in that genomics has an important role in providing data for elucidating amino acid sequences identified through proteomics, and proteomics provides a means of identifying those genes which have functional importance. The identification of future therapeutic targets will be driven by cross-fertilization between these two disciplines through bioinformatics.

15.7 EXPLOITING PROTEOMICS AND GENOMICS IN DRUG TARGETING

Proteomics and genomics provide means of identifying differences between normal and diseased tissue which may be used for targeting of drug substances to these particular tissues.

One of the most exciting new areas of drug delivery is prodrug activation. A perfect prodrug is a molecule which has no intrinsic pharmacological activity until it is converted enzymatically to a new molecular form which displays pharmacological activity.

In principle, prodrug activation simply mirrors activation processes which are used widely in biological systems to regulate important enzymatic cascades. A particularly widespread example in biology is pro-protease activation, in which a small "extension" peptide can be used to restrain or "mask" inherent proteolytic activities which, if they occurred in inappropriate tissue locations, would pose a major problem. The digestive proteases enterokinase, trypsin and chymotrypsin are well-known examples of this phenomenon, although there are now a wide range of examples in which proteolytic activation cascades are known to regulate processes as diverse as virus assembly and 7-transmembrane receptor activation. It has been estimated that over 2% of the expressed human genome is accounted for by proteases of one specificity or another, although only 300 of the expected 2,000 that this would indicate have so far been characterized. Elucidating the biological roles and locations of these novel proteases will provide opportunities for both new therapeutic target identification and protease-activated cell targeting of both macromolecules and small molecule drugs.

In the context of drug delivery, certain cell surface receptor and ion-channel families are particularly appealing as drug delivery targets. Well-characterized examples include the lectin-like receptor gene family as receptors for glycosylated molecules, as well as vitamin- and trace element-uptake systems such as the transferrin-receptor.

In the past, various serendipitous discoveries have capitalized on the differential expression of enzymes by host and viral infected cells. For example, the prodrug Acyclovir, used widely for the treatment of herpes simplex and herpes zoster infections, is selectively activated through phosphorylation by *viral* thymidine kinase to acyclovir monophosphate which is then converted to the triphosphate, which inhibits DNA polymerase, by host cellular enzymes. Similarly several 2',3'-dideoxynucleoside analogs such as Zidovudine (azidothymidine, AZT) and 2',3'-didehydro-3'-deoxythymidine (D4T) have potent antiviral activity against human immunodeficiency virus (HIV). These compounds are selectively phosphorylated intracellularly to the 5'-triphosphate derivatives which inhibit the viral reverse transcriptase.

Drug delivery and targeting is a key area which will benefit from cell and tissue-based information. It seems reasonable to expect similarly sophisticated drug delivery end-points to be achievable through design or screening approaches, given an understanding of the tissue-specific expression of particular activating enzymes, possibly mirroring those already exploited by naturally occurring viruses.

15.8 BIOINFORMATICS

Bioinformatics is the management and analysis of data arising from the fields of proteomics and genomics. The storage of genomic and protein sequences in easily searchable databases to allow comparison of protein and genomic sequences is essential if companies are to maximize the value of their biological data. There are now a number of high quality protein and genetic databases documenting the protein and gene expression of specific cell types under different conditions. Such databases have proved invaluable to companies investigating specific disease states.

With the increasing automation of drug discovery with respect to combinatorial chemistry, high-throughput screening, proteomics and genomics, informatics has developed an increasingly important role. The integration of robotics and informatics with databases correlating molecular properties with biological properties is becoming increasingly important for the management of compound libraries.

Such informatic systems allow companies to readily search compound libraries and identify agents with potential activity against other therapeutic targets. Robotic automation provides a means of extracting these libraries or further screening from storage as necessary. The combination of biological and chemical data in relational databases provides useful data for the computer-based database searching and advanced quantitative structure-activity-relationship studies. The power of these databases in identifying potential lead compounds against new disease states will increase with the integration of proteomic data. For example, knowing that a specific compound class interacts strongly with a particular peptide motif at various receptors/catalytic sites will facilitate the identification of lead compounds for receptors/enzymes with similar motifs.

15.8.1 Adding value to sequence databases through bioinformatics

The efficient exploitation of such exponentially increasing data requires close alignment of bioinformatics with the needs of drug discovery and development. Generic approaches towards the identification of new targets for human drug discovery are now routinely practised within pharmaceutical companies. Early in the process is the "mining" of the currently available DNA sequence databases to identify novel members of gene families with existing "drug target" pedigrees which may be involved in either the development of specific diseases or new strategies for their treatment. Simply trawling these databases for potential targets expressed in diseased tissue has already yielded novel homologs of key enzymes and receptors, many of which have been patented as drug discovery targets. We are still at an early stage of understanding the full complexity of the mammalian and human genetic vocabulary.

A more pharmaceutically oriented approach is to search for novel members of certain key receptor families which are already known from pharmacological studies to be present in a target tissue. This combination of pharmacology and molecular biology is proving particularly interesting, identifying far greater heterogeneity amongst targets than had previously been thought, with both receptor subtypes and the differential splicing of individual genes contributing to this complexity.

The effective management of chemical and biological data underpins the effectiveness of any drug discovery group. All these aspects of drug discovery will impinge on drug delivery and targeting in the future.

15.9 CONCLUSIONS

The advances in drug discovery impinge on drug delivery and targeting by (i) offering through genomics and proteomics means of (a) identifying novel cell specific targeting moieties for drug delivery systems and (b) identifying cellular differences which may facilitate the more effective targeting of delivery systems to specific subsets of cells and (ii) providing wider molecular diversity in the development of new chemical entities potentially allowing the selection of drugs on the basis of their biopharmceutical profile in addition to their affinity and selectivity for a specific therapeutic target. Furthermore, combinatorial chemistry and high-throughput screening will provide targeting molecules for disease-associated surface-expressed receptors and ligands. These may be linked to therapeutic drug molecules to increase epithelial transport by active transport processes and drug targeting selectivity.

15.10 FURTHER READING

Adams, M.D., Kelley, J.M., Gocayne, J.D., Dubnick, M., Polymeropoulos, M.H., Xiao, H., Merril, C.R., Wu, A., Olde, B., Moreno, R.F., Kerlavage, A.R., McCombie, W.R. and Venter, J.C. (1991) Complementary DNA sequencing: expressed sequence tags and human genome project. *Science*, 252:1651–1656.

Ashton, C. (1999) Reinventing drug development. *Chemistry and Industry*, 422–425.

Cronin, M.T., Fucini, R.V., Kim, S.M., Masino, R.S., Wespi, R.M. and Miyada, C.G. (1996) Cystic Fibrosis mutation detection by hybridization to light-generated DNA probe arrays. *Human Mutation*, 7:244–255.

DeRisi, J., Penland, L., O'Brown, P.O., Bittner, M.L., Meltzer, P.S., Ray, M., Chen, Y., Su, Y.A. and Trent, J.M. (1996) Use of a cDNA microarray to analyse gene expression patterns in human cancer. *Nature Genetics*, 14:457–460.

Dyer, M.R., Cohne, D. and Herrling, P.L. (1999) Functional genomics: from genes to new therapies. *Drug Discovery Today*, 4:109–114.

Fields, S. (1997) The future is function. *Nature Genetics*, 15:325–327.

Livak, K.J., Marmaro, J. and Todd, J.A. (1995) Towards fully automated genome-wide polymorphism screening. *Nature Genetics*, 9:341–342.

Lowe, G. (1995) Combinatorial Chemistry. *Chemical Society Reviews*, 309–317.

Sneader, W. (1985) *Drug discovery: the evolution of modern medicines.* John Wiley, Chichester, UK.

Terrett, N.K., Gardner, M., Gordon, D.W., Kobylecki, R.J. and Steele, J. (1995) Combinatorial synthesis – the design of compound libraries and their application to drug discovery. *Tetrahedron*, 51:8135–8173.

Wang, J.H. and Hewick, R.M. (1999) Proteomics in drug discovery. *Drug Discovery Today*, 4:129–133.

15.11 SELF-ASSESSMENT QUESTIONS

1. Outline the principles of combinatorial synthesis.
2. Describe the "split and mix" approach to combinatorial chemistry.
3. Outline the techniques used in proteomics.
4. Outline the techniques uses in genomics.
5. Explain the importance of the interrelationship between proteomics and genomics.
6. Explain the importance of bioinformatics in relation to proteomics and genomics.
7. Describe the potential roles of proteomics and genomics in drug delivery and targeting.
8. Identify two ways in which combinatorial chemistry may impinge on drug delivery and targeting.
9. Describe two types of assay used in high-throughput screening.
10. List three uses of robotics in drug discovery.

16

New Generation Technologies

Hongkee Sah, Yie W. Chien, Haesun Park, Sun-Joo Hwang, Kinam Park and Andrew W. Lloyd

OBJECTIVES

On completion of this chapter the reader should be able to:

- Outline the approaches for achieving cell-specific chemical-based drug delivery using prodrugs
- Describe the use of biosensors in addressing the challenge of chronopharmacology
- Describe the approaches to bioresponsive drug delivery
- Outline the use of microchips for controlled drug delivery
- Describe the use of genetically engineered cell implants in drug delivery

16.1 INTRODUCTION

The interrelationship between drug discovery and delivery becomes increasingly important with respect to the rapid development of pharmaceutically efficacious drugs. The preceding chapters in the last part of this book have highlighted the recent developments in gene therapy, drug discovery, genomics and proteomics as a consequence of the recent developments in molecular biology and chemistry. This chapter concludes this text by examining how the advances in chemistry and biology are providing opportunities for more effective site-specific drug targeting and bioresponsive pulsatile drug delivery. The chapter considers the development of prodrug-based technologies for cell-specific drug delivery, provides an overview of the use of smart polymeric systems, microchips and genetically engineered cell-based implants in addressing the challenges of chronopharmacology, and offers a perspective of the future of drug delivery and targeting in this new millennium.

16.2 RATIONALIZING DRUG DESIGN, DISCOVERY AND DELIVERY

The ability to synthesize large libraries of chemical entities of diverse molecular structures offers the potential to consider the challenges of drug delivery at the earlier stages of pharmaceutical development through rational design, discovery and development. In the discovery process opportunities exist, as illustrated in Chapter 15, to identify cell-specific enzymes and ligands which may be used to target drugs to these cells. The integration of the considerations for drug delivery and targeting into the drug design process may ultimately allow the development of drugs which are not just potent and non-toxic but offer the advantage that their chemical structure dictates the targeting of the drug to its particular site of action through enzyme-based chemical delivery systems using prodrugs.

16.2.1 Prodrugs

Although pharmaceutical companies attempt to design and develop new chemical entities using rational and logical processes, very few of these compounds become clinically useful drugs because unpredictable interactions with biological systems reduce therapeutic efficacy and in many cases lead to undesirable toxicity. As initially discussed in Section 1.3.4.1, prodrug design offers an alternative approach to enhance therapeutic activity through the chemical modification of known compounds to overcome the undesirable physical and chemical properties.

A prodrug is a pharmacaologically inactive compound which undergoes chemical or enzymatic metabolism to the active. Some of the early pharmaceuticals were found to be prodrugs and this finding has led to the subsequent introduction of the metabolite itself into therapy, particularly in cases where the active metabolite is less toxic or has fewer side-effects than the parent prodrug. The administration of the active metabolite may also reduce variability in clinical response between individuals due to differences in pharmacogenetics.

Most chemically designed prodrugs consist of two components; the active drug chemically linked to a pharmacologically inert moiety. The prodrug must be sufficiently stable to withstand the pharmaceutical formulation while permitting chemical or enzymatic cleavage at the appropriate time or site. After administration or absorption of the prodrug, the active drug is usually released by either chemical or enzymatic, hydrolytic or reductive processes. Prodrugs are most commonly used to overcome the biological and pharmaceutical barriers which separate the site of administration of the drug from the site of action (Figure 16.1).

Prodrug design has been used to address a wide range of pharmaceutical problems including:

- unpalatability
- gastric irritation
- pain on injection
- insolubility
- instability.

Prodrug design has also been used widely to address pharmacological problems such as poor drug adsorption and drug distribution. As discussed in Chapter 1, prodrugs may be used to enhance the absorption of poorly adsorbed drugs by increasing the lipophilicity of the drug molecule.

Figure 16.1 A diagrammatic representation of the prodrug concept where a pharmaceutically active drug is converted to an inactive compound to overcome pharmaceutical and biological barriers between the site of administration and the site of action

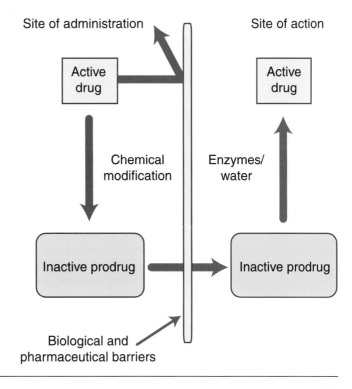

The modification of a drug to a prodrug may also lead to enhanced efficacy by differential distribution of the prodrug to particular body tissues before the release of the active drug.

For example, the administration of the methoxymethyl ester of hetacillin (a 6-side-chain derivative of ampicillin) leads to a more extensive distribution of ampicillin in the body tissues than occurs on administration of ampicillin itself. Conversely, the restriction of tissue distribution which decreases toxic side-effects by restricting the action of a drug to a specific target site in the body may also be achieved through the use of certain prodrug systems as described below. An alternative strategy is to utilize phenotypic differences between cell types to target prodrugs to particular sites within the body through site-specific enzyme-based delivery systems.

16.2.2 Site-specific enzyme-based delivery systems

Site-specific prodrugs are designed to ensure that the release of the active drug only occurs at its site of action thereby reducing toxic side-effects due to high plasma concentrations of the drug or non-specific uptake by other body tissues by utilizing enhanced enzyme or chemical activity of a particular cell type. This has led to the development of systems for site-specific delivery to tumor cells which exploit the unique microenvironment of the tumor.

Improved selective localization of anticancer agents to neoplastic tissue may be achieved using non-toxic prodrugs which release the active drug within the tumor as a result of enhanced enzyme activity in the cell. For example, the prodrug cyclophosphamide is initially activated by hepatic cell enzymes to generate 4-hydroxycyclophosphamide which is then specifically converted to the alkylating cytotoxic phosphoramide mustard in the target cells.

As the blood supply to large solid tumors is disorganized, the internal regions are often non-vasculated and the cells, termed hypoxic, deprived of oxygen. The absence of molecular oxygen enhances the reductase activity in hypoxic tissues providing an alternative means of targeting the internal regions of solid tumors using a selective chemical prodrug-delivery system. Certain aromatic, heterocyclic nitro-containing compounds can be reduced in hypoxic environments to produce intermediates which then fragment into alkylating species. For example, the 2-nitro-imidazole compound misonidazole is selectively cytotoxic to cultured hypoxic cells. An alternative approach utilizes the bioactivation of aromatic nitrogen mustards through the reduction of a substituent group in the aryl ring.

More recently it has been suggested that bioreductive technologies may have applications in the treatment of other disease states. For example, it has been suggested that the essential role of hypoxia in rheumatoid arthritis offers opportunities to specifically deliver anti-inflammatory agents to arthritic joints using bioreductive prodrugs.

As indicated in Chapter 15, the development of genomics and proteomics will undoubtedly provide further information of the differential experessions of enzymes in diseased and normal tissues. This will allow the future development of prodrug-based chemical delivery systems to target specific cell types through the use of the upregulated enzymes in diseased tissues to release the active drug.

16.2.3 Redox-based drug delivery

Although lipophilic prodrugs may be used to overcome the impenetrability of the blood-brain barrier to highly polar drugs, the increased lipid solubility may enhance uptake in other tissues with a resultant increase in toxicity. Furthermore, therapeutic levels of lipophilic prodrugs in the brain can only be maintained if there is an equivalent constant plasma concentration. These problems may be overcome by utilizing a drug delivery system which relies on "trapping" a prodrug in the brain by oxidizing the prodrug to a less membrane permeable derivative. This approach was first used to enhance the CNS penetration of the nerve gas antagonist pralidoxine using a non-polar prodrug which crosses the blood-brain barrier but is then rapidly oxidized to the active form and trapped in the CNS.

More recently a general approach using the dihydropyridine-pyridinium salt redox systems has been developed for the site-specific and sustained delivery of drugs with poor CNS penetration or which undergo rapid CNS metabolism. Both phenylethylamine and dopamine have been used to illustrate the principles of this technology and *in vivo* work has been described in animal studies. The delivery system for phenylethylamine is summarized in Figure 16.2. The 1,4-dihydro-prodrug is prepared by reduction of a quaternized nicotinic acid derivative of phenylethylamine. On administration the prodrug is delivered directly to the brain, where it is oxidized and trapped as the quaternary ammonium salt. Sustained release of the biologically active phenylethylamine and elimination of the carrier molecule occur through enzymatic hydrolysis in the CNS. The metabolism and elimination of the drug from the periphery removes excess drug and metabolic products during and after onset of the required action. This overcomes the need to maintain plasma levels which may cause systemic side-effects.

16.2.4 Antibody-directed enzyme prodrug therapy (ADEPT)

It is also possible to target drugs to specific cells through their specific surface ligands using antibody-directed enzyme prodrug therapy (ADEPT) (Figure 16.3). The approach has been used most extensively to target drugs to tumor cells by employing an enzyme, not normally present in the extracellular fluid or on cell membranes, conjugated to an antitumor antibody which localizes in the tumor via an antibody–antigen interaction on administration. Following clearance of any unbound antibody conjugate from the systemic circulation, a prodrug, which is specifically activated by the enzyme conjugate, is administered. The bound enzyme–antibody conjugate ensures that the prodrug is only converted to the cytotoxic parent compound at the tumor site thereby reducing systemic toxicity. For example, using cytosine deaminase to generate 5-fluorouracil from the 5-fluorocytosine prodrug at tumor sites increases the delivery to

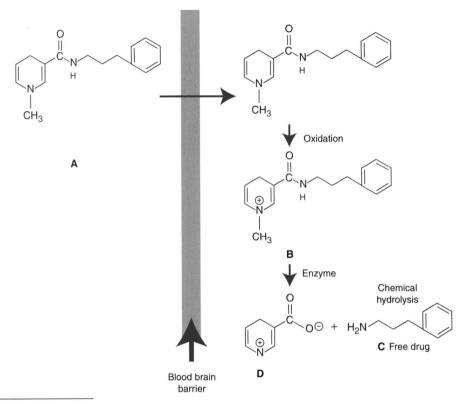

Blood brain
barrier

Figure 16.2
Dihydropyridine-
pyridinium salt redox
system for site-specific
and sustained delivery
to the brain. The
prodrug **A** is delivered
directly to the brain,
where it is oxidized
and trapped as the
prodrug **B**. The
quaternary ammonium
salt is slowly cleaved
by chemical/enzymatic
action with sustained
release of the
biologically active
phenylethylamine **C**
and the facile
elimination of the
carrier molecule **D**.
Elimination of the drug
from the general
circulation is by
comparison
accelerated, either as **A**
or **B** or as cleavage
products

the tumor by 17 fold compared to that achieved on administration of
5-fluorouracil alone.

The ADEPT approach has been recently investigated as a means of
overcoming the side-effects of using taxol to treat breast cancer by utilizing a β-lactamase enzyme antitumor antibody conjugate and a
cepham sulfoxide derivative of taxol (PROTAX). The localized β-lacta-
mase enzyme, which is not normally found in any other tissues,
ensures selective release of taxol at the tumor site. The prodrug is
almost as effective as taxol on cultured human breast cells which have
been treated with the enzyme-bound antibody; however, PROTAX
alone is significantly less toxic to cancer cells and is therefore less likely
to be cytotoxic to normal tissue.

16.2.5 Gene-directed enzyme prodrug therapy (GDEPT)

As described in Chapter 14, the development of molecular biology has
led to the ability to transfect cells with suicide genes. Suicide genes
encode for nonmammalian enzymes which can be used to convert a
prodrug into a cytotoxic agent. Cells which are genetically modified to
express such genes essentially commit metabolic suicide on administration of the appropriate prodrug. Typical suicide genes include
herpes simplex thymidine kinase and *Escherichia coli* cytosine deaminase. Although any gene delivery vector may be employed to deliver
the gene (see Section 14.1), much of the pioneering work in this field
has been undertaken using viral vectors. To ensure tumor-specific

Tumour

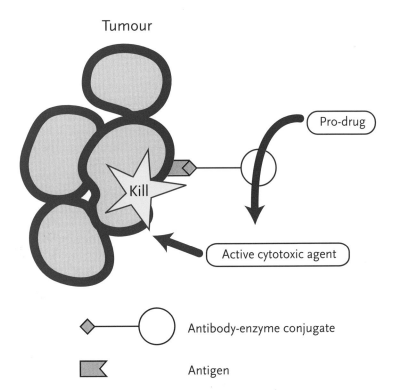

Figure 16.3 A schematic diagram showing the principles of antibody-directed enzyme-prodrug therapy (ADEPT)

transcription of the suicide gene, the suicide gene is encoded downstream of a tumor-specific transcription unit such as the proximal ERBB2 promoter. As the ERBB2 oncogene is overexpressed in approximately a third of all breast and pancreatic tumors this ensures only tumor cells express the suicide gene. For example, *in vitro* studies have been undertaken using a chimeric minigene construct, consisting of the proximal ERBB2 promoter linked to a gene coding for cytosine deaminase, incorporated into a double-copy recombinant retrovirus. *In vitro* studies, using pancreatic and breast cell lines, have shown that treatment of cells expressing ERBB2 with the viral vector and 5-fluorocytosine causes significant cell death, whereas cells which do not express ERBB2 are unaffected.

These chemical approaches to advanced drug targeting are embryonic and their future development will be dependent on the "fruits" of the genomic and proteomic revolutions. Even though it may ultimately be possible to develop site-specific chemical drug delivery systems for a wide range of therapeutic applications, there will still be a need to address the challenges of chronopharmacology in order to achieve better therapeutic control.

16.3 THE CHALLENGE OF CHRONOPHARMACOLOGY

The challenge of chronopharmacology was introduced in Chapter 1 (Section 1.5.2) and highlighted the needs to control drug delivery to accommodate:

- circadian rhythms;
- fluctuating metabolic requirements;
- complex endogenous feedback controls.

Such control requires means of sensing and responding to changes in biological stimuli. This can be achieved by having either a separate biosensor which electronically controls drug release from a drug delivery device or a combination system in which the stimulus has a direct effect on the release of drug from the system. Both these approaches are described in detail below.

16.3.1 Biosensors

A biosensor is a sensing device that is integrated within or intimately associated with a physical transducer. Such a system quantifies electronic signals arising from the interaction between a biosensor and an analyte of interest. Catalytic biosensors use enzymes, microorganisms, or whole cells to catalyze a reaction with the target analyte, while affinity biosensors utilize antibodies, receptors, or nucleic acids to bind with the target analyte.

The integration of biosensors with drug delivery systems allows the controlled release of a drug substance in response to the levels of biological modulator. For example, the use of a glucose biosensor may be used to control the release of insulin from an implanted device or perhaps even an iontophoretic delivery device (see Chapter 8).

The MiniMed Model 2001 implant pump described in Chapter 4 (Section 4.6.2.2) is an open-loop system that does not measure blood glucose levels in diabetic patients. Following physicians' recommendation, patients have to frequently test glucose concentrations by collecting blood or urine samples. A closed-loop system, which automatically monitors the change in glucose levels and accordingly dispenses an accurate dose of insulin, would present an ideal insulin therapy for long-term routine patient care. Concerted research efforts to develop an implantable glucose monitor have been driven by the necessity for such an ideal insulin therapy. A presently available external potentiometric glucose sensor has glucose oxidase affixed on the top of a pH electrode. The enzymatic action on glucose leads to the formation of gluconic acid and hydrogen peroxide. The potential change induced by the pH change is then quantified by a transducer. An amperometric sensor also depends on the enzyme-catalyzed oxidation of glucose, but measures the change in current as a function of the concentration of hydrogen peroxide.

Synthetic Blood International (Kettering, OH) is one of the companies focusing on the development and commercialization of an implantable glucose monitor. Its implantable device consists of a titanium-encased battery and microprocessor, a silicone-sheathed platinum electrode and glucose oxidase immobilized in a semipermeable membrane. Figure 16.4 illustrates the major components of the implantable glucose monitor that would be surgically placed under the skin in diabetic patients. The implantable monitor is about the size of a pacemaker and is connected to an external telemetry device. The

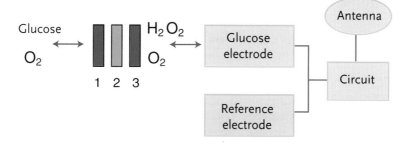

1 Polycarbonate membrane
2 Immobilized glucose oxidase
3 Cellulose acetate membrane

Figure 16.4 Schematic illustration of the implantable glucose monitor under development at Synthetic Blood International. The biosensing mechanism is based on the glucose oxidase-catalyzed oxidation of glucose drawn from tissue fluids. After the enzymatic metabolism, the ratio of hydrogen peroxide to oxygen is detected and expressed by a change in electric current. This signal is transmitted to the receiver outside the body

structure of the inner enzyme layer attenuates the amount of glucose that permeates through. When the immobilized enzyme is in contact with glucose, it produces gluconic acid and hydrogen peroxide at the expense of oxygen. The resultant change in the ratio of hydrogen peroxide to oxygen affects the current in the sensor, and its signal is transmitted to the receiver outside the body. An accurate blood glucose concentration can be inferred from the levels of glucose in tissue fluids. The implantable glucose monitor is expected to be a convenient, reliable alternative to daily finger sticks or pen-sized external glucose monitors frequently used to check glucose levels in diabetic patients.

Although state-of-the-art biosensor technology allows rapid detection of low concentrations of biological molecules, the biofouling of implanted sensors still represents a major challenges. The conditioning of biosensors with serum proteins following implantation reduces the sensitivity and longevity of such devices. Such foreign bodies also elicit an acute inflammatory response which may ultimately result in encapsulation of the implant in a fibrous matrix (see Section 4.3).

Various approaches are presently being investigated to reduce the biofouling and bioincompatibility of such devices including the use of biocompatible coatings. These coatings include systems such as the biomimetic phosphorylcholine-based technologies developed to improve the biocompatibility of medical implants and the poly(ethylene oxide) technologies described in Chapter 5 as means of increasing the circulation times of liposomes.

An alternative approach is to have an external biosensor. The patch-based glucose biosensor is an example of this approach. This system uses electroosmosis to sample serum glucose levels through the skin using a patch-device containing a glucose biosensor.

Even though several glucose biosensors are already in clinical studies, their commercialization is still a formidable task and awaits many years' multidisciplinary research effort. Presently more than 90% of the biosensor industry focuses on glucose sensing systems, but future biosensor technology will offer a more diversified therapeutic horizon including the detection of neurotoxins and the screening of specific diseases.

16.3.2 Stimuli-sensitive intelligent hydrogels

To create biomimetic systems that can release a drug in response to biological needs, many researchers are now focusing on the development of hydrogel-based drug delivery systems. A hydrogel is defined as an entangled network of polymer chains in which a solvent pervades. The degree of cross-linking in a hydrogel determines the flexibility and elasticity of the polymeric network. The dimension of the polymeric network, as well as the content of a solvent present inside, strongly depends upon polymer–polymer and polymer–solvent interactions. Physical forces involved in the noncovalent interactions can be classified into two categories. The first category is represented by electrostatic interactions including ion–ion, ion–dipole interactions, and hydrogen bonding. Dipole–dipole, dipole-induced dipole interactions, and London dispersion forces are grouped together under the general term of van der Waals forces. These forces constitute the second category. If strong attractive forces exist between polymer and water, absorption of water by the polymeric network is thermodynamically favored. This results in the swelling and expansion of the polymeric network. By contrast, if the polymer is poorly solvated, each polymer unit prefers to stick together in order to minimize its exposure to the solvent. In this case the polymeric network tends to collapse or shrink, liberating the solvent out of the polymeric network.

Intrigued by the idea that a drug delivery system may make use of such changes in physical properties of a polymeric network, researchers around the world orchestrated considerable efforts to develop innovative hydrogels. Their research has aimed at the discovery of hydrogels that display a sudden change in properties in response to environmental stimuli including pH, temperature, ionic strength, electromagnetic radiation, electric fields, shear, sonic radiation, enzyme substrates or affinity ligands. Variations in the chemical structure of a hydrogel and the composition of a solvent make it possible to fabricate such responsive hydrogels. For example, a hydrogel can either swell a hundred times in volume or collapses in response to a subtle change in temperature as little as a 1 °C. Other hydrogels do not swell or collapse, but their physical property changes from sol to gel or vice versa. Due to the softness and flexibility of hydrogels, a hydrogel-based implantable device would provide minimal friction to surrounding tissues and house delicate materials, especially proteins or cells, without causing damage to them. The low interfacial tension between the hydrogel surface and biological fluids would minimize protein adsorption and cell adhesion, thereby displaying excellent biocompatibility.

16.3.2.1 Temperature-sensitive gels

Temperature-sensitive gels have previously been described for nasal (Section 9.7.2.2), ophthalmic (Section 12.3.3.4) and vaginal (Section 11.7.6) drug delivery applications. The SmartGel, previously mentioned in the context of vaginal drug delivery, is an example of temperature-sensitive hydrogels. It is a viscoelastic soft gel at room temperature but becomes much firmer at body temperature. This interesting property allows the gel to be used as a shoe insert to tailor the shape of the shoe to the need of an individual wearer. Table 16.1 illustrates polymeric materials that are used to fabricate temperature-sensitive hydrogels for medical applications. An aqueous solution of poly(N-isopropylacrylamide) has a critical transition temperature at 32 ~ 37 °C. Below the critical transition temperature, the polymeric solution is transparent. Above the critical transition temperature, however, polymer strands interact with one another to make a gel structure. A similar change is also observed with the graft copolymer of poly(N-isopropylacrylamide) and polyacrylamide. Its interesting gellation tendency is utilized to immobilize cells inside the gel matrix. For example, a polymeric solution containing islets of Langerhans (insulin-releasing pancreatic cells) is loaded into a pouch with a semi-permeable membrane. When the pouch is implanted, the solution becomes a gel to serve as a matrix to immobilize the cells. Responding to rising glucose levels in diabetic patients, the islets would secrete insulin to maintain a normal glycemic level. It was demonstrated that free islets of Langerhans dispersed in a solution tended to aggregate and lost their viability quickly, while the cells immobilized in the gel matrix remained intact and viable much longer.

Graft copolymers of poloxamers and either poly(acrylic acid) or chitosan change from a sol to a gel at temperature above 37 °C. The appearing gel forms a stable matrix that can retain a drug for its sustained release. The triblock copolymer consisting of poly(ethylene oxide)–poly(l-lactide)–poly(ethylene oxide) (PEO–PLLA–PEO) is also temperature-sensitive but shows an opposite gellation property. At low concentrations, the close association of PLLA blocks results in the formation of micelles. At room temperature, gellation is followed by a further increase in the polymer concentration due to packing of the micelles. Interestingly, the gel is changed into a sol at an elevated temperature such as 45 °C. Upon subcutaneous injection of the polymeric solution into the body (37 °C), a gel is formed immediately. If a drug is dissolved in the polymeric solution prior to the injection, the gel would function as a sustained release matrix for the entrapped drug. The critical gel–sol transition temperature is conveniently modified by varying the length of each block and molecular weight of the triblock polymer.

Table 16.1 Polymers used for fabricating temperature-responsive hydrogels

Polymers	Biodegradability
Poly(methyl vinyl ether)	nonbiodegradable
Poly(N-isopropylacrylamide)	nonbiodegradable
Poly(N-isopropylacrylamide) and poly(acrylic acid) graft copolymer	nonbiodegradable
Poly(N-isopropylacrylamide) and poly(methacrylic acid) graft copolymer	nonbiodegradable
Poly(N-isopropylacrylamide) and Pluronic graft copolymer	nonbiodegradable
Poloxomer[a] and polyacrylic acid graft copolymer (so-called Smart Hydrogel)	nonbiodegradable
Poloxomer and chitosan[b] graft copolymer	biodegradable/bioerodible
Poly(ethylene oxide) - poly(l-lactide)[b] block copolymer	biodegradable/bioerodible
Poly(ethylene oxide) - poly(l-lactide) - Poly(ethylene oxide) block copolymer	biodegradable/bioerodible

[a]Poloxomer (such as Pluorincs) represents the triblock copolymer of poly(ethylene oxide)–poly(propylene oxide)–poly(ethylene oxide); poly(ethylene oxide) and poly(propylene oxide) are bioerodible. [b]Poly(l-lactide) and chitosan are biodegradable.

16.3.2.2 pH-sensitive gels

Many polyanionic materials, such as poly(acrylic acid), are pH sensitive and the degree of swelling of such polymers can be modulated by changing the pH. An application of such technology has been in the development of biomimetic secretory granules for drug delivery applications.

Secretory granules within certain cells consist of a polyanionic polymer network encapsulated within a lipid membrane. The polymer network, which contains biological mediators such as histamine, exists in a collapsed state as a consequence of the internal pH and ionic content which is maintained by the lipid surrounding the granule. Release of histamine from such granules is initiated through the fusion of the granule with the cell membrane exposing the polyanionic internal matrix to the extracellular environment. The change in pH and ionic strength results in ion exchange and swelling of the polyanionic network which in turn causes release of the endogenous mediators.

An environmentally responsive, hydrogel microsphere coated with a lipid bilayer has recently been shown to act as a secretory granule mimic (Figure 16.5). Methylene-bis-acrylamide/methacrylic acid anionic microgels were prepared by precipitation polymerization and loaded with doxorubicin and condensed by incubating in buffer at pH 5. The condensed particles were then coated with a lipid bilayer. Disruption of the lipid bilayer by electroporation was shown to cause the microgel particles to swell and release their drug.

The use of these systems in conjunction with temperature-sensitive lipids offers potential to target drugs to areas of inflammation or to

Figure 16.5 A schematic diagram showing the release of drug from a biomimetic secretory granule on disruption of the external lipid bilayer

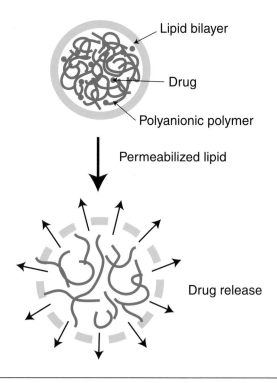

Lipid bilayer

Drug

Polyanionic polymer

Permeabilized lipid

Drug release

achieve site-specific, pulsatile drug delivery through the localized external application of ultrasound or heating to disrupt the lipid bilayers.

16.3.3 Bioresponsive drug delivery systems

In addition to the ability to be a stable matrix for the sustained release of drug and cell implant vehicles, implantable hydrogels have the potential to act like chemical valves that respond to external stimuli. This concept may be visualized by an example of an electrical stimulus-sensitive hydrogel. If it is fabricated into a porous membrane of which edges are fixed in place, the presence and removal of the stimulus would start and stop the exchange of a drug with body fluids. For example, if the implant is exposed to the stimulus, pores in the hydrogel membrane would become wide-open to turn on the chemical valve. Subsequently, the contents of the implant are discharged at the site of implantation. The removal of the stimulus turns off the valve to contract the membrane pores, thereby stopping the flow of the contents. The release of a drug from such an implant, therefore, is at the operator's control. Such implants have potential to release a drug in a pulsatile manner, according to patients' biological needs. The focus of such research has been towards the delivery of insulin in response to changes in glucose levels.

16.3.3.1 Glucose-sensing hydrogels

Hydrogels can be made to undergo sol–gel phase transformation depending on the glucose concentration in the environment. Preparation of glucose-sensitive phase-reversible hydrogels demands two fundamental requirements: glucose-specificity and reversible cross-linking (i.e. physical cross-linking).

A highly specific interaction between glucose and concanavalin A (Con A) was used to form physical cross-links between glucose-containing polymer chains. Since Con A exists as a tetramer at physiological pH and each subunit has a glucose binding site, Con A can function as a cross-linking agent for glucose-containing polymer chains. Because of the non-covalent interaction between glucose and Con A, the formed cross-links are reversible (Figure 16.6). Individual free glucose molecules can compete with the polymer-attached glucose molecules. Thus, the maintenance of the cross-links depends on the relative concentration of free glucose in the environment. The gel is formed by mixing glucose-containing polymers with Con A in the absence of external glucose. In the presence of elevated glucose levels in solution, however, the gel becomes a sol (i.e. the gel dissociates into a solution). As the environmental glucose level decreases again, the competition of free glucose against the polymer-bound glucose decreases and thus the gel is formed again. It has been shown that diffusion of insulin is much slower in the gel state than in the sol state, and insulin release can be controlled as a function of the glucose concentration in the environment.

Glucose-sensitive phase-reversible hydrogels can also be prepared without using Con A. Polymers having phenylboronic groups (e.g.

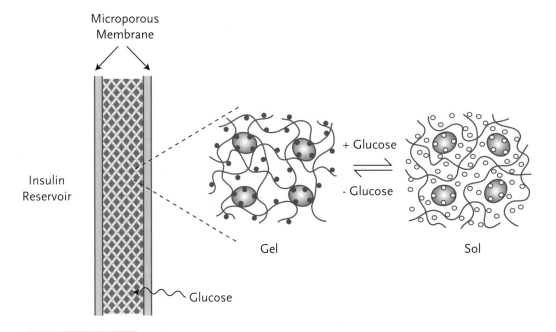

Microporous
Membrane

Insulin
Reservoir

+ Glucose

- Glucose

Gel

Sol

Glucose

Figure 16.6 Sol-gel phase-transition of a glucose-sensitive hydrogel. Large circles represent Con A, a glucose-binding protein. Small closed and open circles represent a polymer-attached glucose and a free glucose, respectively. Diffusion of insulin through the solution (sol) can be an order of magnitude faster than that through the hydrogel (gel)

poly (3-(acrylamido)phenylboronic acid) and its copolymers and polyol polymers (e.g. poly (vinyl alcohol)) form a gel through complex formation between the pendant phenylborate and hydroxyl groups. Glucose, having pendant hydroxyl groups, competes with polyol polymers for the borate groups. Since glucose is monofunctional (i.e. has only one binding site for the borate group), it cannot function as a cross-linking agent as polyol polymer does. Thus, as the glucose concentration increases, the cross-linking density of the gel decreases and the gel swells to release more insulin. With higher glucose concentrations, the gel becomes a sol. The glucose exchange reaction is reversible, and borate–polyol cross-linking is re-formed at a lower glucose concentration. Instead of long chain polyol polymers, shorter molecules, such as diglucosylhexanediamine, can be used as a cross-linking agent. Since the phenylboronic acid gel is sensitive to glucose only at alkaline conditions (pH $\geq$ 9), various copolymers containing phenylboronic acid were synthesized to provide glucose sensitivity at physiological pH.

16.3.3.2 Erodible matrix system

Any sol–gel phase reversible system described above can be used as an erodible matrix system. All the components of the system in the sol state are essentially in the dissolved state, and thus they can be released to the environment in the absence of protecting membranes. During the process of gel to sol transition by the addition of glucose, the incorporated insulin can be released as a function of glucose concentration. There are of course other polymeric systems which can be used in glucose-sensitive erodible insulin delivery.

As discussed in Section 16.3.2.1, some polymers made of relatively hydrophobic monomers phase separate from aqueous solution upon

polymers have been synthesized from N,N′-dimethylaminoethyl
methacrylate and ethylacrylamide monomers providing pH sensitivity and temperature sensitivity, respectively. The uniqueness of poly
(N,N′-dimethylaminoethyl methacrylate and ethylacrylamide) is that
the critical transition temperature increases as the polymer becomes
ionized (i.e. the pH becomes lower). Thus, the insoluble polymer
matrix at a certain temperature becomes water-soluble as the pH of the
environment becomes lower. This unique property has been used for
glucose-controlled insulin release as illustrated in Figure 16.7. In the
presence of glucose, gluconic acid generated by glucose oxidase protonates dimethylamino groups of the polymer. This induces shift of the
critical transition temperature to a higher temperature for the polymers at the surface of the insulin-loaded polymer matrix. This leads to
the dissolution of the polymer from the surface and thus the release of
insulin. An erodible matrix system based on the shift of the critical
transition temperature can also be made using polymers containing
phenylboronic acid groups. Poly(N,N-dimethylacrylamide-co-3-(acrylamido)phenylboronic acid) shifts its critical transition temperature in

Figure 16.7 Sequence
of insulin release from
pH/temperature-
sensitive polymer
matrix. Both glucose
oxidase and insulin are
loaded inside the
matrix. The decrease in
pH by gluconic acid
results in ionization of
the polymer, which in
turn increases the
lower critical solution
temperature. This
makes the polymer
water-soluble, and
erosion of the polymer
matrix at the surface
releases the loaded
insulin

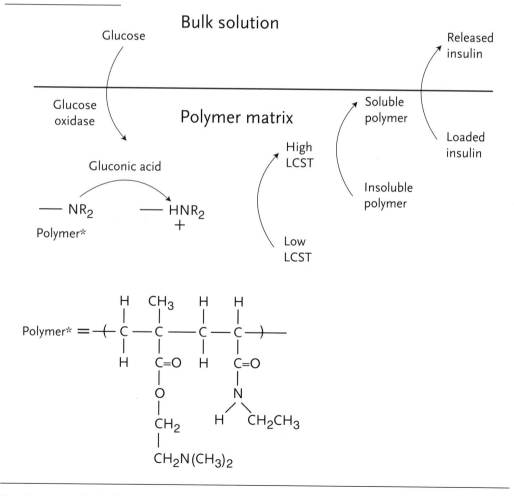

response to changes in glucose concentration. Addition of glucose to such a polymer system can increase the critical transition temperature by 15° around the body temperature. Thus, the system can be designed to become water-soluble in the presence of glucose at the body temperature. Insulin which is loaded inside the polymer can be released as a function of glucose concentration in the environment.

16.3.3.3 pH-sensitive membrane system

Membranes made of cross-linked polyelectrolytes (i.e. polymers with ionizable groups) display large differences in swelling properties depending on the pH of the environment. When a polymer is charged, it dissolves more in aqueous solution. When polymer molecules are cross-linked, the cross-linked network (i.e. a hydrogel) swells more instead of dissolving more. Cationic polyelectrolytes, such as poly(N,N'-diethylaminoethyl methacrylate) (PDAEM), dissolve more, or swell more if cross-linked at low pH due to the ionization. On the other hand, polyanions, such as poly(acrylic acid) (PAA), dissolve more at high pH.

Membranes made of PDAEM have been used for self-regulated insulin delivery. Addition of glucose leads to the lowering of pH, which in turn results in ionization and thus swelling of the membrane (Figure 16.8). When a membrane swells, it tends to release more drugs than the membrane in the non-swellable state. Thus, the PDAMEM membrane can be used to deliver insulin as the environmental glucose concentration increases. Polyanions can also be used for self-regulated insulin delivery. A glucose-sensitive hydraulic flow controller can be designed using a porous membrane system consisting of a porous

Figure 16.8 Self-regulated insulin release membrane made of poly(N,N'-diethylaminoethyl methacrylate) hydrogel membrane. As glucose enters the membrane, glucose oxidase entrapped inside the membrane transforms glucose into gluconic acid, which in turn reduces the pH of the hydrogel membrane. This causes swelling of the membrane followed by more release of insulin through the membrane

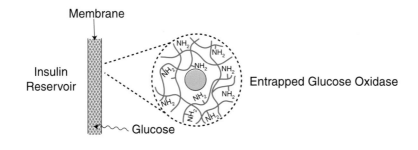

filter grafted with a polyanion (e.g. poly(methacrylic acid-co-butyl methacrylate)) and immobilized glucose oxidase (Figure 16.9). The grafted polyanion chains are expanded at pH 7 due to electrostatic repulsion among charges on polymer chains. Glucose oxidase converts glucose to gluconic acid which lowers the pH and protonates the carboxyl groups of the polymer. Due to the reduced electrostatic repulsion, the polyanion chains then collapse (i.e. shrink) and pores of the membrane become open and insulin is released.

16.3.3.4 Immobilized insulin system

In these types of systems, insulin molecules are attached to a support or carrier through specific interactions which can be interrupted by glucose itself. This generally requires introduction of functional groups to insulin molecules. In one approach insulin was chemically modified to introduce glucose, which has a specific binding site for the Con A lectin. The glycosylated insulin-Con A system exploits complementary and competitive binding behavior of Con A with glucose and glycosylated insulin. The free glucose molecules complete with glucose–insulin conjugates bound to Con A, and thus, the glycosylated insulin is desorbed from the Con A in the presence of free glucose (Figure 16.10). The desorbed glucose–insulin conjugates are released to the surrounding tissue and the studies have shown that the glucose–insulin conjugates are bioactive.

In another approach, insulin was modified to introduce hydroxyl groups so that the hydroxylated insulin can be immobilized by forming a complex with phenylboronic acid groups on the support

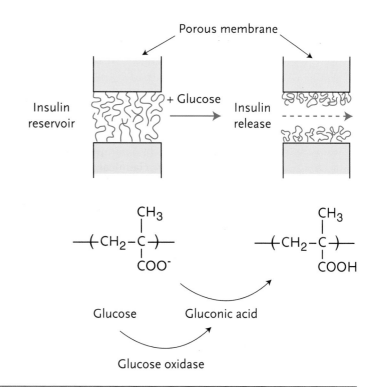

Figure 16.9 Anionic polymer chains grafted to the surface undergo conformational changes in response to pH changes. At physiological pH, poly(methacrylic acid) (PMAA) chains are expanded due to electrostatic repulsion of carboxylate ions. As the pH decreases as a result of gluconic acid formation, the carboxylate groups are protonated and the electrostatic repulsion is reduced. This in turn causes shrinkage of the polymer chains to open pores for insulin release

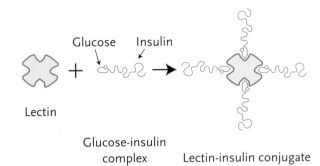

Figure 16.10
Desorption-controlled
release of insulin from
the insulin–Con A
complex. In this
approach, each insulin
molecule is modified
with a glucose
molecule

Glucose   Insulin

Lectin

Glucose-insulin
complex   Lectin-insulin conjugate

High blood
glucose level

Glucose

Release of ---→ Low blood
glucose-insulin complex   glucose level

Porous poly(HEMA) membrane

(Fig.16.11). The support can be hydrogel beads made of polymers containing phenylboronic acid, e.g. poly(m-methacrylamidophenylboronic acid). The hydroxylated insulin can be displaced by the added glucose and the displaced insulin can be released.

Sometimes insulin can be covalently grafted to the support as shown in Figure 16.12. In the example, insulin was grafted to the support through a disulfide bond. In the presence of glucose, electrons generated by glucose oxidase are transferred to the disulfide linkage via flavin adenine dinucleotide (FAD) to result in reductive cleavage of the disulfide bond. The cleaved insulin is then released to the environment. While the approaches taken in the immobilized insulin systems are highly elegant, there is an inherent drawback of this approach. The approach requires modification of insulin to create a new chemical entity which would require full regulatory approval.

16.3.4 Microchip delivery systems

The recent developments in medical microelectronics offers alternative methods of achieving chronopharmacological control using micropumps, valves and flow channels. The Massachusetts Institute of Technology has recently developed a 17 mm by 17 mm by 310 μm device containing 34 reservoirs. Controlled release from the device involves no moving parts with release from the individual reservoirs being initiated by applying an electric potential between the anode membrane and a cathode. The anode membrane undergoes electrochemical dissolution causing the release of solid, liquid or gel from the

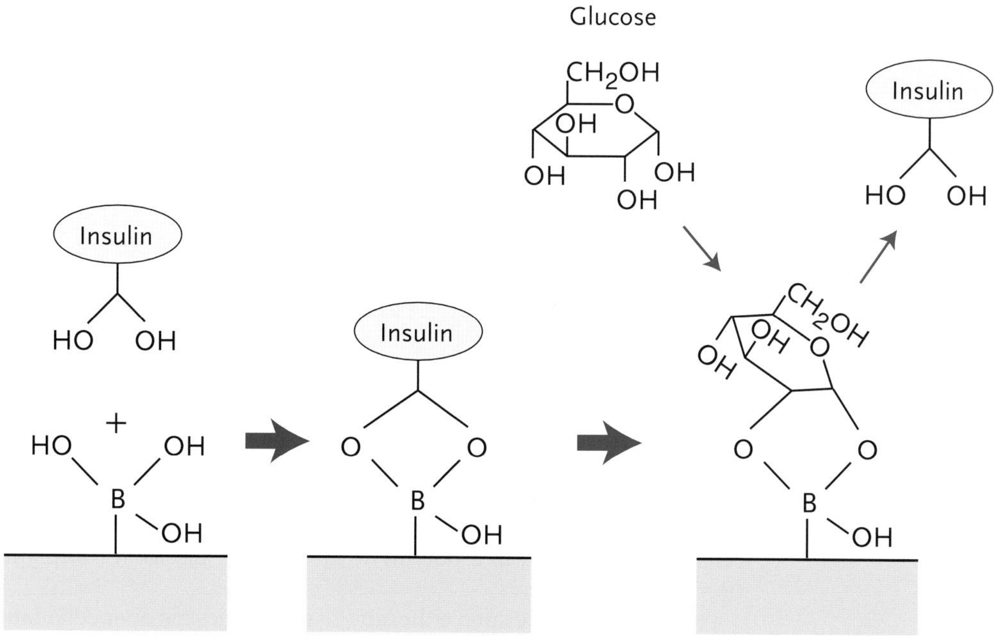

Glucose

Figure 16.11 Release of hydroxylated insulin from the phenylboronic acid support as a result of displacement by glucose

reservoir. The proof-of-principle release studies have demonstrated the controlled, pulsatile release of chemical substances from the device. Future integration of this technology with microchip-based bioanalytical technologies should facilitate the development of microchips in which a microbiosensor controls the release of drug in response to a biological stimulus, allowing both controlled pulsatile release and bioresponsive drug release from the same device.

16.3.5 Genetically-engineered cell implants

An alternative approach to obtain pharmacological control is the use of genetically-engineered cell implants which use the endogenous control systems to regulate delivery of a therapeutic protein.

As described in Chapter 14, a first-choice approach for gene therapy is to introduce a functional gene, using viral or nonviral vectors, into impaired cells that cannot produce necessary proteins. For example, the deficiency in adenosine deaminase in the body gives rise to severe combined immunodeficiency (SCID). It is anticipated that the disease could be treated by introducing the enzyme-coding gene into bone marrow progenitors. This genetic modification enables the body to generate the required enzyme.

Recent advance in genetic engineering technology has made it possible to regulate gene expression including transcription and translation in a variety of cell types. Such success has led to development of a second-type gene therapy making use of "surrogate" cells. Genetic modification of heterologous cells, rather than impaired cells, by viral or nonviral vectors endows the surrogate cells with a missionary function to provide the body with necessary proteins. Examples of the cells

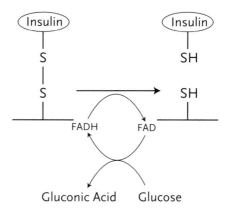

Figure 16.12 Release of immobilized insulin in respond to addition of glucose. The disulfide bond is cleaved by electrons resulting from glucose transformation to gluconic acid by glucose oxidase. This approach requires a coenzyme flavin adenine dinucleotide (FAD)

that are used include fibroblasts, endothelial cells, lymphocytes, keratinocytes, glial cells and mammary cells. These genetically modified cells may be housed in a polymeric implantable device for implantation into the patient.

However, to make such a therapy reality, concerns over cell viability inside the implantable device have to be adequately addressed. The implant's polymer composition and morphology would have to be optimized in order to maximize the life-span of the cells and to minimize host immune responses. The vascularization of the implant would be another determinant that plays an important role regarding cell viability because it enables the implant to receive nutrients necessary for their survival, to eliminate metabolic by-products and to provide the systemic entrance of therapeutic proteins.

16.4 EPILOGUE

This book has highlighted the significant advances in drug delivery and targeting technologies over the past three decades. As drug delivery and targeting technologies advance, the requirements for the next generation of advanced drug delivery systems grows increasingly more demanding, forcing the development of more sophisticated systems. Previous technologies of sustained or zero-order release alone are not adequate to treat diseases requiring long-term care. Effective bioresponsive, modulated advanced drug delivery systems are now the "Holy Grail" of workers in this field. Fortunately the recent advancement of chemistry and biology provides the pharmaceutical scientist with the tools to develop more effective drug delivery systems which target the site-of-action of the drug and address the challenges of chronopharmacology. The future of drug delivery and targeting will rely on the integration of these disciplines and a wider appreciation of the need to address the challenges of drug delivery and targeting at an earlier stage in the drug discovery process. As a consequence, advanced drug delivery research will require a new generation of multidisciplinary pharmaceutical scientists to address these challenges in this new millennium.

16.5 FURTHER READING

Chien, Y.W. (1992) *Novel Drug Delivery Systems*, 2nd edn. Marcel Dekker, New York.

Hisamtsu, I., Kataoka, K., Okano, T. and Sakurai, Y. (1997) Glucose-responsive gel from phenylborate polymer and poly(vinyl alcohol): Prompt response at physiological pH through the interaction of borate with amino group in the gel. *Pharm. Res.*, 14:289–293.

Jaffar, M. and Stratford, I.J. (1999) Bioreductive drugs: selectivity towards hypoxic tissues. *Exp. Opin. Ther. Patents*, 9:1371–1380.

Kier, P.F., Wilson, G and Needham, D. (1998) *Nature*, 394:459–462.

Kost, J. (1990) *Pulsed and Self-regulated Drug Delivery*. CRC Press, Boca Raton, FL.

Lemmer, B. Ed. (1996) *From the biological clock to chronopharmacology*. GmbH Scientific Publishers, Struttgart, Germany.

Lloyd, A.W. and Smith H.J. (1998) Pro-drugs. In *Introduction to the Principles of Drug Design and Action* (H.J. Smith, ed.), 3rd edn. Harwood Academic Publishers, Amsterdam. pp. 236–260.

Obaidat, A.A. and Park, K. (1997) Characterization of protein release through glucose-sensitive hydrogel membranes. *Biomaterials*, 18:801–807.

Prokai, L. and Prokai-Tatri, K. (1999) Metabolism-based drug design and drug targeting. *Pharmaceutical Science & Technology Today*, 2:457–462.

Santini, J.T., Cima, M.J. and Langer, R (1999) *Nature*, 397:335–338.

Yuk, S.H., Cho, S.H. and Lee, S.H. (1997) pH/temperature-responsive polymer composed of poly(N,N'-diethylaminoethyl methacrylate-co-ethylacrylamide). *Macromolecules*, 30:6856–6859.

16.6 SELF-ASSESSMENT QUESTIONS

1. What is meant by the terms (i) prodrug, (ii) ADEPT and (iii) GDEPT?

2. Explain how prodrugs may be used to specifically target tumor cells.

3. Describe the principles of redox-based drug delivery systems.

4. Outline the role of biosensors in addressing the challenge of chronopharmacology. What are the present limitations of using electrical biosensors?

5. Explain the potential uses of (i) temperature-sensitive and (ii) pH-sensitive hydrogels in advanced drug delivery.

6. Describe the approaches to the development of glucose-sensitive hydrogels.

7. Give examples of erodible matrix systems which may have application in the bioresponsive delivery of insulin.

8. Outline the use of microchip technologies in advanced drug delivery.

9. Describe the role of genetically engineered cell implants in bioresponsive drug delivery.

10. Outline the future directions of advanced drug delivery in the new millennium.

Appendix

Answers to Selected Self-Assessment Questions

CHAPTER 1

Question 9

Use the Henderson-Hasselbach Equation to demonstrate that a weak base (pKa = 7.5) should have better absorption from the small intestine (pH = 6.5) than from the stomach (pH = 1).

Solution

In the small intestine, $[B] = 0.1[BH^+]$, i.e. the concentration of ionized drugs is 10 times greater than unionized drug.

In the stomach, $[B] = 0.000000316 [BH^+]$, i.e. the concentration of ionized drugs is 3.16×10^7 times greater than unionized drug.

Thus at the pH of the small intestine, the drug is much less ionized than in the stomach and is therefore more readily absorbed.

CHAPTER 4

Question 2

A new steroidal drug is allowed to pass through a siloxane membrane (surface area = 23.64cm², thickness = 0.85cm). The drug concentration inside the reservoir compartment is 0.0004 g/cm³. The amount of steroid passing *from* the reservoir through the membrane in 4 hours is 40 μg. Provided that the drug release rate be constant, calculate the flux (F) that is defined as the amount of a solute flowing through a membrane per unit time.

Solution

As drug release rate is constant:
Flux $= 40/(4 \times 23.64)$
$= 0.423$ μg/cm²hr

Question 10

The release rate (dM/dt) of a drug from an osmotic pump can be described as Cd (dV/dt) where Cd is the drug solubility in its reservoir compartment. The effective surface area, permeability coefficient, thickness, and osmotic reflection coefficient of the semi-permeable membrane used for the pump are 3.0cm², 0.7×10^{-4} cm²/day, 500 μm, and 0.8, respectively. Initially, the pump has a reservoir compartment with a drug having Cd of 100mg/ml, and the observed $\Delta\pi$ is 100 atm. Now, consider that we have changed the reservoir medium and osmotic agent to increase Cd of the drug from 100 to 300mg/ml and to increase $\Delta\pi$ from 100 to 300 atm, by how much will the release rate of the drug be increased?

Solution

As dV/dt is proportional to $\Delta\pi$ increasing both Cd and $\Delta\pi$ by 3 fold will result in an overall 9 fold increase in release rate of the drug.

Index

Note: page numbers in *italics* refer to figures and tables

albumin *(contd.)*
  microparticulates   67, 70
  microspheres   139
ALEC   275
alginate microspheres   180
alginic acid   265
alkaline phosphatase, vaginal activity   307
alprenolol   159
alveolar clearance with pulmonary drug delivery
    282–283
alveolar region of lungs   271, 272
  drug delivery/fate   283–284
  drug targeting   287
  epithelium   272, *273*, 274
  tight junctions   284
alveoli   272
Alzet mini-osmotic pumps   109–110
AmBisome   134
amenorrhea, hypothalamic   37
amino acids
  absorption   16
  carrier-mediated transport   359
  peptide synthesis   401
  transporters   16, 157, 172
amino-polyethylene glycol-phosphatidylcholine
    391
aminopeptidases   40, 41
amorphous forms   29
cAMP   246
Amphocil   134
amphoterocin B   134
  emulsion   345
  liposomal carriers   140, 141, 348
ampicillin
  distribution   422
  solubility   159–160
  solvates   29
Androderm   227
anesthetics, volatile   270
angina pectoris   52
  drug franchises   53
angiotensin converting enzyme (ACE) inhibitors
  oligopeptide transporter   173
  transporters   17
anthracycline, liposomal   135
anti-anginal drugs, market analysis   56
anti-asthma therapies
  delivery devices   58, 288
  locally-acting   286–287
  market analysis   57–58
  pulmonary delivery   270
anti-idiotypic antibodies   127
anti-infective agents, vaginal preparations   302
anti-inflammatory drugs, market analysis
    56–57

anti-insulin (Mab83–7 and Mab83–14)   367
antibiotics   238
  aerosol delivery   281
  systemic administration for ocular conditions
    332
antibodies
  bispecific   129
  nasal cavity   251
  see also monoclonal antibodies
antibody-directed enzyme/prodrug therapy
    (ADEPT)   70, 128, 425–426, *427*
anticancer therapies
  market analysis   57
  market size   55
  price   56
  selective localization   424
antigen-presenting cells   323, 392, 394
antigens, vaginal delivery   318
antihypertensive drugs   56
antipyrine   154
antisense DNA, nasal delivery   238
antisense genes   392
antisense oligonucleotides   3, 157
antitransferrin (OX26) receptor   367, 368
  peptide nucleic acids   368
α1–antitrypsin   390
  deficiency   393
α-antitrypsin gene   390
antiviral delivery systems
  intravitreal   348
  vaginal   321–322, 326
aphthous ulcers, oral cavity   186
apical plasma membrane   13, 14, 15
apoproteins, non-serum   275
apoptosis   393, 412
apoptotic autolytic cascade   412
aprotinin   163, 266
aqueous humor   332
area postrema   358
area under the curve (AUC)   4, 5
Arrow implantable pump   113
arthritis   56–57
  rheumatoid arthritis   424
asialofetuin   379
asialoglycoprotein   380
asthma
  bronchoconstriction   279
  market analysis of drugs   57–58
  mucociliary clearance   250
  mucus hypersecretion   281
  mucus viscoelasticity   245
  nocturnal   36
  particle deposition in airways   279
  prevalence   58
  pulmonary gene therapy   393